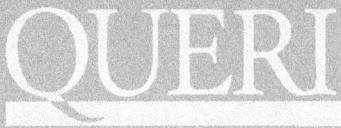

Family Involved Psychosocial Treatments for Adult Mental Health Conditions: A Review of the Evidence

February 2012

Prepared for:
Department of Veterans Affairs
Veterans Health Administration
Quality Enhancement Research Initiative
Health Services Research & Development Service
Washington, DC 20420

Prepared by:
Evidence-based Synthesis Program (ESP) Center
Minneapolis VA Medical Center
Minneapolis, MN
Timothy J. Wilt, MD, MPH, Director

Investigators:
Principal Investigator:
Laura Meis, PhD

Co-Investigator:
Joan Griffin, PhD

Research Associates:
Maureen Carlyle, MPH
Nancy Greer, PhD
Agnes Jensen, BS
Roderick MacDonald, MS
Indulis Rutks, BS

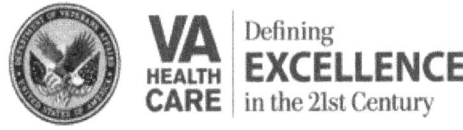

VA HEALTH CARE | Defining EXCELLENCE in the 21st Century

PREFACE

The Quality Enhancement Research Initiative's (QUERI's) Evidence-based Synthesis Program (ESP) was established to provide timely and accurate syntheses of targeted healthcare topics of particular importance to Veterans Affairs (VA) managers and policymakers, as they work to improve the health and healthcare of Veterans. The ESP disseminates these reports throughout VA.

QUERI provides funding for four ESP Centers and each Center has an active VA affiliation. The ESP Centers generate evidence syntheses on important clinical practice topics, and these reports help:

- develop clinical policies informed by evidence,
- guide the implementation of effective services to improve patient outcomes and to support VA clinical practice guidelines and performance measures, and
- set the direction for future research to address gaps in clinical knowledge.

In 2009, the ESP Coordinating Center was created to expand the capacity of QUERI Central Office and the four ESP sites by developing and maintaining program processes. In addition, the Center established a Steering Committee comprised of QUERI field-based investigators, VA Patient Care Services, Office of Quality and Performance, and Veterans Integrated Service Networks (VISN) Clinical Management Officers. The Steering Committee provides program oversight, guides strategic planning, coordinates dissemination activities, and develops collaborations with VA leadership to identify new ESP topics of importance to Veterans and the VA healthcare system.

Comments on this evidence report are welcome and can be sent to Nicole Floyd, ESP Coordinating Center Program Manager, at nicole.floyd@va.gov.

Recommended citation: Meis L, Griffin J, Greer N, Jensen A, Carlyle M, MacDonald R, Rutks I, Wilt T. Family Involved Psychosocial Treatments for Adult Mental Health Conditions: A Review of the Evidence. VA-ESP Project #09-009; 2012

TABLE OF CONTENTS

APPENDIX E. FOREST PLOTS FROM POOLED ANALYSES FOR ALSOHOL AND DRUG USE STUDIES

EXECUTIVE SUMMARY

BACKGROUND

Since 2008, the President has signed two new laws expanding VA authority to provide family services for Veterans' mental health care and creating a need to identify efficacious and promising family involved interventions for improving Veterans' mental health outcomes. With one exception, prior reviews have traditionally focused on one condition at a time, limiting comparisons across conditions and preventing a synthesis of the evidence for all mental health conditions, including those with few randomized controlled trials (RCTs; e.g., Posttraumatic Stress Disorder or PTSD). Finally, prior reviews are potentially less relevant to VA populations due to their focus on studies conducted in non-Veteran populations.

Consistent with prior work defining empirically supported psychological treatments, we conducted a systematic review of the published evidence evaluating if (and which) family involved treatments improve patient outcomes (i.e., efficacy) and if (and which) family involved treatments are superior to alternative interventions (i.e., specificity or comparative effectiveness, especially those therapies that include solely the patient, not family members). This topic was nominated by Sonja Batten, PhD, Office of Mental Health Services, and is primarily intended to help refine clinical guidelines by providing information as to whether family treatments improve the outcomes for Veterans receiving care for mental health conditions and if they provide incremental benefits beyond treatment solely involving Veterans. To evaluate findings of greatest validity and relevance to the United States (and especially Veteran) populations, we included studies if they were RCTs conducted in the United States, and we focused on patient outcomes (i.e., final outcomes), including symptoms of mental health conditions and family/couple functioning. Intermediate outcomes of interest included treatment adherence, treatment attendance, patient satisfaction, and social support for patients.

We addressed the following key questions:

Key Question #1. What is the efficacy of family involved interventions in improving outcomes for adult patients with mental health conditions [i.e., how do family involved psychosocial treatments compare to no psychosocial treatment: (a) waitlist/no treatment or (b) medication management only]?

Key Question 2. What is the effectiveness of family involved interventions compared to alternative interventions in improving outcomes for adult patients with mental health conditions [i.e., how do family involved interventions compare to (a) any individually-oriented psychosocial intervention or (b) any alternative family involved intervention]?

METHODS

We searched MEDLINE (Ovid) and PsycINFO for RCTs and systematic reviews published from 1980 to November, 2011 using standard search terms. We limited the search to articles involving subjects over age 18 and published in the English language. Search terms included: family, couples, home nursing, legal guardians, couple therapy, family therapy, and marital therapy. Additional citations were identified from reference lists. Titles, abstracts, and articles were reviewed by trained research personnel. Due to existing prior reviews and the volume of potentially eligible articles identified at the time of full text review, we narrowed our inclusion criteria to studies published after 1995. We excluded studies conducted outside of the United States.

Study characteristics, patient characteristics, final outcomes, and intermediate outcomes were abstracted onto tables for each mental health condition of interest by a trained research associate and verified by a second research associate under the supervision of the Principal Investigator, a Veterans Affairs psychologist. Our primary outcomes included patient-centered mental health outcomes (i.e., symptom severity, relapse rates, and days abstinent from drugs and/or alcohol) and couple/family functioning (i.e., couple/family adjustment, conflict, communication, and intimate partner violence) for participants with mental health conditions. Intermediate outcomes included treatment adherence, treatment attendance, utilization of mental health care, patient satisfaction, and social support for patients. Pooled analyses were performed where possible, but due to heterogeneity of interventions and outcomes across studies, most findings were narratively summarized. We assessed risk of bias for individual studies according to established criteria for randomized controlled trials, taking into consideration whether the treatment was manualized and whether the treatment was monitored for quality and consistency (i.e., treatment integrity).

Strength of evidence was determined for findings reviewed.

DATA SYNTHESIS

We constructed evidence tables for study characteristics and for outcomes, organized by mental health condition. We analyzed studies to compare their characteristics, methods, and findings. Findings from VA or active service populations were identified and highlighted. We compiled a summary of findings for each question based on qualitative and semi-quantitative synthesis of the findings.

PEER REVIEW

A draft version of this report was reviewed by members of our technical expert panel, nominated peer reviewers, as well as clinical leadership. Reviewer comments were addressed and our responses were incorporated in the final report.

RESULTS

We screened 2469 titles, of which 444 articles potentially met eligibility criteria. From these, 5 systematic reviews and 51 publications, which represented 39 unique RCTs, met eligibility criteria and were included. The findings are described below. The number of studies reviewed for each key question sum to over 39 trials due to trials with more than two conditions (e.g., family treatment, individual treatment, and wait list control). Most studies were of fair quality (10 good, 20 fair, 9 poor), reported multiple outcomes, and may have limited long-term or site applicability. Many reported a large number of comparisons, including non-significant differences between treatment groups. Some of the benefits noted for treatments evaluated in single trials below may be due to chance or reporting bias and their broad clinical applicability should also be viewed with caution. Overall, the majority of studies reviewed compared a family intervention to another active treatment, limiting our conclusions for KQ1.

KEY QUESTION #1. What is the efficacy of family involved interventions in improving outcomes for adult patients with mental health conditions [i.e., how do family involved psychosocial treatments compare to no psychosocial treatment: (a) waitlist/no treatment or (b) medication management only]?

We identified 8 RCTs that compared a family involved intervention to either waitlist/no treatment or medication management only and assessed the following mental health conditions: substance use disorders (1 trial), bipolar disorder (2 trials), PTSD (2 trials), sexual functioning (2 trials), and depression (1 trial). *Low* strength of evidence (one trial for each bullet point) was found regarding the impact of the following interventions on selected patient or intermediate outcomes (e.g., treatment utilization) over waitlist/drug treatment.

SUBSTANCE USE DISORDERS (1 TRIAL)

Family involvement in aftercare planning

- No significant differences were found between conditions on substance use outcomes.

- 92% of patients whose families were involved in aftercare treatment planning initiated substance use treatment after a hospital stay for detoxification. This was a 30% improvement over patients hospitalized for detoxification whose families did not participate in aftercare planning ($r = 0.36$).

BIPOLAR DISORDER (2 TRIALS)

Family therapy

- Neither a general family therapy nor a disorder specific family therapy, delivered in multiple family groups, improved recovery rates over medication management alone.

- Among participants with high levels of family impairment:

  o Disorder specific psychoeducational group family therapy led to significantly fewer depressive episodes per year (mean = 1.4; d = 1.0), 14% percent less time in a mood episode (d = 0.82), and 1.7 fewer mood episodes, yearly (d = 0.92). All effect sizes were considered moderate to large in magnitude.

  o General family therapy led to 0.9 fewer depressive episodes per year (d = 0.70); additional comparisons were non-significant.

3

Marital psychoeducational therapy

- Compared to medication management alone, marital psychoeducational therapy led to higher global functioning (a difference of 7 points on a 100 point scale; Global Assessment Scale) and greater medication adherence (a difference of 0.5 points on a 6 point scale).

- No significant differences were found between conditions on symptoms of bipolar disorder.

SCHIZOPHRENIA (0 TRIALS)

The efficacy of behavioral family therapy and supportive family therapy was established for schizophrenia prior to the timeframe of studies included in our review (i.e., studies published since 1995). The lack of RCTs comparing family treatments to waitlist is consistent with the more advanced nature of this literature. Prior reviews have concluded that family involved therapy leads to lower rates of relapse and hospitalization than waitlist or drug only treatment.

PTSD (1 TRIAL)

Support groups for family

Eighteen months after participation in Coffee and Family Education and Support groups (CAFES), the average number of patient mental health visits increased by 4 visits versus those assigned to waitlist.

SEXUAL FUNCTIONING (2 TRIALS)

Couples sex therapy in addition to medication for erectile dysfunction

- One trial found subjects assigned to couples sex therapy plus medication reported greater satisfaction with treatment than those assigned to medication alone. Differences between conditions on erectile functioning up to two months after treatment were not significant.

- A second trial found no significant difference in erectile functioning between those assigned to four weeks of couples cognitive behavioral sex therapy plus medication versus those assigned to medication alone after 4 weeks of treatment.

OTHER CONDITIONS EXAMINED IN SINGLE TRIALS (2 TRIALS)

Depression (1 trial)

Compared to waitlist, brief, disorder specific, cognitive behavioral couple therapy significantly improved depression symptoms and marital satisfaction for most comparisons in a small RCT (N = 35).

Binge Eating Disorder (1 trial)

A trial of group cognitive behavioral therapy (CBT) for binge eating disorder found that CBT with or without spouse involvement resulted in better symptom improvement than waitlist.

Key Question #2. What is the effectiveness of family involved interventions compared to alternative interventions in improving outcomes for adult patients with mental health conditions [i.e., how do family involved interventions compare to (a) any individually-oriented psychosocial intervention or (b) any alternative family involved intervention]?

For KQ2, we identified 33 RCTs addressing the following mental health conditions: substance use disorders (21 trials; 15 compared family involved treatments to individual behavioral treatment [KQ2A] with many conducted by a single investigative team), bipolar disorder (5 trials; 2 for KQ2A), schizophrenia (4 trials; 1 for KQ2A), PTSD (1 trial for KQ2A), nicotine dependence (1 trial for KQ2A), and binge eating disorder (1 trial). We found *low* to *moderate* strength evidence for the following conclusions:

SUBSTANCE USE DISORDERS

Behavioral Couple Therapy (BCT) for Substance Use Disorders (21 trials)

Disorder-specific, BCT for substance use disorders compared to individual therapy (9 trials)

- BCT or Behavioral Family Therapy (BFT) lead to 4 fewer days of substance use per month and 44 fewer days per year than individual cognitive behavior therapy (ICBT), up to one year after treatment. Additionally, across 8 of 9 studies included in pooled analyses, participants reported a significantly slower rate of relapse when assigned to BCT or BFT versus individual therapy.

- BCT led to higher relationship adjustment scores (12.5%) one year after treatment, with those receiving BCT reporting relationship adjustment in the satisfied range and ICBT patients reporting scores in the distressed range.

- Effects were similar for men, women, drug use disorders, and alcohol use disorders

- Mixed findings indicated that BCT may result in lower rates of intimate partner violence and higher rates of session attendance than ICBT

- Veterans participating in BCT demonstrated comparable or better rates of percent days abstinent (PDA) from alcohol use (post-treatment: 98.0%; short-term follow-up: 87.6%; long-term follow-up: 82.7%) than average rates of PDA reported in the alcohol use disorder (AUD) trials included in our pooled analyses. However, without direct comparisons between Veteran and non-Veteran samples and between BCT and ICBT, we could not assess whether treatment response for Veterans differs from treatment response for non-Veterans.

Community Reinforcement and Family Training (CRAFT; 3 trials)

CRAFT led to 30-48% greater rates of treatment initiation among patients than non-CRAFT family interventions (e.g., Al-Anon, Johnson Intervention).

A series of single RCTs found significant benefits for specific family interventions over comparators. These findings fall within the category of 'possibly efficacious' interventions. In each case, findings within the trial itself were often mixed. Given only one trial for each intervention (and the fact that not all comparison groups were individual therapy), our confidence in the consistency or applicability of these findings to other settings or compared to individual therapy is *low* or *insufficient* (low or insufficient strength of evidence). One trial each indicated:

Alterations and Alternatives to BCT for Substance Use Disorders

Adding relapse prevention to BCT (2 trials)

- The addition of family involved relapse prevention to BCT alone led to 13.2% more days of abstinence from alcohol up to 18 months after treatment (4 more days per month or 48.2 more days per year). Differences were non-significant at the 30 month follow-up.

- The benefits of adding relapse prevention to BCT were especially pronounced for patients with the most severe substance use and poorest couple functioning.

- A second trial found no benefit from adding relapse prevention to BCT.

Alternatives to BCT (2 trials)

- One study found that the combination of reciprocal relationship counseling (disorder specific intervention), contingency management, and naltrexone use was superior to contingency management plus naltrexone only for improving family functioning but not for improving abstinence from substance use or days in treatment.

- A second study found that subjects in a motivational and psychoeducational intervention that included couple therapy for male heroin users with pregnant intimate partners, actually reported higher heroin use at short-term follow up, compared to a counselor-led drug treatment support group.

BIPOLAR DISORDER (5 TRIALS)

Family Focused Treatment (FFT; 3 trials)

- FFT led to lower relapse rates of relapse than crisis management with limited family involvement, 24 months after randomization (35% relapse versus 54%). Patients in crisis management relapsed an average of 20 weeks sooner than those in FFT.

- FFT led to lower relapse rates (28% vs. 60%) and lower hospitalization rates (12% vs. 60%) than individual therapy one year after the end of active treatment.

- No significant differences were found between FFT and individual therapy on medication adherence.

- One trial found no significant differences in symptoms of bipolar disorder or family functioning between FFT and either cognitive behavioral therapy or interpersonal and social rhythm therapy, suggesting FFT may perform similarly, but not superior, to other empirically supported, highly intensive interventions in improving symptoms of bipolar disorder.

*Family-Focused Treatment-Health Promoting Intervention (FFT-HPI; an adaptation of
Family-Focused Treatment; 1 trial)*

FFT-HPI leads to fewer manic (4.2 points on the Young Mania Rating Scale, YMRS; d = 0.34)
and depression symptoms (5.6 points on the Hamilton Depression Rating Scale, HAM-D; d
= 0.67) among bipolar patients than health education provided to families via video diskettes
(DVD).

*Disorder specific (multifamily groups) versus general family therapy (Problem Centered
Systems Therapy of the Family; 1 trial)*

Differences in rates of recovery or between general family therapy and disorder specific family
therapy, delivered in multiple family groups, were non-significant.

SCHIZOPHRENIA (3 TRIALS)

Multiple Family Groups (MFG; 1 trial)

- MFG as compared to an individually oriented psychosocial intervention, improved negative
  symptoms of schizophrenia (e.g., blunted affect, alogia, anhedonia, inattention, avolition). At
  the one year point of a two year intervention, there was a statistically significant difference
  of one point on a 25 point scale. Those in the MFG condition had a 12% lower rate of
  hospitalization at state level psychiatric hospitals at one year follow-up.

- Differences on rates of overall hospitalization, community hospitalization, or use of crisis
  care were non-significant at post-treatment and one year after treatment.

Assertive Community Treatment (ACT) with and without a biweekly multi-family group

No significant differences were found between groups on hospital admissions, symptoms, or
family outcomes.

Applied Family Management (AFM; 1 trial)

- No significant differences were found in hospitalization rates, time to hospitalization/
  relapse, or symptoms between more intensive AFM and less intensive Supportive Family
  Management (SFM).

- AFM improved family functioning (patient rejection scale) by 0.32 scale points at 1 year
  follow-up (medium effect size, 0.31) and 1.03 scale points (medium effect size, 0.30) at 2
  year follow-up, over less intensive SFM..

- Authors note that due to limited group differences, findings may have limited clinical
  significance.

SCHIZOPHRENIA + SUBSTANCE USE DISORDER (1 TRIAL)

- Subjects with a comorbid substance use disorder and serious mental illness (e.g.,
  schizophrenia, bipolar disorder) demonstrated greater improvements in psychiatric symptoms
  (Brief Psychiatric Rating Scale or BPRS psychosis, medium effect size, 0.32; BPRS total,
  small effect size, 0.17) when assigned to a longer term (9-18 months) psychoeducational

family program than a brief (2-3 month) family intervention.

- Differences in substance use and global functioning across conditions were non-significant.

PTSD (2 TRIALS)

One trial found no significant differences between exposure therapy with Behavioral Family Therapy (disorder specific family intervention) versus exposure therapy only on symptoms of PTSD or social adjustment; however the family-involved arm resulted in poorer rates of dropout than exposure alone.

OTHER CONDITIONS EXAMINED IN SINGLE TRIALS (2 TRIALS)

There were no differences between a family involved intervention and individually-oriented treatment in abstinence from smoking or social support in one trial examining smoking cessation in pregnant women and in days of binge eating, depression scale scores, relationship adjustment scale scores, or treatment attendance in a second examining binge eating disorder.

DISCUSSION

The literature we reviewed examined a broad number of family involved interventions for mental health conditions. Importantly, many of our outcomes of interest, including treatment adherence, social support, treatment satisfaction, couple/family conflict, couple/family communication, and intimate partner violence were rarely presented. This was also true of a primary outcome (family and couple functioning) for bipolar disorder and schizophrenia. Some of the outcomes we describe are intermediate, rather than focused on patient symptoms and functioning. For example, while treatment initiation, participation, and attendance in counseling sessions were of interest, they may be of low-value (and actually indicate ineffective health care resource utilization) in the absence of demonstrated improvements in symptom or functioning outcome, especially if interventions lead to increased resource utilization without clinical benefit. Furthermore, many of the positive findings are based on multiple outcomes reported and long-term maintenance of effects beyond the study period are not well known. The majority of studies reviewed compared family interventions to another active treatment, limiting our ability to draw conclusions about the general efficacy (i.e., compared to waitlist or medication only) of the interventions reviewed. In particular some studies compared one form, type, intensity, and method of family or couple therapy versus another or to a waitlist. Thus the evidence regarding the incremental effectiveness of family or couple therapy compared to treatments that solely involve the patient or more ready access to care is limited especially outside of substance use disorders. Over half of the trials reviewed (56%; N = 22) examined family interventions for substance use disorders. For this condition many of the studies were conducted by a single investigative team and thus generalizability to other populations, settings, and therapeutic teams are not clearly known.

Generally, across the 39 trials, family involved treatments for mental health conditions were as effective as or more effective than alternative psychotherapies, with two exceptions. The addition of approximately 23 weeks of disorder-specific behavioral family therapy after 9 weeks (18 sessions) of exposure therapy for PTSD lead to greater rates of treatment dropout than exposure therapy alone or waitlist. Additionally, male opiod users with pregnant female partners who participated in a combination of motivational enhancement, case management, contingency management, and psychoeducational couple therapy reported greater heroin use at short-term follow-up than patients participating in usual care. With the exception of CRAFT and BCT, many of the trials comparing family therapies to alternative family or individual therapies found no significant differences when interventions were equally as intensive.

Among good to fair quality studies with *moderate* strength of evidence, we reached the following conclusions:

1. Behavioral couple therapy (BCT), a disorder-specific couple therapy, results in lower rates of substance use and greater relationship adjustment than individually-oriented treatments over the year following treatment for drug use and alcohol use in both male and female patients

2. Community Reinforcement and Family Training (CRAFT), a disorder-specific and partner-assisted intervention, conducted solely with the family members of individuals with substance use disorders, leads to better rates of treatment initiation among individuals with substance use disorders than alternative family interventions.

Low strength of evidence from single trials indicated that some additional family interventions improve patient symptoms, family functioning, and treatment initiation (see Executive Summary Table below). The existing evidence is limited by small numbers of good to high quality studies and inconsistency of findings both across and within trials. Our findings and strength of evidence ratings are based solely on the results of our search, which included only US studies since 1995 of family involved psychosocial treatments for mental health conditions that included patient outcomes. Consequently, conclusions do not include behavioral family therapy and supportive family therapy for schizophrenia which were established as efficacious prior to our review. Although a body of evidence supporting family treatment for schizophrenia for prevention or delay of relapse exists, many trials did not meet our search criteria. The quality of reporting in most these studies is poor and the applicability of some results from studies outside the United States, particularly in China, is limited. With the exception of behavioral couple therapy and CRAFT for substance use disorders, the literature in U.S. populations and especially Veterans is not well-developed.

FUTURE RESEARCH

The biggest needs for future research are for high quality RCTs of family interventions with Veterans, including BCT and CRAFT, and studies that replicate the family involved treatments identified above as 'possibly efficacious.' In particular, studies are needed (especially in conditions beyond substance use disorders) that compare family/couples interventions to interventions directed solely at patients in order to evaluate the incremental effectiveness of family/couple therapies. Additionally, there is a need for development and standardized reporting of patient centered outcomes (rather than intermediate or process measures) using measures and analysis strategies that are comparable across studies. The clinical significance of many of the reported outcomes including scale scores is not well established. Determining levels that establish clinical significance (and whether interventions achieve a clinically significant effect) would be of value for practitioners, researchers and health care policy makers. Further work is also needed on groups underrepresented across the literature, but important to the VA. These include studies of women, minorities, non-traditional family constellations (i.e., close friends and same sex couples), and patients with complex conditions and common constellations of problems (i.e., those with multiple comorbidities). Also, some work has found that family therapies are especially beneficial when patients are experiencing high levels of family distress or more severe symptoms. Further work is needed to replicate these preliminary findings. RCTs of family interventions for mental health conditions in the US were especially sparse for PTSD, anxiety disorders, sexual functioning, depression, eating disorders, and personality disorders. Future reviews should also examine the effects of family involved interventions on caregiver outcomes, patient preferences for which family members to include and how to involve them in treatment, and methods of engaging patients and their families in family treatment.

EXECUTIVE SUMMARY TABLE.

Family Interventions since 1996 that Improve Outcomes for US Patients with Mental Health (MH) Conditions

MH Condition	Intervention	Comparator	Outcome	Efficacy Status	Strength of Evidence
Alcohol Use Disorders	Behavioral Couple Therapy	Individual Behavioral Therapy	1) Substance Use	1	Moderate[a]
			2) Relationship Adjustment	1	Moderate[a]
			3) Intimate Partner Violence	3	Low
			4) Attendance	3	Low
	Brief family intervention to promote continuing care	Treatment-as-usual	1) Substance Use	ND	Low
			2) Treatment Initiation	3	Low
	Behavioral Couple Therapy + relapse prevention	Behavioral Couple Therapy	1) Substance Use	3	Low
			2) Relationship Adjustment	ND	Low
	Behavioral Family Treatment	Individual Behavioral Therapy	1) Substance Use	3	Low
			2) Family Functioning	ND	Low
	CRAFT	Alternative Family Treatments	1) Substance Use	ND	Low
			2) Family Functioning	ND	Low
			3) Treatment Initiation	3	Low
Drug Use Disorders	Behavioral Couple Therapy	Individual Behavioral Therapy	1) Substance Use	1	Moderate[a]
			2) Relationship Adjustment	1	Moderate[a]
			3) Intimate Partner Violence	3	Low
			4) Attendance	1	Low[b]
	Behavioral Family Treatment	Individual Behavioral Therapy	1) Substance Use	3	Low
			2) Family Functioning	3	Low
	CRAFT	Al-Anon/Nar-Anon	1) Substance Use	ND	Moderate
			2) Family Functioning	ND	Low
			3) Treatment Initiation	1	Moderate

MH Condition	Intervention	Comparator	Outcome	Efficacy Status	Strength of Evidence
Bipolar	Family-Focused Treatment-Health Promoting Intervention	Health information DVDs reviewed by caregivers	1) Symptoms	3	Low
	Family-Focused Treatment	Crisis management with two in-home family psychoeducation sessions	1) Symptoms	3	Low
			2) Medication Adherence	3	Low
		Problem-focused, psychoeducational Individual therapy	1) Symptoms	3	Low
			2) Medication Adherence	ND	Low
		Cognitive Behavior Therapy	1) Symptoms	ND	Low
		Interpersonal and social rhythm therapy	1) Symptoms	ND	Low
	Marital intervention + medication	Medication only	1) Symptoms	ND	Low
			2) Global Functioning	4	Low
			3) Medication Adherence	4	Low
Schizophrenia	Multiple Family Groups	Standard, individually-oriented care	1) Symptoms	ND	Low
			2) Any Hospitalization	ND	Low
			3) State Hospitalization	3	Low
			4) MH Care Utilization	ND	Low
	Family intervention + in home behavioral family therapy (Applied Family Management)	Family intervention	1) Symptoms	ND	Low
			2) Family Functioning	ND	Low
			3) Patient Rejection by Family	3	Low
			4) MH Care Utilization	ND	Low
			5) Attendance	ND	Low
Schizophrenia & Substance Use Disorder	Psychoeducation + skills oriented training (Family Intervention for Dual Disorder)	Short term psychoeducation	1) Schizophrenia Symptoms	3	Low
			2) Substance Use	ND	Low
			3) Global functioning	3	Low
			4) Medication Adherence	ND	Low
PTSD	Coffee and Family Education and Support	Waitlist	1) Number of MH Visits	4	Low
Depression	Brief problem-focused couple therapy	Waitlist	1) Symptoms	4	Low
			2) Relationship Adjustment	4	Low

Efficacy Status:
1 = Efficacious & Specific = superior to placebo, nonspecific, or alternative intervention in at least two studies conducted by independent research teams.
2 = Efficacious; superior to waitlist in RCTs conducted by two independent research teams.
3 = *Possibly* Efficacious & Specific; criteria met for efficacious and specific from a single study.
4 = *Possibly* Efficacious; criteria met for efficacious from a single study.
ND = No significant differences found

Strength of Evidence:
High = High confidence evidence reflects true effect. The effect and confidence in the estimate of effect is unlikely to change with further research.
Moderate = moderate confidence that evidence reflects true effect. The effect and confidence of the effect may change with further research.
Low = Low confidence evidence reflects true effect. The effect and confidence of the effect will likely change with further research.

[a]Seven of the nine trials comparing these conditions were written by or based on data collected by Dr. Fals-Stewart. See Substance Use Disorders Results for KQ2 for discussion.
[b]Several studies also found non-significant differences, leading to low strength of evidence.

ABBREVIATIONS TABLE

AA	Alcoholics Anonymous
ABCT	Alcohol Behavior Couple Therapy
ABIT	Alcohol Behavior Individual Therapy
ABMT	Alcohol Focused Spouse Involvement Plus Behavioral Marital Therapy
ACQ	Area of Change Questionnaire
ACT	Assertive Community Treatment
AFM	Applied Family Management
AL-NAR FT	Alcoholics Anonymous / Narcotics Anonymous Facilitation Therapy
ASI	Addiction Severity Index
AUD	Alcohol Use Disorder
BBCT	Brief Behavioral Couple or Marital Therapy
BCT	Behavioral Couple or Marital Therapy
BDI-II	Beck Depression Inventory 2nd Edition
BFT	Behavioral Family Therapy
BFTI	Brief Family Treatment Intervention
BMRS	Bech-Rafaelsen Mania Scale
BMT	Behavioral Marital Therapy
BPRS	Brief Psychiatric Rating Scale
CAFES	Coffee and Family Education and Support
CAPS	Clinician Administered Posttraumatic Stress Disorder Scale
CBQ	Couples Behavior Questionnaire
CBT	Cognitive Behavioral Therapy
CC	Collaborative Care
CM	Contingency Management
CRAFT	Community Reinforcement and Family Training
CRT	Community Reinforcement Training Intervention
CSQ	Client Satisfaction Questionnaire
CTS	Conflict Tactics Scale
DAS	Dyadic Adjustment Scale
DSM	Diagnostic And Statistical Manual of Mental Disorders
DVD	Video Diskette
ED	Erectile Dysfunction
EDEQ	Eating Disorder Examination Questionnaire
EDITS	Erectile Dysfunction Inventory of Treatment Satisfaction
EE	Expressed Emotions
ESP	Evidence-based Synthesis Program
FES	Family Environment Scale
FFT	Family Focused Training
FFT-HPI	Family-Focused Treatment-Health Promoting Intervention
FIDD	Family Intervention For Dual Disorders
FPE	Family Psychoeducation
FSO	Family or Significant Other
GAS	Global Assessment Scale

HAM-D	Hamilton Depression Rating Scale
HOPE	Helping Other Partners Excel
HSR&D	Health Services Research & Development Service
ICBT	Individual Cognitive Behavior Therapy
ICD	International Classification of Diseases
IIEF	International Index For Erectile Function
IOE	Impact of Events Scale
IPT	Interpersonal Psychotherapy
IPSRT	Interpersonal And Social Rhythm Therapy
ITT	Intention to Treat
KQ	Key Question
LIFE-RIFT	Longitudinal Interval Follow-Up Evaluation - Range of Impaired Function Tool
MAT	Locke Wallace Marital Adjustment Test
MFG	Multiple Family Group
MH	Mental Health
MHS	Marital Happiness Scale
MMSE	Mini-Mental State Exam
M-PTSD	Mississippi Scale for Combat-Related Posttraumatic Stress Disorder
MSANS	Modified Scale for The Assessment Of Negative Symptoms
NA	Not Applicable
ND	No Significant Difference
NR	Not Reported
NS	Not Significant
OIF/OEF	Operation Iraqi Freedom/Operation Enduring Freedom
PACT	Psychoeducational Attention Control Treatment
PAIR	Personal Assessment of Intimacy in Relationships
PDA	Percentage of Days Abstinent
PDHD	Percentage of Days of Heavy Drinking
PDPSU	Percentage of Days Primary Substance Use
PL	Public Law
PORT	Patient Outcomes Research Team
PSBCT	Parent Skills with Behavioral Couple Therapy
PTSD	Posttraumatic Stress Disorder
QOL	Quality of Life
RCT	Randomized Control Trial
RHS	Relationship Happiness Scale
RP	Relapse Prevention
SA	Substance Abuse
SADS-C	Schedule For Affective Disorders And Schizophrenia –Change Version
SAS	Social Adjustment Scale
SAS-FV	Social Adjustment Scale III, Family Version
S-BCT	Standard- Behavioral Couple Or Marital Therapy
SC	Standard or usual care
SFM	Supportive Family Management
SO	Significant Other

SPSI	Social Problem Solving Inventory
STEP-BD	Systematic Treatment Enhancement Program For Bipolar Disorder
SUD	Substance Use Disorder
SV	Spousal Violence
RCT	Randomized Control Trial
TAU	Treatment As Usual
TLFB	Time Line Follow Back
TX	Treatment
US	United States
VA	Veterans Affairs
VS	versus
VISN	Veterans Integrated Service Networks
YMRS	Young Mania Rating Scale

EVIDENCE REPORT

INTRODUCTION

Since 2008, the President has signed two new laws establishing or expanding VA authority to provide family services for Veterans' mental health care. The first law, Public Law 110-387: Veterans' Mental Health and Other Care Improvements Act of 2008, was signed into law on October 10, 2008. Section 301 of the Act amends title 38 of United States Code (U.S.C.) § 1701(5)(B) and 38 U.S.C. § 1782(a) and (b). This law expands VA authority to provide enhanced family mental health services, such as consultation, professional counseling, marriage and family counseling, and training to families of patients with Service Connected and Non-Service Connected injuries or conditions when 1) no Veteran treatment would otherwise occur without the family member's involvement, 2) the Veteran's treatment would be less or not effective without family member's involvement, 3) or, the treatment can be delivered most efficiently when the family member is included in treatment. The second law, Public Law 111-163: Caregivers and Veterans Omnibus Health Services Act, signed in May, 2010, allows, among other things, the VA authority to provide these same services to family caregivers of Veterans and directs the VA to provide additional benefits (e.g., financial stipends and health care benefits) to a select group of eligible caregivers, namely those providing essential care to Veterans injured in Operation Iraqi Freedom (OIF) and Operation Enduring Freedom (OEF). Of note, current eligibility criteria for VA family-related services do not extend to close friends or intimate partners who do not reside with the Veteran. These new laws, along with the VA's adoption in primary care of Patient-Aligned Care Teams, or a patient-centered medical home model, recognize the important role families have on a treatment team and their influence over a patient's care and related outcomes. Synthesis of the scientific literature on the effectiveness of involving family or intimate partners (referred to hereafter as family, encompassing both intimate partners, spouses, and other family members) in psychosocial interventions to treat or improve a broad range of mental health conditions, family problems, marital strain, and physical health conditions, including an examination of both patient outcomes and caregiver and family outcomes, is essential to shaping the VA's provision of family involved care but beyond the scope of a single review. The focus of the present review is on one of these vital areas for synthesis: the effectiveness of family involved interventions in treating mental health conditions. This synthesis is intended to help clarify the evidence for potential best practices within the VA in family involved mental health care to guide both policy and clinical practice. While these family or couple interventions likely also affect caregivers, the focus of this review is specifically on patient outcomes (versus caregiver or family member's personal functioning), including patients' family functioning.

TYPES OF FAMILY TREATMENTS FOR MENTAL HEALTH CONDITIONS

While individual psychotherapies for mental health problems have long been the standard for mental health care, family problems are pronounced among patients with mental health conditions. Among OEF/OIF Veterans recently returning from deployment, interpersonal problems have been identified as increasing at a greater rate than any other health-related problem,[1] and relationship distress in intimate relationships can facilitate or hinder treatment seeking.[2] Consequently, family involvement has been explored for a number of conditions, including depression,[3] substance use,[4] bipolar disorder,[5] schizophrenia,[6] panic disorder with agoraphobia,[7] and posttraumatic stress disorder (PTSD).[8] Family interventions for mental health conditions can take multiple forms, as outlined by Baucom and colleagues,[9] and may fall across any given category or combination of categories.

Partner or Family Assisted Treatment[9]

In this case, family member(s) act as surrogate therapists or coaches to help the patient. Typically, the family aids the patient in completing out-of-session homework within a cognitive-behavioral treatment, and relationships between the patient and family are not a focus of treatment. This category of family involvement capitalizes on prior work establishing robust associations between social support, instrumental support, and treatment adherence across multiple medical conditions.[10]

Disorder Specific Couple or Family Treatment[9]

For interventions taking this approach, family behavior and relationships that are theorized to fuel disorder symptoms are addressed. Family relationships are targeted only to the extent to which they directly influence the patient's disorder or treatment. Such interventions, especially for schizophrenia or bipolar disorder, often target expressed emotions (EE) or related constructs. EE includes family members' expressed criticism, hostility, and emotional over-involvement toward the patient and is tied to poor medication adherence, including among patients with schizophrenia,[11] and greater relapse rates and symptom severity among patients with schizophrenia, eating disorders, depression, PTSD, and bipolar disorder,[12-15] EE likely reflects disturbances within the entire family system, including family organization, emotional climate, and transactions.[16] Supported mechanisms underlying EE include a family member's attributions of patient's negative behavior to controllable factors, personal factors, and beliefs that the patient is not making appropriate efforts at self-improvement.[16, 17]

Additionally, behavior patterns between family and patients and specific to a given disorder can be conceptualized as maintaining the condition, with reciprocal associations postulated between mental health symptoms and family functioning.[18, 19] For example, environmental contingencies have been theorized to maintain use for substance use disorders[20] and avoidance of trauma cues for individuals with PTSD.[21] Additionally, for those with substance use disorders, relationship distress may increase substance use cravings, reinforce the use of substances to cope with distress,[19] or even motivate patients to remain sober due to fears of relationship dissolution.[22]

General Marital OR Family Treatment[9]

Interventions taking this approach directly address general family or relationship distress, under the assumption that improving family functioning will reduce patient stressors and improve patient functioning.[9]

PRESENT STUDY

With one known exception,[9] prior reviews have focused on a discrete number of mental health conditions at a time (i.e., a review of family treatments for depression). To the best of our knowledge, the most recent comprehensive review that included family involved interventions for any mental health condition was published in 1998.[9] A comprehensive review is called for to update the evidence, to serve VA needs, and to facilitate comparisons of the evidence across conditions. Additionally, such a review can highlight family interventions for mental health conditions that may not have been addressed in recent prior reviews due to too few RCTs to warrant a disorder specific review (i.e., sexual functioning disorders, PTSD). Prior reviews are potentially less relevant to VA populations due to their focus on studies conducted both nationally and internationally. Studies conducted outside the US (i.e., family interventions within Eastern societies) may be less relevant to US Veterans, given important cultural differences in family structure and function. Finally, given the VA's interest in including families in order to improve the quality of care provided in the VA, an important question to address is the comparative efficacy of family involved interventions versus individual-only treatment approaches.

In the only known comprehensive review of family involved psychosocial treatments for mental health conditions, Baucom and colleagues[9] established categories for evaluating the efficacy of a couple/family intervention, based upon Chambless and Hollon's[23] definition of empirically supported treatments (i.e., "clearly specified psychological treatments shown to be efficacious in controlled research with a delineated population," p. 7). They define an *efficacious* treatment as one in which the intervention has demonstrated superiority over waitlist control in studies conducted by two independent research teams. An *efficacious and specific* intervention has demonstrated superiority in at least two studies conducted by independent research teams over a placebo, nonspecific, or alternative intervention. They modify these labels with *possibly* (i.e., possibly efficacious and possibly efficacious and specific) when the above criteria are met by a single study. Using these criteria, the conclusions from the 1998 review are outlined in Table 1.

Table 1. Empirically Supported Couple and Family Treatments for Mental Health Conditions (Baucom 1998[9])

Mental Health Condition	Intervention	Efficacy Status
Schizophrenia	Behavioral Family Therapy[24-28]	1
	Supportive Family Therapy[29] [30-32]	1
	Family systems[33]	3
Alcohol Use Disorders	Community Reinforcement Approach[34-36]	3
	Behavioral Marital Therapy[37, 38]	3
Female orgasmic disorder	Sexual skill training for primary female orgasmic disorder[39, 40]	3
	Masters and Johnson for female orgasmic disorders[41]	3
Mixed female sexual dysfunctions	Behavioral Marital Therapy + Masters and Johnson[42]	3
Female hypoactive sexual desire	Marital + orgasm consistency training[43]	3
Depression	Behavioral Marital Therapy[44, 45]	4
Obsessive Compulsive Disorder	Family-assisted exposure therapy[46]	4
	Partner-assisted exposure therapy[47, 48]	4
Agoraphobia	Partner-assisted exposure therapy[49-53]	4
	Partner-assisted Cognitive-Behavioral Therapy[54]	4
	Partner-assisted exposure + couple communication training[55]	4

Efficacy Status:
1 = Efficacious & Specific; superior to placebo, nonspecific, or alternative intervention in at least two studies conducted by independent research teams.
2 = Efficacious; superior to waitlist in RCTs conducted by two independent research teams.
3 = *Possibly* Efficacious & Specific; criteria met for efficacious and specific from a single study.
4 = *Possibly* Efficacious; criteria met for efficacious from a single study.[9, 23]

Baucom and colleagues[9] concluded that family involved treatments for schizophrenia were clearly efficacious for reducing relapse rates. These family treatments often incorporated elements from all three types of approaches to family involvement (family assisted interventions, disorder specific interventions, and family/couple therapy). These findings are largely consistent with larger reviews of empirically supported treatments.[23] Chambless and Ollendick[56] reviewed the American Psychiatric Association's Task Force and various other work groups' recommendations for psychosocial interventions considered efficacious and possibly efficacious, using similar criteria and including family treatments. Their review largely overlaps with Baucom and colleagues'[9] conclusions, with a few exceptions. First, one group[57] identified behavioral marital therapy as efficacious for depression among patients with marital discord and a second[58] identified behavioral marital therapy as possibly efficacious for depression. Second, multiple work groups identified the Community Reinforcement Approach and behavioral couple therapy for alcohol use disorders as either efficacious or possibly efficacious.

OBJECTIVES

The present study provides an update to prior work conducted by Baucom[9] and others[56] by examining the effectiveness of family involved psychosocial treatments in US samples for mental health conditions. Due to our focus solely on mental health conditions and US studies, our findings are not intended to be a strict replication and extension of Baucom and colleagues'[9] prior review. We conducted a systematic review of randomized controlled trials (RCTs) of psychosocial interventions, addressing a mental health condition through a family intervention. Given prior work already conducted in this area, we focused on only those studies conducted after 1995. To optimize relevance to Veterans and the VA, in addition to a focus on US studies, we limited our review to improvements in patient functioning, including patient symptoms and family/couple functioning (primary outcomes) and treatment adherence, treatment attendance, patient satisfaction, and social support for patients (intermediate outcomes). Figure 1 provides our analytic framework, depicting our population, interventions, comparators, and outcomes of interest. We were interested in reviewing the evidence of the efficacy of family involved interventions (compared to no psychosocial intervention), as well as the degree to which family involved interventions are superior to an alternative individually-focused or family involved intervention (i.e., specificity).

We sought to address two specific questions:

Key Question #1. What is the efficacy of family involved interventions in improving outcomes for adult patients with mental health conditions [i.e., how do family involved psychosocial treatments compare to no psychosocial treatment: (a) waitlist/no treatment or (b) medication management only]?

Key Question #2. What is the effectiveness of family involved interventions compared to alternative interventions in improving outcomes for adult patients with mental health conditions [i.e., how do family involved interventions compare to (a) any individually-oriented psychosocial intervention or (b) any alternative family involved intervention]?

**Family Involved Psychosocial Treatments for Adult Mental Health
Conditions: A Review of the Evidence**

Figure 1. Analytic Framework

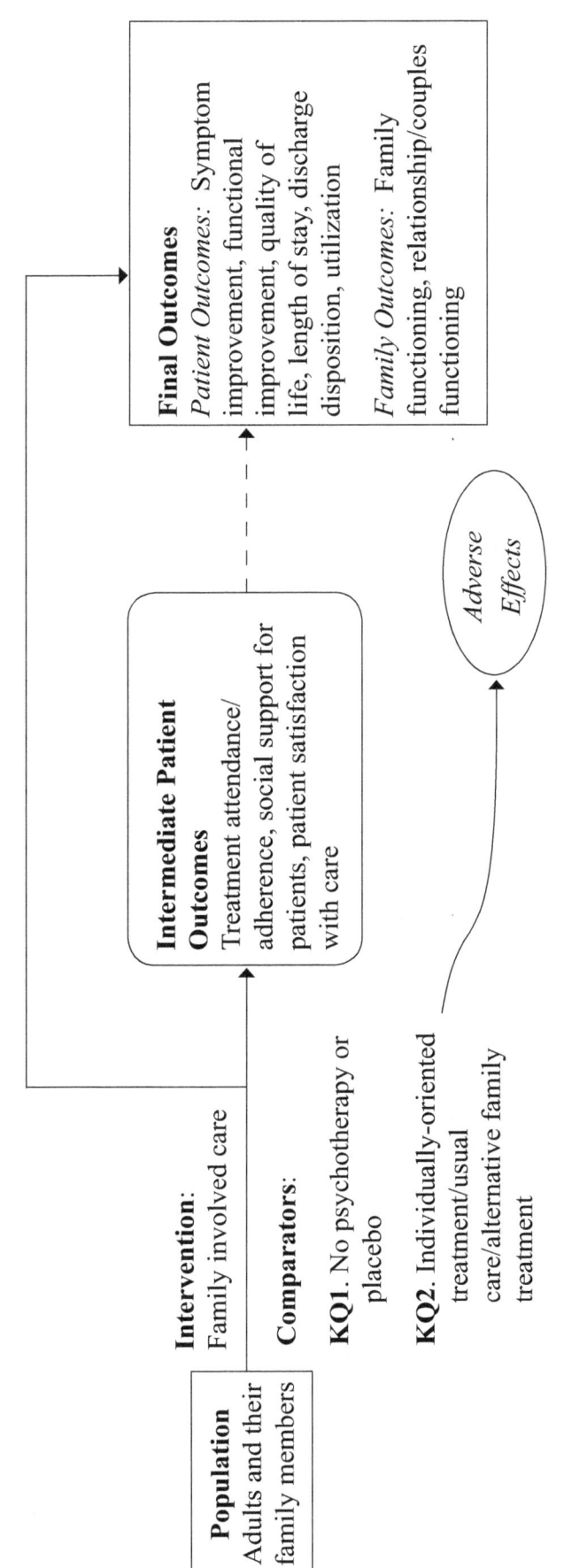

METHODS

TOPIC DEVELOPMENT

This project was nominated by Sonja Batten, PhD, Office of Mental Health Services. The key questions and scope were refined with input from a technical expert panel.

SEARCH STRATEGY

We searched MEDLINE (Ovid) and PsycINFO for randomized controlled trials (RCTs) and systematic reviews published from 1980 to November, 2011 using standard search terms. We limited the search to articles involving adolescents and adults and published in the English language. Search terms included: family, couples, home nursing, legal guardians, couple therapy, family therapy, and marital therapy. The search strategies are presented in Appendix A.

We obtained additional articles from systematic reviews, reference lists of pertinent studies, and suggestions from members of our technical expert panel.

STUDY SELECTION

Titles and abstracts were reviewed by researchers trained in the critical analysis of literature. Full text versions of potentially eligible articles were retrieved for review. Although our search identified studies of patients with both mental health and physical health conditions published from 1980 to the present, due to the volume of eligible articles identified by our search, we narrowed our inclusion criteria at the time of full-text review to include the following:

- RCT conducted in the United States or systematic review or meta-analysis of RCTs.
- Study involves a patient age 18 and over with a DSM-III or DSM-IV **mental health** condition.[59, 60]
- Intervention must involve family members or caregivers of the adult patient (patient may or may not be present for the intervention).
- Study reports intermediate patient outcomes or final outcomes of interest as outlined in the analytic framework (Figure 1).
- Control group must be used; control group may be no treatment/placebo or an alternative active treatment (e.g., usual care, individually-oriented treatment, or another family/ couple-oriented intervention).
- Study published in a peer-reviewed publication after 1995.

DATA ABSTRACTION

We abstracted the following study characteristics for each included study: author, date of publication, funding source, sample characteristics (gender, age, race/ethnicity, marital status, education, Veteran status, family characteristics, and recruitment method), inclusion and exclusion criteria (mental health condition, how the condition was assessed, family/caregivers involved, specific inclusion and exclusion criteria), treatment groups, intervention characteristics (format, whether manualized, number of sessions, treatment length, approach, and treatment integrity), outcomes assessed (list of patient, family/couple, and intermediate outcomes assessed), and study quality (allocation concealment, blinding, analysis approach, description of withdrawals). We extracted final outcomes (patient outcomes and family/couple functioning measures) and intermediate outcomes, by mental health condition, for each treatment arm, where reported, and noted whether the analysis included all patients randomized or study completers only. Final patient outcomes of interest were: symptom improvement, global functioning, quality of life, length of stay, disposition at discharge, and health care utilization. The family/couple functioning outcome of interest in all studies was global function or satisfaction. We also were interested in intimate partner violence, communication skills and relationship conflict, observational data of communication skills among couples, and sexual satisfaction. Sexual satisfaction was abstracted under patient symptom improvement for studies of treatment for sexual dysfunction and as a measure of couples functioning in the studies of treatment for substance abuse. Intermediate outcomes of interest were treatment attendance, adherence, social support for the patient, and satisfaction with care. We assessed outcomes at a number of different time points in order to determine initial and persistent changes in behavior. When available, we examined behavior at baseline, after treatment (post-treatment), short-term follow-up (up to 6 months), and long-term follow-up (up to 12 months or longer) across treatment arms. All abstraction was done by trained research personnel and verified by a second research associate under the supervision of the Principal Investigator.

QUALITY ASSESSMENT

We assessed study quality of included trials (all were randomized, controlled trials) according to the following criteria: 1) adequate allocation concealment, 2) blinding of key study personnel, 3) analysis by intention-to-treat, and 4) reporting of number of withdrawals/dropouts by group assignment.[61] We also considered whether the treatment protocol was manualized and whether the quality and consistency of the treatment protocol was evaluated (i.e., treatment integrity) as part of the quality assessment for individual studies. Studies were rated as good, fair, or poor quality. A rating of good generally indicated that the treatment was manualized and integrity was assessed. In addition, the trial reported adequate allocation concealment, blinding, analysis by intent-to-treat, and reasons for dropouts/attrition. Studies were generally rated poor if the treatment was neither manualized nor assessed for quality, the method of allocation concealment was inadequate or not defined, blinding was not defined, analysis by intent-to-treat was not utilized, and reasons for dropouts/attrition were not reported and/or there was a high rate of attrition.

DATA SYNTHESIS

We constructed evidence tables showing the study characteristics and results for all included studies, organized by clinical condition. We critically analyzed studies to compare their characteristics, methods, and findings. We compiled a summary of findings for each key question and drew conclusions based on qualitative synthesis of the findings or pooled analyses where feasible.

RATING THE BODY OF EVIDENCE

We assessed the overall strength of evidence using the method reported by Owens et al.[62] The overall evidence was rated as: (1) high, meaning high confidence that the evidence reflects the true effect; (2) moderate, indicating moderate confidence that further research may change our confidence in the estimate of effect and may change the estimate; (3) low, meaning there is low confidence that the evidence reflects the true effect; or (4) insufficient, indicating that evidence either is unavailable or does not permit a conclusion.

PEER REVIEW

A draft version of this report was reviewed by members of our technical expert panel and VA clinical leadership. Their comments and our responses are presented in Appendix C. Responses were also incorporated into the final report.

RESULTS

LITERATURE FLOW

We reviewed 2,469 titles and abstracts from the electronic search. After applying our initial inclusion/exclusion criteria at the abstract level, 2,025 references were excluded. We retrieved 444 full-text articles for further review and another 397 references were excluded. Inclusion criteria added at the full-text review stage included limiting the scope of the review to patients with mental health conditions and articles published after 1995. Four articles were identified by hand search. We therefore identified a total of 51 references for inclusion in the current review representing 39 unique projects. We grouped the studies by mental health condition and addressed the key questions for each condition. Table 2 details the number of publications and number of unique projects per condition.

Table 2. Number of Publications and Number of Unique Trials for Each Mental Health Condition

Mental Health Condition	Publications	Unique Trials
Substance Use Disorders	26	22
Schizophrenia Spectrum	8	4
Bipolar	10	6
Depression	1	1
Eating Disorders	1	1
Nicotine Dependence	1	1
Posttraumatic Stress Disorder (PTSD)	2	2
Sexual Dysfunction	2	2
Total	**51**	**39**

Figure 2 details the exclusion criteria and the number of references excluded at the abstract and full-text review stages.

Figure 2. Literature Flow Diagram

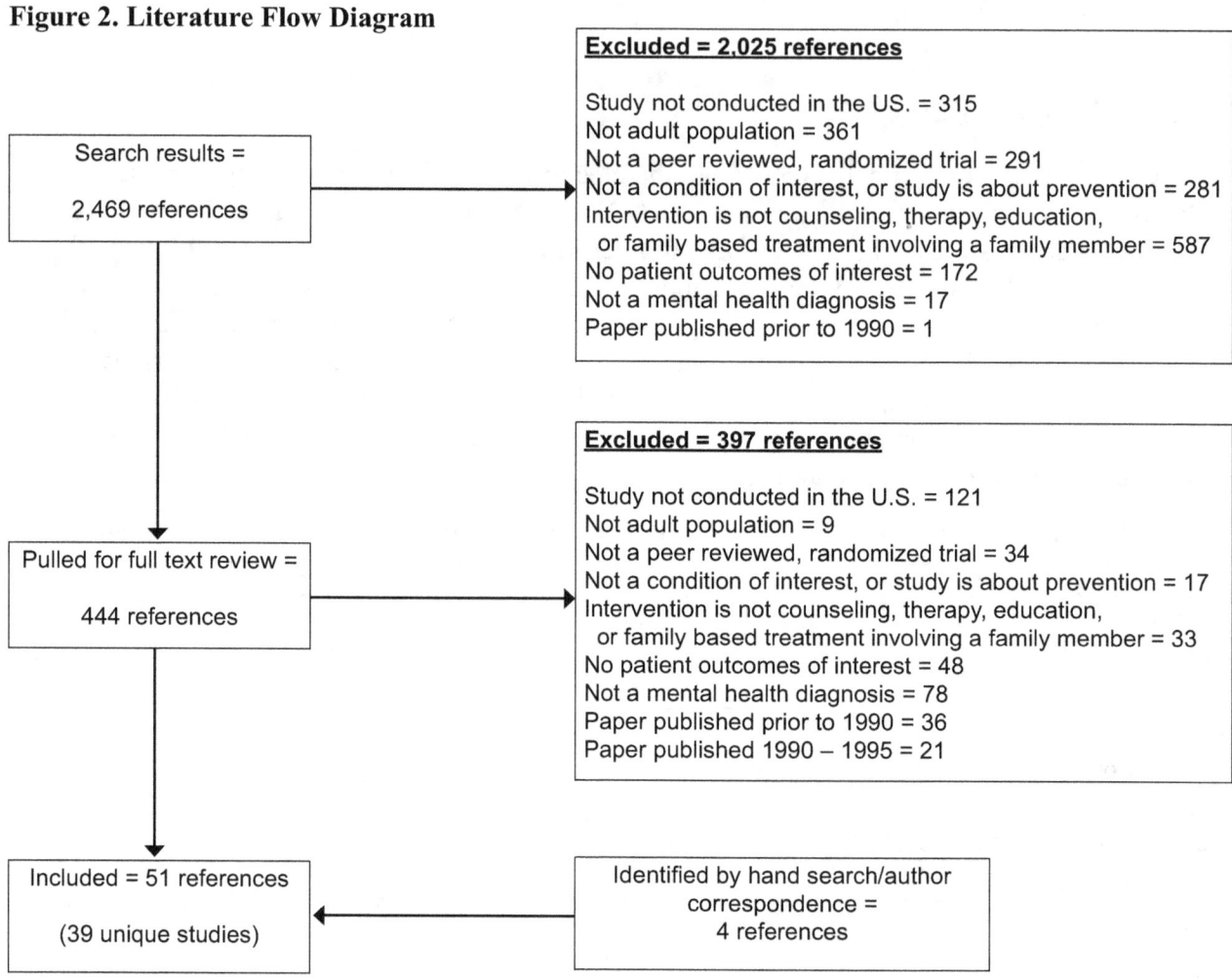

OVERVIEW OF TRIALS

Substance Use Disorders

The largest set of studies that met our criteria was from the substance use disorder (SUD) literature. Detailed descriptions of the study characteristics and outcomes are provided in Appendix D, Tables 1 to 4. We found twenty-six papers that met our criteria for substance use disorders, representing twenty-two unique RCTs. As summarized in Table 3 below, the 22 RCTs were nearly split between trials for treatment of alcohol (n=11) and drug use (n = 9) and two studies included treatment for either alcohol or drug use.[63, 64] Most studies (16 of 22) verified the SUD by a structured interview using DSM criteria.[60]

Population Studied

Subject and intervention characteristics are summarized in Tables 3 and 4. There were a total of 1623 patients studied, ranging from 29 to 184 participants in a single trial. Samples sizes for treatment conditions were small. Over 60% of the twenty-two trials (n=14) had an intervention condition arm with 30 or fewer subjects. The average patient and family member were each 38 years old. Patients were racially diverse (69% non-white, on average) and typically male (77%) with a female participating family member or intimate partner (76%). All subjects were married or cohabitating in all but four of the trials reporting marital status. Two trials[4, 65] were conducted with Veteran samples; none reported whether the family member was a Veteran. Eleven trials limited their participants to men,[4, 63, 65-73] including five alcohol use disorder (AUD) trials,[4, 65, 71-73] five drug use disorder trials,[66-70] and one trial that included those with drug use or alcohol use disorders.[63] Three trials limited patients to women.[74-76] These included two AUD trials[74, 75] and one drug use disorder trial.[76] The remaining seven trials included both men and women.[64, 77-82] Of these, two were AUD trials,[79, 81] four were drug use disorder trials,[77, 78, 80, 82] and one trial included subjects with either alcohol or drug dependence.[64]

Table 3. Summary of Baseline Characteristics, Substance Use Disorders Studies (22 trials)

Characteristics	Number/mean (range)	Number of trials reporting
Total number of patient/family dyads randomized	1623 (29-184)	19
Total number of patients from dyads analyzed	1589 (28-184)	19
Total number of family randomized for family only studies (patient not involved in intervention)	252 (32-130)	3
Total number of family only analyzed (patient not involved in intervention)	252 (32-130)	3
Marital status, % married	82% (17-100%)	16
Patient gender, % male	80%	20
Family member gender, % female	76%	17
Race, % non-white patients	31.5% (2-59.5%)	18
Veterans, %	100	2
Age of patients, years	38.0 (27.7-47.8)	19
Age of family members, years	37.8 (28.8-55.3)	13

Although we had a broad definition of family for inclusion in our review, most of the studies examined the effects of including a spouse or romantic partner in treatment. Of the twenty-two trials, 15 included a spouse or partner (wife/female partner = 10; husband/male partner = 3; either husband or wife/romantic partner = 3) of the subject.[4, 63, 65-67, 69-76, 78, 79] Seven trials did not restrict to wives or partners, allowing adult children, partners, or friends to participate.[64, 68, 77, 80-83] One of these trials specified any family member who was *not* a spouse or partner was eligible.[82]

Inclusion of Patients with Comorbid Conditions

Rates of co-occurring conditions among participants were not typically reported. However, in 15 trials, individuals with co-occurring serious mental health conditions defined as an organic mental, paranoid, psychotic disorders or schizophrenia, were typically excluded from participation. Patients at risk of harming oneself or others, including those with suicidal/homicidal ideation or history of domestic violence were excluded in three trials and one study reported excluding anyone with a psychiatric condition that may affect informed consent for treatment.

Intervention

By far the most commonly investigated family involved intervention (17 of 22 trials) was behavioral couples, marital, or family therapy (BCT/BMT/BFT), a dyadic (one patient and one family member/intimate partner), disorder-specific, couple/family treatment, designed to address a SUD through 1) cognitive behavioral strategies to promote abstinence, involving the family member, and 2) traditional behavioral couple therapy techniques to enhance communication, problem solving skills, and relationship satisfaction.[9] For simplicity, we use BCT in this review to refer to behavioral couple therapy for SUDs that includes either a spouse or an unmarried intimate partner (BCT or BMT). BFT refers to the same intervention, but including other family members. BCT/BFT were typically delivered in an outpatient setting, and with only two exceptions,[4, 64] participants were recruited from outpatient settings, the community, or the media, rather than following an inpatient stay. The length of the intervention varied, ranging from 10 to 56 weeks. The other psychological interventions reviewed included motivational enhancement treatment with psychoeducation and couple therapy (Helping Other Partners Excel or HOPE)[70] and community reinforcement training with families (i.e., CRAFT), an intervention delivered solely to the families of patients with SUDs to enhance communication, build skills, and develop coping strategies that would encourage the family's loved one to enter treatment.[80, 81, 83] HOPE and CRAFT were conducted in outpatient settings, and treatments ranged from 2 to 24 weeks.

Table 4. Summary of Heterogeneity, Substance Use Disorders Studies (22 trials)

		Number of trials reporting
Subjects diagnosed with:	Alcohol use disorders only	11
	Drug use disorders only	9
	Either drug or alcohol use disorders	2
Diagnosis verified by structured interview:	Yes	16
	Not reported	6
Family intervention with:	Wife/female intimate partner	11
	Husband/male intimate partner	3
	Husband/wife or male/female intimate partner	2
	Any identified family member	5
	Anyone but spouse	1
Family intervention compared to:	Waitlist	0
	Drug treatment only	2
	Treatment as usual or individual treatment(s)	14
	Other family treatment (s)	6
Subject gender:	Men	12
	Women	3
	Both men and women	7

Comparison Interventions and Study Designs

Family involved treatments were compared to one (11 trials[4, 64, 66-68, 70, 76, 79, 80, 82, 84-86]), two (9 trials[63, 65, 71-74, 77, 81, 83, 86, 87]), or three (2 trials[69, 78]) comparison interventions. Comparison interventions included 1) medical observation only (1 trial[64]); 2) individual treatment(s) only (10 trials[66-68, 70, 75-77, 79, 80, 82]); 3) individual and alternative family involved treatment(s) (8 trials[63, 69, 71, 73, 74, 78, 81, 83]); or 4) only an alternative family involved treatment (3 trials[4, 65, 72]).

Comparison to Medical Observation

As noted, one study compared a family involved treatment to medical observation only and was reviewed for Key Question 1. In this study, authors tested the effect of a family intervention on the utilization of continuing care after patients were discharged following hospital admission for alcohol detoxification. Male and female participants admitted to an inpatient detoxification unit for alcohol use (with or without comorbid drug dependence) and a family member were randomized into either treatment as usual (consisting of assisting the patient with withdrawal symptoms, monitoring risks for developing serious problems during withdrawal, but no family involvement) or a brief family intervention. The family intervention included two meetings with participants and family members (either a spouse or parent) to review continuing care plans both prior to and after discharge and develop strategies for successful outcomes. This intervention was delivered by phone and in-person, depending on what was most convenient for the family member.

Comparison to Individual Treatment Only

Fifteen trials compared family involved treatments to individual behavioral treatment.[63, 66-71, 73-79, 82] These trials were reviewed to assess evidence for Key Question 2A.

Seven of the fifteen trials were two-armed trials that directly compared BCT to individual cognitive-behavioral therapy (ICBT).[66-68, 75, 76, 79, 82] An additional six trials compared BCT to ICBT and another family involved treatment(s) or variation of BCT. Three of the six trials[63, 73, 74] compared BCT to ICBT plus a psychoeducational program serving as an attention control condition. Two of these trials had the same psychoeducational program (Psychoeducational Attention Control Treatment or PACT)[63, 74] while the other was slightly different, but had common strategies and education targets with the PACT treatment.[73] Two other trials also included a comparison of BCT to ICBT and PACT, but also included a fourth arm to compare standard BCT to a briefer version of the therapy (B-BCT).[69, 78] Another three-arm trial[71] compared BCT to ICBT, but also a variation of BCT that included a parent training intervention. Results from these trials that compared a family involved intervention to an individual treatment were used to assess evidence for Key Question 2A.

The remaining two trials[70, 77] did not use BCT, but instead another family involved treatment. One was three-arm trial that included male and female participants with a substance abuse diagnosis who were assigned either to 1) naltrexone with ICBT; 2) naltrexone, ICBT, plus contingency management (incentives for participants to remain in treatment); 3) naltrexone, ICBT, contingency management, and reciprocal relationship counseling for the patient and a family member, friend, spouse, or child.[77] The second non-BCT trial was a two-armed trial that compared group motivational enhancement therapy with psychoeducation and couple therapy (Helping Other Partners Excel, HOPE) to a counselor-led drug treatment support group for men with drug use disorders.[70]

Comparison to Alternative Family Treatment(s) Only

Six trials compared family involved treatments to one or more alternative family treatments.[4, 65, 72, 80, 81, 83] Evidence from these trials were used to assess evidence for Key Question 2B. Two of these trials[4, 72] compared Behavioral Marital Therapy (BCT) to BCT plus a relapse prevention condition. O'Farrell and colleagues[4] conducted a two armed trial that directly compared these two conditions; the trial by McCrady et al.[72] was a three-armed trial that compared BCT to BCT plus relapse prevention or to BCT plus a self-help group for family members. Another trial that compared family involved treatments was also by O'Farrell et al.[65] In that two-armed trial, a combination of BCT and ICBT was compared to BCT and interactional treatment, a therapy approach that does not pre-plan therapy sessions, but instead focuses on mutual support, sharing of feelings, and problem solving through discussion. The remaining three studies were unique in that they targeted the family members of patients with a drug use disorder, not the patient with the disorder, directly.[80, 81, 83] Each of these three trials compared a family intervention to alternative treatments for families. In Kirby and colleges two-armed trial,[80] family members (spouses, parents, siblings) were randomized into either a 12-step self-help group counseling program or a community reinforcement training (CRT) which included individual counseling for a family member to enhance communication, build skills, and develop coping strategies that were specific to the subject's drug use disorder. The other two trials were similar. A variation of the community reinforcement training, called the community and reinforcement and family training (CRAFT) was tested. Like Kirby et al.,[80] both compared CRAFT to a 12-step self-help group counseling program. In the trial by Meyers et al.,[83] these two conditions were also compared to a CRAFT plus aftercare, which consisted of additional group therapy with family members for 6 months after the CRAFT intervention. In the trial by.[81] CRAFT and the self-help conditions were compared to a Johnson Institute intervention, where families confront the alcoholic about their abuse and describe their own experiences and observations about the abuse in order to encourage treatment engagement.

Outcomes

The most common patient outcomes reported were self-reported days of abstinence within a specified period of time, self-reported quantity and/or frequency of substance use, and initiation of treatment (utilization of care). The degree of symptom relief was commonly measured by the percentage of days abstinent (PDA) from alcohol or drugs or the percentage of heavy drinking days (PDHD), typically using the Time-Line Follow Back procedure (TLFB).[88] Tables 5 and 6 provide an overview of our findings. The most frequently reported family outcome was family or couple functioning, most often measured by the Dyadic Adjustment Scale (DAS). Length of time that participants were followed for assessments was variable, but typically included at the least a post-treatment or short-term assessment and in many cases assessments every 3 months for 12 months after treatment termination.

Table 5. Main Findings, Substance Use Disorders Studies (Alphabetical Order by First Author)

Study, Year Interventions	Patient Outcomes[a]		Family Outcomes			
	Symptoms	Utilization	Family Functioning	Couple Functioning	Intimate Partner Violence	Communication/ Conflict
Carroll, 2001[77] 1) Counseling for significant other+ ICBT+Contingency Management + Naltrexone vs. 2) ICBT + Contingency Management + Naltrexone vs. 3) ICBT and Naltrexone	Cond. 1) vs. 2): *Post: ns* Cond. 1)& 2) vs. 3): *Post: ns*		Cond. 1) vs. 2): *Post: +*			
Fals-Stewart, 1996,[66] 2000,[84] 2002[85] 1) Behavioral couple therapy vs. 2) Individual treatment - behavioral therapy	**(1996)** *Post: ns Short term: ns Long term: ns* **(2000)** *Long term: +*			Marital Happiness Scale : **(1996)** *Post: + Short term: ns Long term: ns* **(2000)** *Long term: +* % days separated: *Post: + Short term: + Long term: ns*	**(2002)** *Long term: +*	**(1996)** *Post: + Short term: ns Long term: ns*
Fals-Stewart, 2001[67] 1) Behavior Couple Therapy treatment package vs. 2) Individual based methadone maintenance (standard treatment)	*Post: +*			*Post: +*		
Fals-Stewart, 2003[68] 1) Naltrexone + Behavioral Family Therapy vs. 2) Naltrexone + individual based therapy	*Post: + Long term: +*		*Long term: +*			
Fals-Stewart, 2005[69] 1) Standard Behavioral couple therapy vs. 2) Individual based therapy vs. 3) Brief Behavioral couple therapy vs. 4) Psychoeducational attention control treatment	Cond. 1) vs. 2)[b] *Post: ns Short term: ns Long term: +* Cond. 3) vs. 2) *Post: + Short term: + Long term: +* Cond. 1) vs. 4) *Post: + Short term: + Long term: +* Cond. 3) vs. 4) *Post: ns Short term: ns Long term: ns*			Cond. 1) vs. 2)[b] *Post: + Short term: + Long term: +* Cond. 3) vs. 2) *Post: + Short term: + Long term: +* Cond. 1) vs. 4) *Post: + Short term: + Long term: +* Cond. 3) vs. 4) *Post: + Short term: + Long term: +*		

Study, Year Interventions	Patient Outcomes[a]		Family Outcomes			
	Symptoms	Utilization	Family Functioning	Couple Functioning	Intimate Partner Violence	Communication/ Conflict
Fals-Stewart, 2006[74] 1) Behavioral couple therapy vs. 2) Individual based therapy vs. 3) Psychoeducational attention control treatment	Cond. 1) vs. 2) Post: ns Short term: ns Long term: ns Cond.1) vs. 3) Post: ns Short term: ns Long term: ns			Cond. 1) vs. 2) Post: + Short term: + Long term: + Cond.1) vs. 3) Post: + Short term: + Long term: + Cond. 2) vs. 3) Post: ns Short term: ns Long term: ns	Cond. 1) vs. 2) Long term: + Cond.1) vs. 3) Long term: +	
Fals-Stewart, 2008[78] 1) Standard Behavioral couple therapy vs. 2) Individual based therapy vs. 3) Brief Behavioral couple therapy vs. 4) Psychoeducational attention control treatment	Cond. 1) vs. 2)[b] Post: + Short term: + Long term: + Cond.1) vs. 3) Post: ns Long term: ns Cond. 3) vs. 2) Post: ns Long term: + Cond. 3) vs. 4) Post: ns Long term: +			Cond. 1) vs. 2)[b] Post: + Short term: + Long term: + Cond.1) vs. 3) Post: ns Long term: ns Cond. 3) vs. 2) Post: + Long term: + Cond. 3) vs. 4) Post: + Long term: +		
Fals-Stewart, 2009[79] 1) Behavioral Couple Therapy vs. 2) Individual based treatment	Post: ns Short term: + Long term: +			Post: + Short term: + Long term: +		
Jones, 2011[70] 1) HOPE: Helping Other Partners Excel vs. 2) Usual care	Short term: -			Short term: -		
Kelley, 2002[63] 1) Behavior Couple Therapy vs. 2) Individual Behavioral Therapy vs. 3) Psychoeducational attention control treatment	Cond. 1) vs. 2) & 3) Post: + Short term: + Long term: +			Cond. 1) vs. 2) & 3) Post: + Short term: + Long term: +		
Kirby, 1999[80] 1) Individual counseling and Psychoeducation vs. (community reinforcement training intervention) 2) Self help (Narcotics Anonymous)	Post: ns	Post: ns	Post: ns			

Study, Year Interventions	Patient Outcomes[a]		Family Outcomes			
	Symptoms	Utilization	Family Functioning	Couple Functioning	Intimate Partner Violence	Communication/ Conflict
Lam, 2009[71] 1) Behavioral Couple Therapy vs. 2) Individual based treatment vs. 3) Parent Skills with Behavioral Couple Therapy	Cond. 1) vs. 2)[b] Post: ns Short term: ns Long term: ns Cond. 1) vs. 3) Post: ns Short term: ns Long term: ns Cond. 2) vs. 3) Post: ns Short term: ns Long term: ns			Cond. 1) vs. 2)[b] Post: + Short term: ns Long term: ns Cond. 1) vs. 3) Post: ns Short term: ns Long term: ns Cond. 2) vs. 3) Post: ns Short term: ns Long term: ns	Cond. 1) vs. 2) Post: ns Short term: ns Long term: ns Cond. 1) vs. 3) Post: ns Short term: ns Long term: ns Cond. 2) vs. 3) Post: ns Short term: ns Long term: ns	
McCrady, 1996,[72] 1999,[86] 2004[87] 1) Alcohol focused spouse involvement + behavioral marital therapy (ABCT) vs. 2) ABCT+ AA/Al Anon vs. 3) ABCT + relapse prevention	(1996) Cond. 1) vs. 2) Post: ns Cond. 1) vs. 3) Post: ns Cond. 2) vs. 3) Post: ns (1999) Cond. 1) vs. 2) Short term: ns Cond. 1) vs. 3) Short term: ns Cond. 2) vs. 3) Short term: ns (2004) Cond. 1) vs. 2) Long term: ns Cond. 1) vs. 3) Long term: ns Cond. 2) vs. 3) Long term: ns			(1999) Cond. 1) vs. 2) Short term: ns Cond. 1) vs. 3) Short term: ns Cond. 2) vs. 3) Short term: ns (2004) Cond. 1) vs. 2) Long term: ns Cond. 1) vs. 3) Long term: ns Cond. 2) vs. 3) Long term: ns		

Family Involved Psychosocial Treatments for Adult Mental Health Conditions: A Review of the Evidence

Study, Year Interventions	Patient Outcomes[a]		Family Outcomes			
	Symptoms	Utilization	Family Functioning	Couple Functioning	Intimate Partner Violence	Communication/ Conflict
McCrady, 2009[75] 1) Alcohol Behavior Couple Therapy vs. 2) Alcohol Behavior Individual Therapy	% PDA[c] Post: ns Long term: ns % PDHD Post: ns Short term: ns Long term: ns % complete abstinence Short term: ns Long term: ns % no drinking Short term: ns Long term: ns	ns		+		
Meyers, 2002[83] 1) Community Reinforcement and Family Training (CRAFT) vs. 2) Al-Anon or Narcotics Anonymous facilitation therapy vs. 3) CRAFT + aftercare	Cond. 1) vs. 2) Short term: ns Long term: ns Cond. 1) vs. 3) Short term: ns Long term: ns Cond. 2) vs. 3) Short term: ns Long term: ns	Cond. 1) vs. 2) Short term: + Cond. 1) vs. 3) Short term: ns Cond. 1) vs. 3) Short term: +				
Miller, 1999[81] 1) CRAFT vs. 2) Al-Anon vs. 3) Johnson Institute intervention		Cond. 1) vs. 2) Short term: + Long term: + Cond. 1) vs. 3) Short term: + Long term: + Cond. 2) vs. 3) Short term: ns Long term: ns	Cond. 1) vs. 2) Short term: ns Cond. 1) vs. 3) Short term: ns Cond. 2) vs. 3) Short term: ns			Cond. 1) vs. 2) Short term: ns Cond. 1) vs. 3) Short term: ns Cond. 2) vs. 3) Short term: ns
O'Farrell (1998a)[4] 1) Behavioral Couple Therapy + Relapse Prevention vs. 2) Behavioral Couple Therapy	Post: ns Short term: + Long term: + Final: ns			Post: ns Short term: ns Long term: ns Final: ns		Post: ns Short term: ns Long term: ns Final: ns

Family Involved Psychosocial Treatments for Adult Mental Health Conditions: A Review of the Evidence

Study, Year Interventions	Patient Outcomes[a]		Family Outcomes			
	Symptoms	Utilization	Family Functioning	Couple Functioning	Intimate Partner Violence	Communication/ Conflict
O'Farrell (1998b)[65] 1) Behavioral Marital Therapy vs. 2) Interactional Couple Therapy vs. 3) Individual treatment only				Cond. 1) vs. 2) *Post: ns* Cond. 1) vs. 3) *Post: ns* Cond. 2) vs. 3) *Post: ns*		
O'Farrell (2008)[64] 1) Brief Family Treatment Intervention vs. 2) Treatment as usual	*Short term: ns*	*Post: +* *Short term: ns*				
O'Farrell (2010)[82] 1) Behavioral Family Counseling + Individual Based Treatment vs. 2) Individual Based Treatment	PDA: *Post: ns* *Short term: ns* PDPSU: *Post: ns* *Short term: ns*		*Post: ns* *Short term: ns*			
Walitzer, 2004[73] 1) Behavior Couple Therapy (alcohol-focused) vs. 2) Individual group counseling vs. 3) Alcohol focused spouse involvement in behavior change	Mean days abstinent: Cond. 1) vs. 2) *Post: ns* *Short term: ns* *Long term: ns* Cond. 3) vs. 2) *Post: +* *Short term: ns* *Long term: ns* Mean days heavy drinking: Cond. 1) vs. 2) *Post: +* *Short term: +* *Long term: ns* Cond. 3) vs. 2) *Post: +* *Short term: +* *Long term: ns*			1) vs. 2) *Post: ns* *Short term: ns* *Long term: ns* Cond. 3) vs. 2) *Post: ns* *Short term: ns* *Long term: ns*		
Winters, 2002[76] 1) Behavior Couple Therapy vs. 2) Individual Behavioral Therapy	*Post: +* *Short term: +* *Long term: ns*			*Post: +* *Short term: ns* *Long term: ns*		

Note: Symbols denote differences between condition 1 and condition 2 unless otherwise noted: + effects favor condition 1; − effects favor the comparator treatment; = no differences; *ns* = differences between conditions are non-significant (p > 0.05). Post refers to post-treatment assessment; short-term refers to the last assessment conducted within 6 months of treatment ending; long term refers to the last assessment conducted within 12 months of treatment ending; final refers to the last assessment conducted after 12 months of treatment ending

[a]No patient outcomes reported for global functioning.
[b]Mean comparisons not conducted by author, but in secondary analysis for this review.

cAfter adjusting for relationship functioning, both short and long term.

Table 6. Intermediate Findings, Substance Abuse Disorder Studies (Alphabetical Order by First Author)

Study, Year Interventions	Intermediate Outcomes		
	Attendance	Adherence	Satisfaction
Carroll, 2001[77] 1) Counseling for significant other+ ICBT+ Contingency Management + Naltrexone vs. 2) ICBT + Contingency Management + Naltrexone vs. 3) ICBT and Naltrexone	Cond. 1) & 2) vs. 3): + Cond. 1) vs. 2): ns	Naltrexone adherence: Cond. 1) & 2) vs. 3): ns Cond. 1) vs. 2): ns	
Fals-Stewart, 1996,[66] 2000,[84] 2002[85] 1) Behavioral Couple Therapy vs. 2) Individual treatment - behavioral therapy	ns		ns
Fals-Stewart, 2001[67] 1) Behavior Couple Therapy treatment package vs. 2) Individual based methadone maintenance (standard treatment)	ns		ns
Fals-Stewart, 2003[68] 1) Naltrexone + Behavioral Family Therapy vs. 2) Naltrexone + individual based therapy	+	Naltrexone adherence: +	ns
Fals-Stewart, 2005[69] 1) Brief Behavioral Couple Therapy 2) Standard Behavioral Couple Therapy vs. 3) Individual based therapy vs. 4) Psychoeducational attention control treatment	ns		ns
Fals-Stewart, 2006[74] 1) Behavioral Couple Therapy vs. 2) Individual based therapy vs. 3) Psychoeducational attention control treatment	ns		ns
Fals-Stewart, 2008[78] 1) Brief Behavioral Couple Therapy vs. 2) Standard Behavioral Couple Therapy vs. 3) Individual based therapy vs. 4) Psychoeducational attention control treatment	ns		ns
Fals-Stewart, 2009[79] 1) Behavioral Couple Therapy vs. 2) Individual based treatment	ns		ns
Kelley, 2002[63] 1) Behavior Couple Therapy vs. 2) Individual Behavioral Therapy vs. 3) Psychoeducational attention control treatment	ns		

Family Involved Psychosocial Treatments for Adult Mental Health Conditions: A Review of the Evidence

Study, Year Interventions	Intermediate Outcomes		
	Attendance	Adherence	Satisfaction
Kirby, 1999[80] 1) Individual counseling and Psychoeducation vs. (community reinforcement training intervention) 2) Self help (Narcotics Anonymous)	+		
Lam, 2009[71] 1) Parent Skills with Behavioral Couple Therapy vs. 2) Behavioral Couple Therapy vs. 3) Individual based treatment	ns		
McCrady, 1996,[72] 1999,[86] 2004[87] 1) Alcohol focused spouse involvement + behavioral marital therapy (ABCT) vs. 2) ABCT + AA/Al Anon vs. 3) ABCT + relapse prevention	ns	Patient homework completed ns (1996) + (1999)	
McCrady, 2009[75] 1) Alcohol Behavior Couple Therapy vs. 2) Alcohol Behavior Individual Therapy	+		
Meyers, 2002[83] 1) Community Reinforcement and Family Training (CRAFT) vs. 2) CRAFT + aftercare vs. 3) Al-Anon or Narcotics Anonymous facilitation therapy	ns		
Miller, 1999[81] 1) CRAFT vs. 2) Johnson Institute intervention vs. 3) Al-Anon	Cond. 1) vs. 2): + Cond. 3) vs. 2): +		
O'Farrell, 1998a[4] 1) Behavioral Marital Therapy + Relapse Prevention vs. 2) Behavioral Marital Therapy		Anti-abuse contract: Post: ns Short term: ns Long term + Final: ns	
O'Farrell, 2010[82] 1) Behavioral Family Counseling + Individual Based Treatment vs. 2) Individual Based Treatment	+		
Walitzer, 2004[73] 1) Behavior Couple Therapy (alcohol-focused) vs. 2) Individual group counseling vs. 3) Alcohol focused spouse involvement in behavior change	ns		
Winters, 2002[76] 1) Behavior Couple Therapy + Individual Behavioral Therapy vs. 2) Individual Behavioral Therapy	ns		ns

Note: Symbols denote differences between condition 1 and condition 2 unless otherwise noted: + effects favor condition 1; – effects favor the comparator treatment; ns = differences between conditions are non-significant (p > 0.05)

Bipolar Disorder

We included 6 unique RCTs (10 publications) of family interventions for subjects with bipolar disorder. Detailed descriptions of the study characteristics and outcomes are provided in Appendix D, Tables 5 to 8. Subject and intervention characteristics are summarized in Tables 7 and 8. Table 9 is an overview of our findings.

Population Studied

Baseline characteristics of the study subjects are summarized in Table 7. There were a total of 625 subjects; two trials had less than 50 subjects and 3 trials had more than 100 subjects. The mean age in all 6 studies was less than 50 years. The majority of subjects were white, less than half were male, and approximately half were married. No study specifically enrolled Veterans.

Table 7. Summary of Baseline Characteristics, Bipolar Disorder Studies

Characteristic	Mean (range) except as noted	Number of trials reporting*
Total number of patients randomized	Total=625 (40-293)	6
Gender, % male	42 (37-54)	6
Age of subjects, years	38 (26-48)	6
Race, % white	87 (60-94)	4
Veterans, %	NR	0
Marital status, % married	52 (15-67)	5

*6 trials were presented in 10 articles

Five studies examined family involved interventions with patients with either bipolar I mood disorder, (3 studies[89-91]) or bipolar I or II mood disorder (2 studies[92, 93]). One study did not specify a bipolar type but included patients with "major affective disorder or bipolar disorder, manic, depressed, or mixed."[94] In five studies, the intervention targeted patients with these disorders,[89-92, 94] while the sixth directly targeted the caregivers of individuals with either condition.[93] Two studies enrolled participants predominantly while they were inpatients,[89, 90] while the remaining studies enrolled participants predominantly while they were outpatients. Few requirements for participating family members were reported. In one study, the family member was a spouse or intimate partner.[94] One study required that caregivers (family or other individual in close contact, supporting the patient financially, or involved in their treatment) had to have at least one physical or mental health problem.[93]

Inclusion of Comorbid Conditions

Rates of co-occurring conditions among participants were not typically reported. However, the five studies that enrolled patients[89-92, 94] excluded individuals with a current alcohol or drug dependence disorder. Individuals with other co-occuring mental health diagnoses were not explicitly excluded although two studies did exclude patients with organic central nervous system disorder.[91, 94] In two studies, the patient had to be either taking[91, 92] or willing to take[92] mood stabilizing medications.

Intervention

The interventions included general marital or family therapy,[89, 94] disorder-specific family therapy,[90-92] and a combination of disorder-specific family intervention and family-assisted treatment.[93] In the study by Clarkin et al.,[94] the intervention was manualized psychoeducational marital therapy delivered by social workers with experience in family treatment.[94] It is unclear whether the intervention was delivered to individual or multiple couples. In the study reported by Miller et al.,[89] the family therapy program, titled Problem Centered Systems Therapy of the Family, was a 6 to 10 session intervention with a patient and his or her family members, focused on problem solving, communication, roles, affective responsiveness, affective involvement, and behavior control. Several studies[90-92] provided Family-Focused Treatment (FFT), a 9-month psychoeducation program (up to 21 sessions) providing education on bipolar disorder, communication training, and problem-solving skills training delivered to individual patients and their family members. Perlick et al.[93] provided a variant of FFT referred to as Family-Focused Treatment-Health Promoting Intervention (FFT-HPI), a 12-15 session psychoeducational intervention focused on enhancing caregiver skills for managing their relative's illness, defining self-care goals, resolving barriers to patient care and self-care, examination of core beliefs, and problem solving. It is unclear whether the caregivers met individually or in a group. FFT-HPI was explicitly developed to address both patient symptoms and health behaviors of the caregiver. Treatment periods generally ranged from 6 weeks to 9 months. All interventions were delivered in outpatient settings.

Comparison Interventions and Study Design

Comparator groups included medication only (2 trials[89, 94]), individual therapy plus medication (2 trials[91, 92]), multifamily group therapy with medication (1 trial[89]), crisis management with medication (1 trial[90]), ICBT with medication (1 trial[92]), collaborative care with medication (1 trial[92]), and health education.[93]

Table 8. Summary of Heterogeneity, Bipolar Disorder Studies

		Number of trials reporting*
Subjects diagnosed with:	Bipolar I only	3
	Bipolar II only	0
	Bipolar I or Bipolar II	2
	Not specified	1
Diagnosis verified by structured interview		6
Subjects recruited:	Shortly after episode (hospitalization not reported)	1
	While admitted to inpatient or outpatient services	4
	Not reported	1
Family intervention with:	Intimate partner only	1
	Any single family member	1
	Any combination of family members	4
	One couple/family at a time	6**
	Groups of families	1**
Family intervention compared to:	Waitlist	0
	Another treatment	6
Subject gender:	Men	0
	Women	0
	Both men and women	6

*6 trials were presented in 10 articles
**Miller (2004) compared an intervention with one family at time to a multifamily group intervention (represented in both counts)

Outcomes

Five studies assessed subject symptoms using established rating scales[89-91, 93, 94] with one study reporting recovery status,[89] and one study reporting relapse,[91] rather than the actual symptom scores. One study assessed clinical status based on DSM-IV criteria.[92] Global family functioning was reported in one study.[95] Two studies reported measures of global patient function,[94, 95] and two reported hospitalization data.[89, 91] Five studies reported intermediate outcomes related to treatment attendance or medication adherence.[89-92, 94] Three studies reported post-treatment results following 5 months,[93] 9 months,[95] or 11 months[94] of treatment. One study reported results at 12 months, 3 months after treatment programs lasting up to 9 months.[92] Another reported results at 28 months or 22 months after a 6 month treatment program.[89] One study reported data following treatment (9 months) and 3 months post-treatment (12 months total)[90] with 24 month follow-up in a subsequent publication.[5] Finally, one study reported results after an active treatment year (9 months treatment program) and after an additional follow-up year.[91]

Table 9. Main Findings, Bipolar Disorder Studies (Alphabetical Order by First Author)

Study, year Interventions	Patient Improvement			Family/Couple Improvement[a]
	Symptoms	Global Functioning	Utilization	Family Functioning
Clarkin, 1998[94] 1) Medication management + marital intervention vs 2) Medication management only	*ns*	+		
Miklowitz, 2000,[90] 2003[96] 1) Family focused + medication vs 2) Crisis management + medication	+ Survival without relapse: +			
Miklowitz, 2007[92, 95] 1) Family focused therapy vs 2) Inter-personal and social rhythm therapy vs 3) Cognitive behavioral therapy 4) Collaborative care	# months well[b]: *ns* Recovery[c]: +			
Miller, 2004,[89] Solomon, 2008,[97] Miller, 2008[98] 1) Medication + family therapy vs 2) Medication + multiple-family group therapy vs 3) Medication only	Recovery[d]: *ns*		*ns*[e]	
Perlick, 2010[93] 1) Family focused, health promoting vs 2) Health education	+			
Rea, 2003[91] 1) Family focused + medication vs 2) Individual therapy + medication	Relapse, rehospitalization: active treatment year: *ns* post-treatment year: +			

[a]No family outcomes reported for couples' global functioning, intimate partner violence, communication or conflict.
Note: For comparison of condition 1) to condition 2) except where noted + effects favor the intervention; – effects favor the comparator treatment; *ns* = differences between conditions are non-significant (p > 0.05).
[b]Conditions 1, 2, and 3 significantly different from 4; condition 1 not significantly different from 4
[c]Conditions 1, 2, and 3 significantly different from 4; condition 1 also significantly different from 4
[d]No differences between any treatments
[e]Condition 1 not significantly different from condition 3; results reported only for subgroup of patients who recovered

Schizophrenia Spectrum Disorders

For schizophrenia spectrum disorders, 4 unique studies (8 publications) met inclusion criteria for the current review. Detailed descriptions of the study characteristics and outcomes are provided in Appendix D, Tables 9 to 12. Participant and intervention characteristics are summarized in Tables 10 and 11.

Population Studied

Baseline characteristics of the study subjects are summarized in Table 10. There were a total of 810 participants, with data analyzed for 595 of these participants. The mean age in all studies was less than 35 years. The majority of subjects were male and predominantly white. No study excluded patients based on gender. Current marital status was reported in two of four trials, and most subjects were not married (90%). No study reported subjects' Veteran status. Each of the four studies included participation from the subject and any family member; Mueser et al.[99, 100] expanded that definition to include any person in a "caring but non-professional relationship" with subject (e.g., clergy). None of the four studies required the subject and participating family member to reside together; however, two of the studies[99-103] required a minimum four hours per week contact between them.

Inclusion of Comorbid Conditions

Each of the four studies included subjects with a range of schizophrenia spectrum disorders, as verified by structured interview. The complexity of clinical presentation included in the above trials varied. Schooler and colleagues[24, 104] employed the most restrictive inclusion/exclusion criteria, excluding participants with liver damage, chronic organic brain syndrome, or substance dependence,[24, 104] but participants with substance abuse disorders were not excluded (unless diagnosed with schizophreniform disorder). A second trial also did not explicitly exclude participants who met criteria for a substance abuse disorder.[101-103] Both Mueser et al.[99, 100] and McFarlane et al.[29] explicitly studied complicated cases by requiring eligible subjects to have either an active substance abuse disorder,[99, 100] or a 'complicating' factor,[29] including lack of consistent treatment participation, history of violence or suicidality, arrests, criminal convictions, homelessness, moderate to severe substance abuse, or frequent hospitalization. McFarlane et al.[29] however, did exclude acutely violent or suicidal participants, or participants with a major medical illness or physical addiction that required hospitalization, until they were stabilized. Participants were not excluded for any other comorbid mental health diagnosis or co-occurring problem.

Table 10. Summary of Baseline Characteristics, Schizophrenia Spectrum Disorder Studies

Characteristics	Mean (range) except as noted	Number of trials reporting
Total number of subjects randomized	810 (68-528)	4
Total number of subjects analyzed	595 (68-313)	4
Gender, % male	69 (65-77)	4
Age of subjects, years	31 (30-34)	4
Race, % white	74 (71-78)	2
Veterans, %	NR	0
Marital status, % married	10 (6-13)	2

Intervention

All interventions were two years in length, with the exception of Mueser et al.[99, 100] Mueser and colleagues[99, 100] compared a brief treatment lasting 2-3 months to an intervention lasting 9-18 months. All of the studies were conducted in an outpatient setting; however, two of the four studies recruited subjects after an acute psychotic episode or hospitalization,[24, 29] while the other two recruited subjects from community mental health agencies.[99-103]

Two of the interventions[29, 101-103] utilized multi-family groups. Multi-family groups combine disorder specific family intervention (emphasizing improvement of communication) with general family therapy goals (formal problem solving) and building of a social support network. The subject was included in the multi-family groups. Psychoeducation was a component to both interventions, to better understand the subjects' mental illness and engage family members in the subjects' recovery. McFarlane and colleagues[29] examined Asserted Community Treatment (ACT), which included an initial family education and engagement component, one home visit, and multi-family groups.

Schooler and colleagues assigned subjects to either Applied Family Management (AFM) or Supportive Family Management (SFM).[24, 104] Both AFM and SFM included an initial psychoeducational workshop, case management, and monthly support group meetings for both subjects and families over a two year period. The more intensive AFM added behavioral single family treatment conducted in the home. Subjects who stabilized (16-24 weeks) were further randomized into three double blind medication dosages of fluphenazine decanoate (continuous moderate or 'standard' dose, continuous low dose, or targeted dose only when symptomatic) and entered a two year maintenance phase.

Mueser et al.[99, 100] utilized both the disorder specific and general family therapy approaches in their Family Intervention for Dual Disorders, which combines behavioral single family therapy with a family education component through the 9-18 month intervention. A multi-family support group was available after the active intervention up to the 36 month point.

A commonality with all interventions was that even if an initial "family only session" was provided, the subject was present and included in subsequent family therapy sessions.

Table 11. Summary of Heterogeneity, Schizophrenia Spectrum Disorder Studies

		Number of trials reporting
Subjects diagnosed with:	Schizophrenia only	0
	Schizoaffective disorder only	0
	A range of possible schizophrenia spectrum disorders	4
Diagnosis verified by structured interview		4
Subjects recruited:	Following a recent hospitalization	2
	From community mental health setting	2
Family intervention with:	Intimate partner only	0
	Any single family member	4
	Any combination of family members	0
	One couple/family at a time	0
	Groups of families	0
Family intervention compared to:	Waitlist	0
	Another treatment	4
Subject gender:	Both men and women	4

Comparison Interventions and Study Design

In one study, with follow up for one year post-treatment,[101-103] the comparison condition was standard care which consisted of individual case management and medication management services.

Three interventions[24, 29, 99, 100, 104] compared more to less intense family intervention. In McFarlane et al. (1996), the intervention and comparison groups both participated in manualized Asserted Community Treatment (described above), but the comparison group did not include multi-family groups. Additional family interaction with the treatment team occurred throughout the two year intervention only in the event of a crisis. Schooler et al.[24] included case management and monthly family group meetings in the comparison condition (Supportive Family Management) throughout the two year intervention. Mueser et al.[99, 100] provided only brief psychoeducation (2-3 months) in the comparison group; however, a multi-family support group was available after the active intervention up to the 36 month point.

Outcomes

Patient outcomes assessed included hospitalization,[24, 29, 102, 103] service utilization,[102, 103] symptom severity,[101] global functioning,[29] and time to relapse/rescue medication (medication added with prodromal relapse signs and discontinued after stabilization).[24] Mueser and colleagues[100] reported on numerous dual diagnosis patient outcomes including substance use, psychiatric functioning, problem solving, and knowledge of disease. Family outcomes were assessed in two studies[29, 104] using the Social Adjustment Scale and the Patient Rejection Scale.[104] All studies reported outcomes post-treatment, with the exception of McDonell and colleagues,[103] who reported one year-post-treatment outcomes, and Mueser and colleagues,[100] who included 36 month outcomes. Table 12 is an overview of our findings.

Table 12. Main Findings, Schizophrenia Spectrum Disorder Studies (Alphabetical Order by First Author)

Study, year Interventions	Patient Improvement			Family/Couple Improvement	
	Symptoms	Global Functioning	Utilization	Family Functioning	Couple Functioning
Dyck, 2000,[101] 2002,[102] McDonell, 2006[103] 1) Multiple Family Group vs. 2) Standard Care	+		State Hospitalization: + Any Hospitalization: ns Crisis/urgent care: ns		
McFarlane, 1996[29] 1) Assertive Community Treatment + Multiple Family Group vs 2) Assertive Community Care + Crisis Care only	ns	ns	ns	ns	
Mueser, 2009[99] and in press[100] 1) Family Intervention for Dual Disorders vs 2) Family Psychoeducation	Schizophrenia symptoms: + substance use: ns	+			
Schooler, 1997[24] 1) Applied Family Management vs 2) Supportive Family Management	ns		ns	SAS/Social: NS PRS + SAS Friction: +	SAS/Sexual: ns

Note: For comparison of condition 1) to condition 2) except where noted + effects favor the intervention; – effects favor the comparator treatment; *ns* = differences between conditions are non-significant (p > 0.05).
SAS = Social Adjustment Scale (family friction, social/leisure and sexual/romance factors); PRS = Patient Rejection Scale

Posttraumatic Stress Disorder

There were two studies which met our search criteria examining family involved interventions for PTSD. Detailed descriptions of the study characteristics and outcomes are provided in Appendix D, Tables 13 to 16.

Population Studied

The two studies included a total of 233 participants. All patients in the trial conducted by Glynn and colleagues[8] were recruited from the Los Angeles VA (either inpatient or outpatient care). Participants for Weine[105] trial were recruited from the community. For Glynn and colleagues[8] (N = 36) the average patient was 47 years old, 45% were white, and all participants were Vietnam Veterans with combat-related PTSD (100% male). Ninety percent participated in the family intervention with their wife or intimate partner. For Weine and colleagues[105] (n = 197), all patients were Bosnian refugees, screening positive for PTSD, and not currently in mental health treatment. The average patient was 38 years old, most were married (82%), and half were male (48%). Veteran status was not reported. All adult family members were invited to participate and descriptive information on family members' relationship to patients was not described. Most family members were female (60%) with mean age of 36 years.

Inclusion of Comorbid Conditions

Glynn and colleagues[8] excluded participants with a number of conditions, including organic brain disorder, psychotic disorders, severe dissociative conditions, current substance dependence, or overt physical aggression to self or others in the past year. Weine[105] excluded participants with active psychosis, substance intoxication or withdrawal, or an acute confusional state. Participants were not excluded for any other comorbid mental health diagnosis or co-occurring problem.

Intervention

The family involved treatment condition in Glynn and colleagues' trial[8] included 9 weeks of exposure therapy (18 sessions) followed by PTSD-specific behavioral family therapy, which included psychoeducation about PTSD, anger management, and communication training (disorder-specific family treatment;[9] 34 sessions). Weine and colleagues[105] examined a 9 session (16 week) family involved support group intended to increase the access of Bosnian refugees with PTSD to mental health services (Coffee and Family Education and Support; CAFES; disorder specific family therapy[9]). Both trials were delivered through outpatient treatment.

Comparison Interventions and Study Design

Glynn and colleagues[8] compared the family involved treatment (exposure therapy with BFT) to two conditions: 1) exposure therapy alone (18 sessions, 9 weeks) or 2) wait list followed by behavioral family therapy (16 sessions) for interested dyads. Weine and colleagues[105] compared CAFES to a no treatment control group.

Outcomes

Primary outcomes relevant for the present study examined by Glynn and colleagues[8] included a composite of symptoms of PTSD assessed through structured clinical interview and self-report, social adjustment, and rates of treatment dropout. Outcomes were assessed at post-treatment and 6 months post-treatment. Weine and colleagues[105] examined the number of mental health visits attended by participants who screened positive for PTSD at 6, 12, and 18 months post-treatment. Main findings are reviewed in Table 13.

Table 13. Main Findings, Post Traumatic Stress Disorder Studies (Alphabetical Order by First Author)

Study, year Interventions	Patient Improvement			Family/Couple Improvement[a]	
	Symptoms	Global Functioning	Utilization	Family Functioning	Couple Functioning
Glynn, 1999[8] 1) Exposure Therapy + Behavioral family therapy vs. 2) Exposure Therapy vs. 3) Wait list	ns	ns			+
Weine, 2008[105] 1) Coffee and Family Education and Support vs. 2) No treatment control			+		

Note: For comparison of condition 1) to condition 2) except where noted + effects favor the intervention; − effects favor the comparator treatment; ns = differences between conditions are non-significant (p > 0.05).
[a]No family outcomes reported for intimate partner violence, communication or conflict.

Sexual Functioning Disorders

There were two studies which met our search criteria examining family involved interventions for sexual functioning disorders. Detailed descriptions of the study characteristics and outcomes are provided in Appendix D, Tables 17 to 20. Main outcomes are summarized in Table 14.

Population Studied

The two studies included a total of 97 participants. For both studies, all patients were males with erectile dysfunction (ED) who participated with their female intimate partner. Both samples were highly similar in terms of age (Aubin et al.,[106] mean age = 52 years; Banner et al.,[107] mean age = 57years) and race (Aubin:[106] 86% white; Banner:[107] 85% white). For the trial conducted by Aubin and colleagues,[106] eight-six percent were married. Rates of marriage were not reported by Banner and colleagues.[107] Veteran status was not reported in either study.

Inclusion of Comorbid Conditions

Both studies included only participants in heterosexual relationships of at least 6 months (Banner,[107]: 6 months; Aubin[106]: 12 months) and whose intimate partners did not have a sexual functioning disorder. Aubin and colleagues[106] included participants with ED, regardless of the etiology of the condition (50% not due to a medical condition; findings not stratified by etiology of ED). They excluded participants who reported a history of gender identity disorder, screened positive for depression, reported intimate partner violence, reported an extra-marital affair in the last year, discussed separation in the last year, and reported sexual dysfunction among intimate partners. Banner and colleagues[107] only included patients whose ED was not due a medical condition. They also excluded patients diagnosed with a number of medical conditions which could cause ED, participants with significant mental health conditions, and participants whose intimate partner had one of a number of sexual functioning disorders.

Intervention

The family involved treatment Aubin and colleagues[106] examined consisted of 12 weeks (8 sessions) of medication (Sildenafil) plus outpatient sex therapy that included a combination of existing couple and sex therapy techniques including communication skills, sensate focus, sexual fantasy training, and cognitive restructuring. Banner and colleagues[107] examined medication (Sildenafil) plus cognitive-behavioral sex therapy. They assigned participants to either medication plus cognitive-behavioral sex therapy or medication only for four weeks. At four weeks, they then provided cognitive-behavioral sex therapy to those in the medication only condition with continuing symptoms. Due to contamination across conditions after 4 weeks, only outcome data at 4 weeks are presented.

Comparison Interventions and Study Design

Aubin and colleagues[106] compared the family involved treatment to 12 weeks of medication management (Sildenafil), including 8 brief, typically individual, 15 minute, medication pick up visits to discuss any medical concerns. Banner and colleagues[107] compared the family involved intervention to medication management (Sildenafil) that included a pre-treatment information session.

Outcomes

Primary outcomes for both studies included the International Index for Erectile Function (IIEF)[108] and the Dyadic Adjustment Scale (DAS)[109] although DAS findings were not reported by Banner and colleagues.[107] Aubin and colleagues[106] also assessed relationship functioning using the Personal Assessment of Intimacy in Relationships scale (PAIR),[110] as well as treatment satisfaction through the Erectile Dysfunction Inventory of Treatment Satisfaction (EDITS).[111] Assessments were conducted at post-treatment and 2 months after treatment completion. Banner and colleagues[107] also assessed patient global functioning through the Beck Depression Inventory,[112] and Beck Anxiety inventory.[113]

Table 14. Main Findings, Sexual Functioning Disorders Studies (Alphabetical Order by First Author)

Study, year Interventions	Patient Improvement[a]		Family/Couple Improvement[b]
	Symptoms	Global Functioning	Couple Functioning
Banner, 2007[107] 1) Sildenafil + couple sex therapy vs 2) Sildenafil + couple sex therapy for treatment non-responders	*ns*		
Aubin, 2009[106] 1) Sildenafil + couple sex therapy vs 2) Sildenafil only	*ns*		*ns*

Note: For comparison of condition 1) to condition 2) except where noted + effects favor the intervention; − effects favor the comparator treatment; *ns* = differences between conditions are non-significant (p > 0.05).
[a]No patient outcomes were reported for health care utilization.
[b]No studies reported family/couple outcomes for intimate partner violence, communication, or conflict.

Other Conditions

We identified one trial each of family involved interventions for depression, eating disorders, and smoking cessation. The findings are summarized in Table 15. Subject characteristics treatment descriptions and outcomes are presented in Appendix D, Tables 21 to 24.

Depression

The depression study[114] included 35 heterosexual couples in which the woman was diagnosed with depression and the male partner was non-depressed. The mean age of the women was 43.2 years; the mean age of the men was 45.0 years and 94.3 percent of the couples were married. Eighty-eight percent of the sample were non-Hispanic white, 5.6 percent were Hispanic, 3.1 percent were black, and 3.1 percent were Asian. Couples were excluded if there was infidelity in the past 6 months or more than two acts of aggression in the past year. Couples were mildly to moderately distressed with severely discordant couples excluded. The women could be receiving other treatment for depression if they had been in individual psychotherapy for at least 12 weeks or on a stable dose of psychotropic medication for at least 8 weeks. The intervention was brief, problem-focused couple therapy for depression with wait list control as the comparator. Outcomes included measures of depression and relationship satisfaction. Thirty couples completed the 5 week treatment conducted in an outpatient setting. Three month follow-up data were obtained for twenty-seven couples.

Eating Disorders

Overweight women with binge eating disorder were the focus of the study by Gorin et al.[115] Women were excluded if they engaged in purging behaviors more than once per month or met diagnostic criteria for anorexia nervosa, bulimia nervosa, or eating disorder of no specific origin. They also could not be receiving concurrent treatment for weight loss, including appetite suppressants. The women were required to have a spouse or cohabiting partner willing to participate in treatment but marital status was not reported. The mean age of the women was 45.2 years, and 86 percent of the sample was Caucasian. The intervention was group CBT for binge eating disorder with involvement of the spouse or intimate partner. The goal was for both partners to understand binge eating disorder, identify coping resources, agree about a plan of action, and feel confident in their ability to address binge eating disorder (i.e., a disorder specific couple intervention.)[9] The comparators were standard group CBT and wait list control. The primary outcomes were binge eating frequency assessed with both a 7 day calendar recall and the Eating Disorder Examination Questionnaire (EDEQ).[116, 117] The treatment phase was 12 weeks with an additional 6 month follow-up; participants were outpatients.

Nicotine Dependence

The smoking cessation study[118] targeted women, pregnant for 20 weeks or less, who were current smokers or recent quitters. The women were required to be living with an intimate partner and willing to have the partner contacted regarding participation in the study. The mean age of the women was 24 years, 77 percent were white, and 96 percent were married. It was reported that 77% of the women had tried to quit smoking, with a mean of 3 prior attempts. Fifty-two percent of partners were smokers. The intervention was individual counseling calls by a health advisor with partners assisting in a coaching capacity (partner-assisted treatment[9]). The comparators were individual counseling and usual care. Outcomes of interest were support for cessation, general support, and smoking status. The patients were followed to 12 months post-partum, and the study was conducted on an outpatient basis.

Table 15. Main Findings, Depression, Eating Disorders, and Smoking Cessation Studies

Study, year Interventions	Patient Improvement			Family/Couple Improvement[a]	
	Symptoms	Global Functioning	Utilization	Family Functioning	Couple Functioning
DEPRESSION: Cohen, 2010[114] 1) Brief Couple Therapy vs. 2) Wait list control	+				+
EATING DISORDERS: Gorin, 2003[115] 1) Group Cognitive Behavioral Therapy (CBT) with spouse vs. 2) Group CBT vs. 3) Wait list control	ns^b	ns^b			ns^b
SMOKING CESSATION: McBride, 2004[118] 1) Partner assisted + woman-only care vs 2) Woman-only care vs 3) Usual care	ns^b				

Note: For comparison of condition 1) to condition 2) except where noted + effects favor the intervention; − effects favor the comparator treatment; ns = differences between conditions are non-significant (p > 0.05).
[a]No family outcomes reported for intimate partner violence, communication or conflict.
[b]No differences across all treatment conditions

RESULTS BY KEY QUESTION

KEY QUESTION #1. What is the efficacy of family involved interventions in improving outcomes for adult patients with mental health conditions [i.e., how do family involved psychosocial treatments compare to no psychosocial treatment: (a) waitlist/no treatment or (b) medication management only]?

Substance Use Disorders

Detailed descriptions of the outcomes are provided in Appendix D, Tables 2 to 4.

As noted above, no studies that we reviewed compared a family involved intervention to waitlist, but one study directly compared family treatment to medication-only care. O'Farrell and colleagues[64] tested the effect of a family intervention on the utilization of continuing care. Male and female subjects admitted to an inpatient detoxification unit for alcohol use (with or without comorbid drug dependence) and a family member were randomized into either treatment as usual, consisting of assistance with withdrawal symptoms, monitoring risks for developing serious problems during withdrawal, but no family involvement, or a brief family intervention. The family intervention included meeting with subjects and family members (either a spouse or parent) to review continuing care plans both prior to and after discharge. This intervention was delivered by phone and in-person, depending on what was most convenient for the family member. Three months post-discharge, there were no significant differences between conditions in the percent of days using alcohol or drug use. However, those in the brief family condition were twice as likely to enter continuing care programs compared to the usual care group (r = 0.36; medium effect). The authors did not report any family functioning outcomes.

Bipolar Disorder

None of the studies we identified included a wait-list control or no-treatment arm; two studies included a medication only arm.[89, 94] Outcomes are presented in Appendix D, Tables 6 to 8. In one study, it was noted that the psychiatrist provided support, encouragement, and direct advice as needed but avoided the use of psychotherapy.[89] Clarkin and colleagues[94] reported on change in symptoms when medication management plus marital therapy was compared to medication management only. The symptom change in scores over time did not differ significantly for the two treatment groups. However, they did find greater improvement in post-treatment medication adherence (p = 0.008) following marital therapy. Additionally, significantly improved global functioning was also reported (change in Global Assessment Scale, GAS, of 8.6 points in the marital therapy group compared to a change of 1.0 point in the medication only group).

The second study, evaluating Problem Centered Systems Therapy of the Family (PCSTF), reported no differences in recovery, median time to recovery, or relapse after recovery between subjects receiving medication plus family therapy (PCSTF) or multi-family group therapy (MFG) and subjects receiving medication only. There were also no differences in recovery or relapse when level of family impairment was considered. However, there were significant family impairment by treatment interactions for the number of depressive episodes per year, percentage of time in episode, and percentage of time in a depressive episode, indicating family therapy resulted in an improved course of illness for participants with high family impairment.[89, 98] Compared to medication management, the disorder specific psychoeducational family therapy (MFG) led to 1.4 fewer depressive episodes per year (d = 1.0), 14% percent less time in a mood episode (d = 0.82), and 1.7 fewer mood episodes, yearly (d = 0.92). The general family therapy (PCSTF) led to 0.9 fewer depressive episodes per year (d = 0.70) than medication management, additional comparisons between these groups for impaired families were non-significant.

No significant difference in number of medication sessions attended for the entire study population were reported, but significantly greater number of sessions were attended among those in PCSTF than the medication only group when only subjects who recovered were analyzed.[89, 97, 98]

Summary

No studies compared a family intervention to no intervention. Of two studies that compared marital or family therapy to medication only, marital therapy was associated with improved overall functioning and better medication adherence but not with improvement in symptoms. Problem Centered Systems Therapy of the Family was not found to be associated with recovery. However both PCSTF and MFGs were associated with improved depression over medication management only for patients in distressed families. No studies reported a family or couple function outcome.

Schizophrenia Spectrum Disorders

No studies compared a family intervention to no treatment or medication only.

Posttraumatic Stress Disorder

Each of the two studies of family involved interventions for PTSD compared the family involved intervention to a waitlist control. Results are presented in Appendix D, Tables 14 to 16. Glynn and colleagues[8] found that those assigned to either exposure therapy plus behavioral family therapy or exposure therapy alone reported fewer post-treatment PTSD symptoms than waitlist controls, however this difference eroded with time (differences non-significant at 6 month follow-up) and differences between groups on social adjustment were non-significant at each time point. Additionally, those who participated in exposure therapy plus behavioral family therapy were more likely to drop out of treatment than waitlist controls.[8] However, Weine and colleagues[105] found the patients of family members who participated in a family support group (i.e., CAFES) were significantly more likely attend mental health care treatment (the primary study outcome) than no treatment controls. Weine and colleagues[105] also collected data relevant to our key questions on PTSD symptoms and depression. However, differences on these variables across conditions were not presented. Also, the role of family distress in predicting treatment response was not examined.

Sexual Functioning Disorders

Two studies compared a family involved intervention to a medication only condition.[106, 107] Outcomes are reported on Appendix D, Tables 18 to 20. Findings suggested that sex therapy plus medication resulted in greater satisfaction with treatment[106] and cognitive-behavioral sex therapy plus medication did not result in greater erectile functioning on continuous scale scores. Differences were provided in rates of patient exceeding cutoffs indicating clinical improvement of erectile functioning (48% in the sex therapy condition and 29% in the medication only condition), but significance tests of these differences were not provided.[107] All other results indicated non-significant differences between conditions on couple functioning.[106]

Other Conditions

Findings from studies of depression, eating disorders, and smoking cessation are presented in Appendix D, Tables 22 to 24.

Depression

We identified one trial of couple therapy for depression that met our inclusion criteria.[114] Briefly, 35 heterosexual couples (94% of whom were married) were randomly assigned to Brief Couple Therapy (18 couples) or wait list control (17 couples). In each couple, the female was diagnosed with depression; male partners could not meet diagnostic criteria for depression. While single time point, univariate analyses at the 3 month follow-up demonstrated significant differences only in HAM-D[119] and not Beck Depression Inventory 2nd Edition (BDI-II) scores,[120] analyses using hierarchical linear modeling found that BDI-II (d = 0.54) and HAM-D (d = 0.72) scores decreased significantly over the course of the study (both p < 0.01, mean follow-up of 24.2 weeks). It was reported that 67% of women in the treatment group improved (a 50% or greater reduction in BDI-II or HAM-D scores) compared to 17% in the control group and that 47% of the treatment group showed full recovery (BDI-II score below 11 and HAM-D score below 6) compared to 8% of the control group. Scores for marital satisfaction, as measured by the Dyadic Adjustment Scale (DAS),[109] did not differ between treatment and control using the univariate approach. However, using hierarchical linear modeling, greater improvements in marital satisfaction were observed for treatment couples than control couples (p < 0.01). At the 3 month follow-up, the average participant in couple therapy reported relationship adjustment in the satisfied range (above 97.5;[121] mean = 102.1) while those in the waitlist condition reported scores indicating clinically significant relationship distress for the average participant (mean = 92.4).

Summary

One trial met our inclusion criteria and compared disorder-specific brief couple therapy to wait-list control. When examined over time through hierarchical linear modeling, brief couple therapy was associated with greater improvements in symptoms and greater marital satisfaction, though at any given time point, there were no significant differences in depression symptoms or marital satisfaction.

Eating Disorders

We included one study of family involved treatment of eating disorders that included a wait-list control.[115] The study enrolled women ages 18 to 65 years who were diagnosed with binge eating disorder. Participants were randomized to group CBT with spouse involvement, standard CBT, or wait-list control. Wait-list control results were only available at the end of the 12 week treatment period. There was no direct test for differences between the CBT with spouse group and wait-list controls. Data from the two CBT groups were combined and the "active CBT" group was found to have higher post-treatment self-reported abstinence rates (p = 0.02) and greater reductions in self-reported number of days binged (p=0.04) than the waitlist condition. However, scores on the EDEQ,[116, 117] administered as a confirmatory measure of binge eating frequency, did not differ significantly.

Summary

Group CBT for binge eating disorder with spouse involvement was not directly compared to wait-list control. Active CBT (i.e., CBT with spouse or individually) subjects had better symptom improvement than wait-list controls.

KEY QUESTION #2. What is the effectiveness of family involved interventions compared to alternative interventions in improving outcomes for adult patients with mental health conditions [i.e., how do family involved interventions compare to (a) any individually-oriented psychosocial intervention or (b) any alternative family involved intervention]?

Substance Use Disorders

Overview

The remaining 21 SUD trials (25 papers) in our review addressed Key Question 2. Outcomes data are presented in Appendix D, Tables 2 to 4. The majority of studies that addressed Key Question 2 were aimed at three different time points in the trajectory of treatment: treatment initiation or initial engagement, attendance or adherence, and treatment response. Results, therefore, were first organized by these stages. Trials providing data on treatment response are organized by common outcomes of interest: substance use or abstinence, relationship adjustment, and intimate partner violence. Within these categories, we then reviewed studies that addressed any SUD, including an alcohol use disorder (AUD) or a drug use disorder. Lastly, we reviewed the studies that compared different types of family interventions and then results by various sub-groups of interest, including Veteran status, gender, and family composition.

Studies by Fals-Stewart

Fifteen studies compared family involved treatment to an individual treatment. Of these, ten (67%) were either written by Dr. William Fals-Stewart[66-69, 74, 78, 79, 84, 85] or based on data he collected.[63, 71, 76] In 2010, Dr. Fals-Stewart was criminally charged by the State of New York with fraud that allegedly occurred during a scientific misconduct hearing held to review evidence about whether Dr. Fals-Stewart fabricated data in some of his federally-funded studies.[122] Dr. Fals-Stewart died in 2010 soon after criminal charges were filed, and because of his death, associated legal proceedings never reached a conclusion. While his studies have not been retracted by any journal, given the nature of the potential misconduct, we present findings both with and without Dr. Fals-Stewart's work.

Initiation

Three studies examined family interventions to improve patient initiation to SUD treatment.[80, 81, 83] These studies were unique in that they did not directly involve the person with the AUD or drug use disorder in the intervention. Each trial compared one family involved intervention to at least one other alternative family involved intervention (KQ2B). No trials reviewed included an individually-oriented treatment for the subject with an AUD or drug use disorder as a comparator (KQ2A). Consequently, we can make no conclusions regarding the comparative efficacy between family involved interventions versus individually-oriented interventions, targeting patients only, in promoting treatment initiation. All three trials examined community reinforcement training with families (i.e., CRAFT). CRAFT was developed to enhance communication, build skills, and develop coping strategies that would encourage the family's loved one to enter treatment. Kirby and colleagues[80] randomized 30 family members (spouses, parents, siblings) of someone with a drug use disorder into either 1) an earlier version of CRAFT, community reinforcement training (CRT), or 2) a 12-step self-help group counseling program. Miller and colleagues[81] randomized 130 family members of alcoholics into either 1) a version of the CRAFT intervention refined for families of alcoholics, 2) the Johnson Institute intervention, where families confront the alcoholic about their abuse and describe their own experiences and observations about the abuse in order to encourage treatment engagement, or 3) Alcoholics-Anonymous (Al-Anon), a self-help group for families of alcoholics. Meyers et al.[83] randomized 90 family members with a drug-abusing loved into either 1) CRAFT, 2) CRAFT plus 6 months of post-intervention group counseling sessions, or 3) Al-Anon/Narcotics-Anonymous (Narc-Anon), a 12-step program for family and friends of drug users. Across all three studies, the CRAFT intervention was significantly better at promoting initiation of treatment than the non-CRAFT approaches. Miller and colleagues[81] also found that parents were more likely to persuade drinkers into treatment than spouses. Initiation of treatment, however, was narrowly defined. For example, in Kirby and colleague's study,[80] treatment initiation was defined as whether the drug user entered counseling or drug abuse treatment or attended a self-help group. Miller et al.[81] defined initiation as completing an initial 4-hour assessment and at least one treatment session and Meyers et al.[83] viewed a patient completing a baseline assessment and scheduling a substance use treatment session as treatment initiation. These findings suggest that CRAFT may be a useful intervention for promoting treatment engagement, but evidence is limited about whether it is effective in improving treatment attendance or adherence.

Attendance and Adherence (KQ2A and KQ2B)

Eighteen of our twenty-one trials (86%) reported outcomes on treatment attendance. Ten trials reported no statistically significant differences across treatment conditions. Six, however, reported significantly better attendance for those in family involved interventions.[68, 75, 77, 80-82] Four of these six were drug us disorder trials; the other two were AUD trials. All six addressed Key Question 2A, since all compared attendance in a family involved treatment to attendance in an individual treatment. Three compared BFT or BCT to ICBT[68, 75, 82] and another compared reciprocal relationship counseling to ICBT. In two of these trials, patient treatment attendance was significantly better for those in family involved treatments than for those enrolled in only individual treatment (5-8 more session attended; patients were male opioid users only[68] or men and women with any substance use problem[82]). However, McCrady and colleagues[75] found those in ICBT were significantly more likely to complete treatment than those in BCT (24% versus 44% completed; patients were all female alcohol use disorder patients).

In the two other trials, both of which used CRAFT-type interventions[80, 81] the subject in the intervention with the AUD or drug use disorder was not the target for the intervention; therefore, family attendance to intervention sessions was measured. Family members were more likely to attend CRAFT sessions than either a self-help group[80] or the Johnson Institute training sessions.[81] However, there was no evidence to suggest that family attendance to intervention sessions for any of the three family interventions examined affected the primary outcome, patient initiation of treatment.

Two studies[68, 77] of patients receiving outpatient treatment reported differences in adherence to naltrexone (a medication to reduce substance use cravings). Both studies compared medication adherence for those randomized into family involved treatment versus those in individual treatment. Findings were mixed. Carroll and colleagues[77] did not find a significant difference in doses of naltrexone taken by condition, but Fals-Stewart and colleagues[68] did find superior medication adherence in BCT versus ICBT. With only two studies reporting medication adherence data, there is little evidence to suggest that family treatment significantly improves abstinence supporting medication adherence among individual with an SUD.

Treatment Response

As noted, fifteen of the twenty-one AUD and drug use disorder trials that addressed Key Question 2 examined if outcomes from family involved treatments differed from outcomes of at least one individual based treatment.[63, 66-71, 73-79, 82] We first review this evidence across all studies and then separately for studies addressing AUD and drug use disorder symptoms.

The most common symptom-related outcomes were related to either abstinence or days of heavy use, most frequently collected using subject or family members' self-report of abstinence, typically using the Time Line Follow Back (TLFB).[88] These reports were then converted into the percent of days an individual was abstinent (percent days abstinent; PDA) from substances or the percent of days that alcohol or drugs were heavily used (percent days of heavy drinking; PDHD) during the period assessed. Only six used urine tests to assess reliability of self-reported abstinence or use. Participants were typically assessed post-treatment and at three months, six months, nine months, and twelve months after treatment and asked to recall their use since the last assessment. A few studies continued follow-up assessments up to 18 months after treatment. Researchers often used survival analyses and growth curve modeling to assess factors associated with cumulative PDA or time to relapse. For our report we categorize follow-up assessments into three time points: post-treatment, short-term follow up (within 6 months post-treatment), and long-term follow up (at least 12 months post-treatment).

Substance Use Disorder Symptoms (Key Question 2A)

BCT Trials. Thirteen of the fifteen trials compared BCT/BFT to ICBT.[63, 66-69, 71, 73-76, 78, 79, 82] Nine of these trials used PDA from alcohol or drug use as a primary outcome. All but one[79] also included sample sizes for each condition. Consequently, for the remaining eight trials we were able to pool data and compare unadjusted weighted means in order to assess the evidence for these two conditions. Data from the pooled analysis examining PDA among these eight studies are presented below in Figure 3. Note that for one study (Kelley, 2002) we present data separately for the drug use and alcohol use populations. Although results from each individual study did not consistently show significant differences across conditions, on average, we found a 4% difference in mean days abstinent between BCT to ICBT at post-treatment. This translates into 1.2 fewer days of drinking or drug use per month (30 day month) or 14.6 days per year for those in BCT/BFT. At short-term follow up (within 6 months of treatment completion), the mean difference in days abstinent was 11%, a statistically significant difference across conditions. This equates to 3.3 fewer days of drinking/drug use per month (30 day month) or 40 fewer days per year for those in BCT/BFT. This difference is even greater at long-term-follow up (within 12 months of treatment completion), increasing to nearly 12%, which equates to 3.6 fewer days of drinking/drug use per month (30 day month) or nearly 44 fewer days per year for those in BCT/ BFT. The proportion of those abstinent decreased in both groups with each subsequent follow up, but those in the BCT/BFT condition showed less of a decrease in PDA than those in ICBT, suggesting the effects of the intervention eroded more slowly for those in BCT/BFT. Although not part of the pooled analysis, this trend is repeated in all but one of the studies used in the pooled analysis.[63] Using survival analyses and growth curve modeling, all of these studies report a significantly slower rate of relapse for the BCT/BFT condition than for ICBT.

Of the studies not included in the pooled analysis, three used outcomes specific to alcohol use that are described in more detail below,[69, 73, 75] and one used an addiction severity index to assess change,[67] also described below.

Alternatives to BCT Trials. Two of the fifteen trials did not compare BCT/BFT to ICBT.[70, 77] Carroll et al.[77] found no significant differences in the PDA from cocaine or opioid use between those who received naltrexone and reciprocal relationship counseling versus those who received ICBT and naltrexone. Jones et al.,[70] however, found that subjects in HOPE, the motivational and psychoeducational group intervention with couple therapy, actually had <u>higher</u> heroin use at short-term follow up, compared to a counselor-led drug treatment support group for men with drug use disorders. The inconsistency of these data for non-BCT trials provides little evidence to support non-BCT interventions for improving abstinence, especially for drug use disorders.

Figure 3. Differences between BCT and ICBT: Percent Days Abstinent for Alcohol and Drug Use

Study or Subgroup	Couple/Marital Mean	SD	Total	Individual Mean	SD	Total	Weight	Mean Difference IV, Random, 95% CI
1.1.1 Post-treatment								
Fals-Stewart 1996	95.4	15.4	40	91.1	14.1	40	12.3%	4.30 [-2.17, 10.77]
Fals-Stewart 2006	96.3	16.3	46	93.6	17.7	46	10.7%	2.70 [-4.25, 9.65]
Fals-Stewart 2008	94.1	13.4	46	88.3	13	46	17.7%	5.80 [0.40, 11.20]
Kelley 2002 (Drug)	85.9	22.7	22	81.8	26.2	21	2.4%	4.10 [-10.58, 18.78]
Kelley 2002 (EtOH)	90.2	21.9	25	86.6	17.4	22	4.1%	3.60 [-7.65, 14.85]
Lam 2009	92.3	15.2	10	88.3	16.7	10	2.6%	4.00 [-10.00, 18.00]
McCrady 2009	80.5	27.7	50	74.2	35	52	3.5%	6.30 [-5.92, 18.52]
O'Farrell 2010	71.1	37	15	43.6	41.9	14	0.6%	27.50 [-1.35, 56.35]
Winters 2002	94.2	6.4	36	90.2	8	36	46.1%	4.00 [0.65, 7.35]
Subtotal (95% CI)			290			287	100.0%	4.43 [2.16, 6.70]
Heterogeneity: Tau² = 0.00; Chi² = 3.12, df = 8 (P = 0.93); I² = 0%								
Test for overall effect: Z = 3.82 (P = 0.0001)								
1.1.2 Short-term followup (6 months)								
Fals-Stewart 1996	81.5	28.6	40	70.4	24.5	40	11.9%	11.10 [-0.57, 22.77]
Fals-Stewart 2006	85.9	18.1	46	75	20.3	46	26.3%	10.90 [3.04, 18.76]
Fals-Stewart 2008	84.1	26.5	46	70.3	27.1	46	13.6%	13.80 [2.85, 24.75]
Kelley 2002 (Drug)	77.6	25.8	22	63.6	42.3	21	3.7%	14.00 [-7.06, 35.06]
Kelley 2002 (EtOH)	80.6	27.2	25	71.4	26.2	22	7.0%	9.20 [-6.08, 24.48]
Lam 2009	85.1	20.7	10	78.2	22.6	10	4.5%	6.90 [-12.09, 25.89]
McCrady 2009	75.7	34.3	50	61.4	39.5	52	7.9%	14.30 [-0.04, 28.64]
O'Farrell 2010	57.7	40.4	15	46.4	32	14	2.3%	11.30 [-15.14, 37.74]
Winters 2002	81.9	16.3	31	71.9	17.9	32	22.8%	10.00 [1.55, 18.45]
Subtotal (95% CI)			285			283	100.0%	11.21 [7.17, 15.24]
Heterogeneity: Tau² = 0.00; Chi² = 0.81, df = 8 (P = 1.00); I² = 0%								
Test for overall effect: Z = 5.45 (P < 0.00001)								
1.1.3 Long-term followup (12 months)								
Fals-Stewart 1996	73.2	29.8	40	65.1	26.9	40	10.9%	8.10 [-4.34, 20.54]
Fals-Stewart 2003	59.6	26.4	62	49.3	28.4	62	18.1%	10.30 [0.65, 19.95]
Fals-Stewart 2006	79.3	29.7	46	60.2	20.9	46	15.3%	19.10 [8.61, 29.59]
Fals-Stewart 2008	74.1	25.8	46	60.2	27.3	46	14.3%	13.90 [3.05, 24.75]
Kelley 2002 (Drug)	66.9	35.6	22	53.4	24.8	21	5.1%	13.50 [-4.77, 31.77]
Kelley 2002 (EtOH)	70.9	25.6	25	60.4	22.4	22	9.0%	10.50 [-3.22, 24.22]
Lam 2009	77.8	20.2	10	70.2	18.6	10	5.8%	7.60 [-9.42, 24.62]
McCrady 2009	75.4	34.7	50	63.1	37.6	52	8.6%	12.30 [-1.73, 26.33]
Winters 2002	74.2	22.2	33	65.4	26.1	35	12.8%	8.80 [-2.70, 20.30]
Subtotal (95% CI)			334			334	100.0%	11.93 [7.82, 16.04]
Heterogeneity: Tau² = 0.00; Chi² = 3.00, df = 8 (P = 0.93); I² = 0%								
Test for overall effect: Z = 5.69 (P < 0.00001)								

Mean Difference IV, Random, 95% CI
-20 -10 0 10 20
Favors Individual   Favors Couple/Marital

Test for subgroup differences: Chi² = 14.59, df = 2 (P = 0.0007), I² = 86.3%

Horizontal bars for each study represent the study's confidence interval. Confidence intervals extending below 0 indicate non-significant differences. Size of box or diamond reflects sample size.

Fals-Stewart Studies. Given that six of the eight studies included in the pooled analyses were either first-authored by Dr. Fals-Stewart or were based on data he collected, we also conducted the pooled analyses using the two studies that did not include Dr. Fals-Stewart's studies[75, 82] (forest plots shown in Appendix E; Figures 1a and 1b). In this analysis, at post-treatment, there was not a significant mean difference in PDA between those in BCT and ICBT. At the short term follow-up, however, those in BCT had a significantly higher mean PDA than those in ICBT. The difference in mean PDA was 13.6%, which equates to 4 fewer days of drinking/drug use per month or nearly 50 fewer days per year for those in BCT/BFT. Only the McCrady et al.[75] study measured long term outcomes, and there was no significant difference between BCT and ICBT during that follow-up period.

Alcohol Use Disorder Symptoms (Key Question 2A)

Of the fifteen studies that family treatment to individually-oriented treatment, seven trials examined AUDs.[63, 69, 71, 73-75, 79] Kelley et al.[63] included subjects with both AUD and drug use disorders and stratified data by disorder.[63]

BCT. All but one of the seven trials compared BCT to an individual treatment.[73] Five included measures of PDA[63, 71, 74, 75, 79] and three included measures of PDHD[69, 75, 79] during the follow-up period of interest using the TLFB procedure.[88] As noted previously, one trial[79] did not include sample sizes for each condition and was not included in the pooled analysis. As shown in Appendix E, Figure 2, pooled analyses demonstrated no significant difference in PDA between BCT and ICBT post-treatment. However, at both short- and long-term follow up, those in BCT had significantly more PDA than those in individual treatments. Those in BCT, on average, had nearly 11% more days abstinent (3.3 more days abstinent per month; 40 fewer days per year) than ICBT at 6 months and 12.5% more days abstinent at 12 months (3.8 days per month; 45.6 per year). Although there were far fewer studies, this same pattern was found for PDHD: there was no significant difference in PDHD between BCT and ICBT post-treatment, but at both short- and long-term follow up, those in BCT had a significantly lower PDHD than those in ICBT (Appendix E, Figure 3). On average, we found that those in BCT had 10.2% fewer days of heavy drinking than those in ICBT at 6 months (3 days per month; 37 days per year) and nearly 14% fewer days at 12 months (4 days per month; 51 days per year). It should be noted that one of these studies, a trial conducted by McCrady and colleagues,[75] included both PDA and PDHD outcomes, and was the only study not based on data collected by Dr. Fals-Stewart. In that study, neither PDA nor PDHD showed a significant difference across treatment conditions.

One study not included in the pooled analysis was by conducted by Walitzer et al.[73] It was not included because neither the comparator nor the outcomes were similar to the pooled studies. Instead of comparing BCT to ICBT, BCT was compared to individual group counseling and a combination of abstinence, light drinking days, and heavy days of drinking per month were assessed at post-treatment, short-term follow-up, and long-term follow up. Means days abstinent or days light drinking were not significantly different across conditions. The mean days of heavy drinking at post-treatment and short-term follow-up, however, were significantly different, with fewer subjects in the BCT condition drinking heavily compared to individual group counseling. Long-term outcomes were not significantly different across conditions.

Alternatives to BCT. We did not find any studies that met our criteria that tested differences between alternative family treatments to BCT or BFT and individual treatment for AUDs.

Drug Use Disorder Symptoms (Key Questions 2A and 2B)

Of the fifteen studies that compared family treatment to individually-oriented treatment, eight trials examined drug use disorders.[63, 66-68, 70, 76-78] One of these trials[66] had three papers included in our review.[66, 84, 85] A trial conducted by O'Farrell and colleagues[82] included those with drug use disorders and alcohol dependence.[82] Of the eight trials that examined drug use disorders, all but two compared BCT to ICBT. One of the two alternative interventions to BCT and ICBT, described in detail below, compared a combination of motivational enhancement therapy (MET), psychoeducation, and couple therapy to a weekly, counselor-led support group for drug users,[70] The second trial compared a program that included naltrexone, contingency management, and group CBT with reciprocal relationship counseling to a similar program but without reciprocal relationship counseling.[77]

BCT. Five of the eight studies examined BCT and included measures of PDA using the TLFB.[63, 66, 68, 76, 78, 88] As shown in Appendix E, Figure 4, pooled analyses demonstrated a significant difference in PDA between BCT and ICBT for the four studies that included post-treatment assessments and short-term follow ups. Five studies included outcomes at the long-term follow up and these findings were also consistent with earlier time points. We found that, on average, those in BCT/BFT had nearly 4.5% more days abstinent (1.3 days per month; 16 days per year) than ICBT at post-treatment. At 6 months, they had, on average, 11.5% more days (3.5 days per month; 45.4 days per year) and at 12 months they had 10.4% more days abstinent (3 days per month; 38 days per year). All of these studies were conducted by or had data collected by Dr. Fals-Stewart, making it impossible to examine the effects of treatment among non-Fals-Stewart studies.

Alternatives to BCT. As noted, two studies did not compare BCT to ICBT. In the first study, 62 opioid-dependent male partners of pregnant women received either psychoeducation and support in individual group sessions (usual care) or an intervention program called Helping Other Partners Excel (HOPE), which included pregnancy and SUD psychoeducation for couples and motivational enhancement therapy, case management, and contingency management for symptom reduction for subjects.[70] Results showed that, at short-term follow up, those in the HOPE condition had spent more days in outpatient treatment and fewer days on public assistance than those in usual care. However, although days of heroin use were significantly lower for both conditions compared to baseline, these gains were not sustained at the same rate. Those in the HOPE condition, in fact, had significantly more days of heroin use at short-term follow up than those in usual care. Because of the multi-factorial intervention, however, it was not clear if any one part of the intervention reduced the intervention's effectiveness.

In the second non-BCT study, Carroll and colleagues[77] examined male and female subjects with a drug use diagnosis who were assigned either to 1) naltrexone (a medication to reduce cravings for alcohol or drugs) plus group CBT, 2) naltrexone, group CBT, plus contingency management (incentives for subjects to remain in treatment), or 3) naltrexone, group CBT, contingency management, and reciprocal relationship counseling for the patient and a family member, friend, spouse, or child. There were no significant differences in the number of naltrexone doses taken or PDA from cocaine or opioid use between those in the naltrexone-only group and the group that included relationship counseling. The authors did find, however, that those participating in the relationship counseling condition reported significantly improved family functioning over time, as assessed by the Addiction Severity Index, compared to the other two groups.

Alternative Comparison Conditions. Although the majority of studies examining symptom reduction compared BCT to ICBT, six trials included additional conditions which were also compared to BCT and ICBT. These additional conditions included BFT with parenting skills training (1 trial[71]); a psychoeducational attention control treatment (PACT) as an additional comparison condition in trials with BCT and ICBT treatment groups (4 trials[63, 69, 74, 78]); and, an alternative form of BCT.[65] Two additional trials, one for AUDs and one for SUDs, compared standard BCT with a briefer version of the treatment.[41,69]

In the parenting skills study, Lam and colleagues[71] examined a sample of 30 married fathers with an AUD and found, although all three groups showed significant improvement at 12-months compared to baseline, neither attendance rates nor PDA at baseline, post-treatment, or 12-months post-treatment were significantly different across conditions (BCT, ICBT, BCT + parent skills training). Nor did the authors find any significant reductions in interpersonal violence, dyadic adjustment, or relationship satisfaction related to treatment condition.

Across the four studies that compared PACT to BCT and ICBT, the authors found that the pattern of differences between BCT and PACT was similar to the pattern of differences between BCT and ICBT. Specifically, across each study, there were no significant differences between BCT and PACT in PDA at post-treatment, but by 12 months, the difference in PDA between conditions was significant compared to those in PACT. Similar findings were reported for the effect of treatment on couple functioning. Significantly greater improvements in couple functioning were found for those in BCT than those in PACT at post-treatment and at short- and long-term assessments. Two of the studies that included a PACT condition also included both a standard and brief version of BCT.[69, 78] In both of these studies, the standard and brief versions showed significant differences in PDA compared to ICBT and PACT, but few differences between the two versions.

One study examined the effect of different family involved treatments on symptom reduction.[65] BCT was compared to interactional treatment, a therapy approach that does not pre-plan therapy sessions, but instead focuses on mutual support, sharing of feelings, and problem solving through discussion. In this study, which included 36 participants with an AUD, PDA or PDHD were not reported, but relationship functioning, measured as sexual satisfaction was. The data show that subjects in the two treatment conditions did not significantly differ in their reports of sexual satisfaction.

Effectiveness of Interventions on Relapse Prevention for AUDs and Drug Use Disorders (KQ2B)

Two studies, by McCrady and colleagues[72] and O'Farrell and colleagues,[4] specifically compared BCT to BCT plus relapse prevention. McCrady and colleagues compared 1) BCT, 2) BCT with enhancements to prevent relapse (BCT/RP), and 3) BCT plus Al-Anon in their clinical trial of 90 men with AUDs and their spouses/female partners. Relapse prevention training included strategies to anticipate risky situations and identify potential signs for relapse. The addition of relapse prevention to BCT did not significantly increase participant's time before relapse or improvements in relationship functioning at 6 or 18 months after treatment. However, in a sample of 59 male alcoholics and their female spouses, O'Farrell and colleagues[4] found that those who received BCT plus relapse prevention had more PDA at 6 and 12 months than those who received BCT alone. At 18 months after treatment, those assigned to BCT plus relapse prevention reported 13.2% more days abstinent than those in BCT (4.0 more days per month or 48.2 more days per year). However, differences were no longer significant at the 30 month follow-up. Those with the most severe drinking and poorest couple functioning at baseline reported the greatest benefit from BCT plus relapse prevention. Finally, those with the lowest severity of marital problems at baseline were more likely to maintain complete abstinence through 18 months.

No studies specifically examined relapse prevention for those with drug use disorders.

Family Functioning (Family Involved versus Individual Treatment; KQ2A)

The primary family outcome in studies that met our inclusion criteria was family or couple functioning. Twenty-one of the twenty-two trials, including both drug use disorder and AUD trials, reported either family or relationship functioning outcomes. Multiple instruments were used to measure functioning, but the most prevalent was the Dyadic Adjustment Scale (n=9) followed by the Marital/Relationship Happiness Scale (n=4) and the family/relationship sub-scale of the Addiction Severity Index (n=3).

BCT. Overall, nine trials reported differences in relationship adjustment between individuals participating in BCT versus ICBT using the Dyadic Adjustment Scale (DAS) at post-treatment, short-term follow-up, and long-term follow-up assessments. We pooled data to analyze the effect of treatment conditions on DAS scores but, as previously reported, one trial[79] did not include sample sizes for each condition and, therefore, was not included in the pooled analysis. Pooled analyses that included unadjusted weighted means are presented in Figure 4. Again, we reported separate findings for drug use and alcohol use subjects in the 2002 study by Kelley et al. Findings were consistent with findings for PDA. At post-treatment, on average there was a 12% difference in DAS scores, with those receiving BCT having significantly higher couple and family functioning than those in ICBT. The total weighted mean post-treatment for BCT was 112.7 and for ICBT, 100.5, both of which are above the threshold of 97.5 used as a screen for relationship distress (scores range from 0 – 151; Christenson et al.[121]). At short-term follow up (within 6 months of treatment completion), those in BCT had scores 14% higher than those in ICBT, with a total weighted mean of 106.8 for BCT and 93.5 (below the threshold indicating relationship distress) for ICBT. At 12 months, BCT scores were 12.5% higher than ICBT, and while weighted mean scores for BCT remained above 97.5 (mean = 101.2), scores for ICBT were below (mean = 90), consistent with couples experiencing clinically meaningful relationship distress.

Of the trials comparing BCT to ICBT not included in the pooled analysis,[66, 68, 75, 82] all measured different elements of relationship distress, including marital adjustment,[66] family functioning,[68] separation,[75] and relationship happiness,[82] yet none reported significant differences across conditions.

Figure 4. Differences between BCT and ICBT: Relationship Adjustment for AUD and Drug Use Disorder Studies

Study or Subgroup	Couple/Marital Mean	SD	Total	Individual Mean	SD	Total	Weight	Mean Difference IV, Fixed, 95% CI
1.17.1 Post-treatment								
Fals-Stewart 2001	97.9	16.4	17	79.2	18.1	19	5.9%	18.70 [7.43, 29.97]
Fals-Stewart 2005	119.3	11.9	25	104.6	11.6	25	17.7%	14.70 [8.19, 21.21]
Fals-Stewart 2006	123	12.1	46	111.2	18.6	46	18.3%	11.80 [5.39, 18.21]
Fals-Stewart 2008	114.2	15.1	46	101.9	13.6	46	21.8%	12.30 [6.43, 18.17]
Kelley 2002 (Drug)	103.6	22.1	22	88.7	16.4	21	5.6%	14.90 [3.30, 26.50]
Kelley 2002 (EtOH)	115.4	18.2	25	102.2	19.1	22	6.6%	13.20 [2.49, 23.91]
Lam 2009	114.6	16.8	10	98.1	17.9	10	3.3%	16.50 [1.28, 31.72]
Walitzer 04 CAF+BCT	108.4	14.4	19	105.4	26.2	21	4.5%	3.00 [-9.94, 15.94]
Winters 2002	105.3	13.2	36	97.2	16.1	36	16.3%	8.10 [1.30, 14.90]
Subtotal (95% CI)			246			246	100.0%	12.25 [9.51, 15.00]
Heterogeneity: Chi² = 5.74, df = 8 (P = 0.68); I² = 0%								
Test for overall effect: Z = 8.75 (P < 0.00001)								
1.17.2 Short-term followup (6 months)								
Fals-Stewart 2005	112.6	16.2	25	98.4	11.6	25	15.5%	14.20 [6.39, 22.01]
Fals-Stewart 2006	117.2	13.7	46	102.2	14.4	46	28.6%	15.00 [9.26, 20.74]
Fals-Stewart 2008	109.8	16	46	94.1	14.8	46	23.8%	15.70 [9.40, 22.00]
Kelley 2002 (Drug)	93.6	17.2	22	77.8	18.7	21	8.2%	15.80 [5.05, 26.55]
Kelley 2002 (EtOH)	103.9	16.2	25	86.7	19.2	22	9.0%	17.20 [6.97, 27.43]
Lam 2009	105.9	19.6	10	93.9	20.2	10	3.1%	12.00 [-5.44, 29.44]
Walitzer 04 CAF+BCT	107.8	12.7	16	108.3	25.6	15	4.6%	-0.50 [-14.87, 13.87]
Winters 2002	93.4	22.7	31	84.3	23.6	32	7.2%	9.10 [-2.33, 20.53]
Subtotal (95% CI)			221			217	100.0%	14.08 [11.01, 17.15]
Heterogeneity: Chi² = 5.55, df = 7 (P = 0.59); I² = 0%								
Test for overall effect: Z = 8.98 (P < 0.00001)								
1.17.3 Long-term followup (12 months)								
Fals-Stewart 2005	109.3	17.2	25	96	19.3	25	12.1%	13.30 [3.17, 23.43]
Fals-Stewart 2006	112.4	14	46	98	18.8	46	27.0%	14.40 [7.63, 21.17]
Fals-Stewart 2008	106.9	16.5	46	87.3	17.2	46	26.1%	19.60 [12.71, 26.49]
Kelley 2002 (Drug)	90.7	22.3	22	75.8	20.4	21	7.6%	14.90 [2.13, 27.67]
Kelley 2002 (EtOH)	91.4	19.9	25	82.1	20.7	22	9.1%	9.30 [-2.35, 20.95]
Lam 2009	99.8	20.3	10	88.9	22	10	3.6%	10.90 [-7.65, 29.45]
Walitzer 04 CAF+BCT	101.2	15.9	17	113.6	23	14	6.1%	-12.40 [-26.62, 1.82]
Winters 2002	86.2	25.2	33	82.8	25.9	35	8.4%	3.40 [-8.75, 15.55]
Subtotal (95% CI)			224			219	100.0%	12.51 [8.99, 16.03]
Heterogeneity: Chi² = 18.79, df = 7 (P = 0.009); I² = 63%								
Test for overall effect: Z = 6.97 (P < 0.00001)								

Test for subgroup differences: Chi² = 0.83, df = 2 (P = 0.66), I² = 0%

Horizontal bars for each study represent the study's confidence interval. Confidence intervals extending below 0 indicate non-significant differences. Size of box or diamond reflects sample size.

Alternatives to BCT. Two trials[70, 77] did not compare BCT to ICBT. Both included measures of relationship functioning. In the trial conducted by Carroll et al.,[77] those randomized to naltrexone plus CBT plus relationship counseling had significantly higher reports of family functioning post-treatment, as assessed by the Addiction Severity Index sub-scale, than those in the CBT plus naltrexone only condition. In the trial conducted by Jones et al.,[70] however, there were no significant differences in couple functioning, as measured by the Partner Support Questionnaire and the Relationship Assessment Form, across conditions, either during or after treatment.

Family Functioning - Alcohol Use Disorder Studies (KQ2A)

<u>BCT</u>. Seven trials examined treatments for AUDs and six used the DAS as a measure of couple or family functioning. All six compared BCT to ICBT. We pooled data from all but one of these studies;[79] a study that did not provide sample sizes by condition. At post-treatment, there was a significant difference in DAS scores (12.5, p<0.001), with those in BCT reporting significantly higher couple and family functioning (Appendix E, Figure 5). Weighted means at post-treatment were 117.8 for BCT and 106.2 for ICBT, both above the clinical cut-point for relationship distress. This same pattern persisted at short-term follow up: those in BCT had scores nearly 14% higher than those in ICBT (p<0.001), although the weighted means were lower than post-treatment (BCT, mean = 111.4 and ICBT, mean = 98.6). At 12 months, scores were nearly 10% higher (p<0.001), with weighted means indicating that, while BCT patients were still in the satisfied range on relationship adjustment, those in IBCT were, on average, reporting relationship adjustment scores consistent with relationship distress (BCT, mean = 104.9; ICBT, mean = 95.7). Only one of these studies, a study by Walitzer et al (2004), was not first-authored by and did not use data collected by Dr. Fals-Stewart. Although a small study (N = 64 across 3 treatment conditions), this one study did not show any significant differences in DAS scores across conditions.

Two studies that compared BCT to ICBT were not included in the pooled analysis. One, as noted, was due to sample sizes not being available.[79] In this analysis, however, the authors reported that compared to ICBT, those in BCT had significantly higher DAS scores at post-treatment, short-term follow-up, and long-term follow-up. The other was a study by McCrady et al.[75] that assessed separation rates. At long-term follow up, there was no significant difference in separation rates across conditions.

<u>Alternatives to BCT</u>. We did not find any studies that met our inclusion criteria, tested differences in family functioning among patients with only AUDs, and compared a non-BCT/BFT family treatment to individual treatment.

Family Functioning - Drug Use Disorder Studies (KQ2A)

<u>BCT studies</u>. Eight trials examined treatments for drug use disorder s.[63, 66-68, 70, 76-78] Of those, six compared BCT to ICBT [63, 66-68, 76, 78] and four of the six[63, 67, 76, 78] used the DAS to assess relationship functioning. As with AUDs, we pooled data from those trials that included an assessment of DAS and found that those in BCT had significantly higher family functioning at post-treatment, short-term follow-up, and long-term follow-up (Appendix E, Figure 6). Four studies reported post-treatment DAS scores and those in BCT had scores nearly 12% higher than those in ICBT. Weighted mean scores at post-treatment were lower than those for AUD, with the average BCT score being 107.3 and the average for IBCT being 94.7 (consistent with a positive screen for relationship distress). Three studies reported data for short- and long-term outcomes. For short-term, those in BCT conditions had 14.5% higher scores than those in ICBT. The weighted mean score at short-term follow up for BCT was consistent with relationship satisfaction (above the clinical threshold for relationship distress; mean = 101.1), but this was not the case for ICBT, with scores indicating the average participant was experiencing relationship distress (mean = 87.5). The difference across conditions at the long-term follow-up was even larger. Those in BCT or BFT had DAS scores over 15.5% higher of than those in ICBT at least

one year after treatment, although the weighted mean DAS scores had declined with time with both groups now falling within the clinically distressed range on relationship adjustment (BCT, mean = 96.6; ICBT, mean = 83.4). All of the studies in the pooled analysis used data from, or were first-authored by, Dr. Fals-Stewart.

Two studies, both conducted by Fals-Stewart and colleagues,[66, 68] compared BCT to ICBT, assessing relationship functioning through alternate measures. In Fals-Stewart et al.'s 1996 trial,[66] the Locke Wallace Marital Adjustment Test (MAT) was used to assess couple functioning. No significant differences were reported across conditions at any follow up. Likewise, in the Fals-Stewart and colleagues[68] trial, using the Addiction Severity Index to assess family functioning, no significant differences were found across conditions at post-treatment.

Alternatives to BCT. As previously reported, the trials conducted by Jones et al.[70] and Carroll et al.[77] did not compare BCT, but alternatives to BCT. The Carroll et al.[77] trial found significant differences in family functioning, with the family treatment having better outcomes than the individual treatment. Jones et al.,[70] however, found no significant differences in couple functioning across conditions.

Intimate Partner Violence

BCT. Three studies, 2 examining subjects with AUDs and 1 with drug use disorders, assessed whether BCT compared to ICBT reduced intimate partner violence among those with a drug use disorder .[71, 74, 85] Lam found no significant changes across conditions at any time point. In Fals-Stewart et al.'s[85] paper, violent behaviors are reported, but tests of association by condition were not. In Fals-Stewart and colleagues'[74] study, however, those in BCT reported significantly less physical aggression at long-term follow up than those who participated in ICBT.

Alternatives to BCT. We were unable to locate studies meeting our inclusion criteria that examined intimate partner violence outcomes among patients with a SUD that examined alternatives to BCT.

Family Functioning (Comparisons among Different Family Treatments; KQ2B)

Six trials compared family involved treatments to one or more alternative family treatments.[4, 65, 72, 80, 81, 83] All but Meyers and colleagues[83] reported outcomes associated with family or couple functioning. Because study designs and measures used were different across studies, these data were not pooled. Of the two trials that tested variations of the CRAFT intervention,[80, 81] neither reported significant differences in couple or family functioning across conditions at any follow up assessment. McCrady et al.,[87] a 1996 trial of BCT versus BCT + Al/Anon versus BCT + relapse prevention, reported no significant long-term differences in marital happiness across conditions. O'Farrell et al.,[4] a study of BCT versus BCT + relapse prevention, also did not find any significant differences in marital happiness post-treatment or in the short- or long-term follow-up across conditions. However, using repeated measures analysis of covariance to assess the effects of the intervention over time (as opposed to one specific time point), they found that couples randomized to BCT with relapse prevention had greater marital satisfaction over longer periods of time than those randomized to BCT only. In O'Farrell et al.'s[65] trial that analyzed data on sexual satisfaction, no significant differences were found across conditions. No evidence from any of the trials we reviewed, therefore, show that one family involved treatment improves relationship functioning more than another.

Sub-Groups of Interest

Veterans. As noted, only two studies reported Veterans as study participants.[4, 65] In both studies, all participants were Veterans. In one of these studies, comparing BCT to BCT plus relapse prevention, researchers found that the addition of relapse prevention to BCT resulted in more PDA at 6 and 12 months than those who received BCT alone (see above for further discussion). In the other study, also by O'Farrell et al.,[65] there were no differences in sexual satisfaction, a common problem associated with AUDs, between those randomized to BCT and those receiving interactional treatment. With the inconsistency of these findings, there is little evidence about whether BCT is effective with Veteran populations. No evidence exists to evaluate whether Veterans respond differently to BCT than non-Veterans. However, the average PDA reported for Veteran BCT participants in the one trial reporting this information[4] found PDAs (post-treatment: 98.0%; short-term follow-up: 87.6%; long-term follow-up: 82.7%), that were comparable, if not better, than average rates of PDA reported in the AUD trials included in our pooled analyses (post-treatment: 80.5-96.3%; short-term follow-up: 75.7-85.9%; long-term follow-up: 70.9-79.3%).

Women. Overall, four studies examined women with drug use disorders or AUDs.[74-76, 79] One examined drug use disorders in both men and women, but did not stratify the results by gender.[82] McCrady and colleagues[75] found that women in the ICBT group were significantly more likely to attend treatment sessions and complete all sessions than those in the BCT group. Additionally, women with an additional Axis I disorder had significantly higher PDA with BCT than ICBT, women with poor relationship functioning at baseline reported greater declines in substance use when assigned to BCT than ICBT, and women in BCT with drinking behavior that was influenced by their spousal or romantic relationship prior to treatment reported greater declines in substance use than those assigned to ICBT. Women with the best relationship functioning at baseline also had a slower decrease over time in PDA. In growth curve models, Fals-Stewart[74] found that women in BCT increased their alcohol use at a slower rate than women in ICBT or PACT at 12 months, but not post-treatment.

Three of the four studies that limited participation to women reported PDA and two reported mean DAS scores; therefore, we pooled these results (Appendix E, Figures 7 and 8). In order to compare women to men, we also pooled data from trials comparing BCT to ICBT that were limited to men and assessed PDA (4 trials) and DAS (3 trials) (Appendix E, Figures 9 and 10). At each follow-up, women in BCT had significantly greater PDA than those in ICBT. At post-treatment, women in BCT had nearly 4% greater PDA than women in ICBT. This equates to 1.2 fewer days per month (30 day month) or 14.6 days per year. At short-term follow up this difference was 11%, or 3.3 days a month or 40 days per year, and at long-term follow up, the difference increased to almost 14% (4.2 days per month or 51 days per year). The mean difference between BCT and ICBT at post-treatment and short-term follow up was nearly the same for men, but at long-term follow up, the difference between conditions was less for men than women, with almost a 10% difference between BCT and ICBT (3 days per month or 36.5 days per year).

For DAS, women in BCT were also significantly more likely to have higher scores than women in ICBT. At post-treatment, women in BCT had over 10% higher scores than women in ICBT. Weighted mean scores at post-treatment were 115.2 for BCT and 105.1 for ICBT. At short term follow up, women in BCT had 14% higher scores than women in ICBT, with weighted mean scores of 107.6 for BCT and 94.9 for ICBT, with ICBT patients meeting the clinical cutoff consistent with relationship distress. At long term follow up mean DAS scores for women in BCT were nearly 12% higher than for women in ICBT. Weighted mean scores at long term treatment were 101.5 for BCT and for ICBT, 91.4. ICBT patients at the long term follow-up assessment had scores that met the clinical cutoff consistent with relationship distress. For men, the difference in mean scores across conditions was greater, but overall weighted means were lower. At post-treatment, men in BCT had over 14.5% higher scores than men in ICBT. Weighted mean scores at post-treatment were 110.7 for BCT and 96.1 for ICBT. At short term follow up, however, men in BCT had a nearly 16% higher score than men in ICBT, with a weighted mean score of 100.3 for BCT. For ICBT, the weighted mean score was 84.5. At long term follow up, mean DAS scores for men in BCT were 11.7% higher than for men in ICBT. Weighted mean scores at long term treatment were 92.6 for BCT and for 80.9 for ICBT. Men in ICBT conditions had DAS scores at each follow up that met clinical criteria for relationship distress; men in BCT conditions, however, had scores that met the clinical cutoff consistent with relationship distress only at long-term follow up.

Intimate Partner versus Family Involvement. As noted, most of the studies in our review included spouses or romantic partners of someone with an AUD or drug use disorder. Of the seven trials that included family members and did not restrict participation to wives or intimate partners, three were the CRAFT interventions that targeted the family member of individuals with a drug use disorder to encourage the drug use disorder patient's treatment initiation,[80, 81, 83] and one targeted family members as a means of encouraging patients completing hospitalization for substance use detoxification to initiate continuing care and treatment.[64] Although data were typically not stratified by relationship status, Miller and colleagues,[81] as previously noted, did find that parents were better at encouraging drinkers to engage in treatment than spouses. All four studies did show that interventions targeting families broadly, and not restricted to spouses, were effective at promoting treatment initiation. Three other studies[68, 77, 82] that did not restrict therapy to spouses compared a family involved to an individually-oriented treatment. Two trials compared BFT to ICBT.[68, 82] Findings from these two studies, however, were not consistent. Fals-Stewart and colleagues[68] found that, compared to ICBT, participants in BFT attended significantly more sessions, took naltrexone on more days ICBT, and had significantly higher PDA for opioids, cocaine, alcohol and all drugs combined at 12 months post-treatment. They also had significantly longer periods of abstinence from opioids during treatment and higher family functioning at 12 months post-treatment. O'Farrell and colleagues,[82] however, found that, although participants with an SUD in the BFT condition attended more sessions than those in ICBT, subjects did not have greater PDA from drinking or other illicit drugs or fewer days using their primary substance than those in ICBT at post-treatment or 6-month follow up. Similarly, Carroll and colleagues,[77] as described above, found no significant differences in the number of naltrexone doses taken or PDA from cocaine or opioid use between those in the naltrexone and CBT group therapy conditions than those who received naltrexone, group CBT, contingency management, and reciprocal relationship counseling.

Same Sex Couples. One study examined the impact of family involved treatment on same sex couples. Fals-Stewart and colleagues[79] compared BCT to ICBT among men (n=52) and women (n=48) in same sex relationships who were entering outpatient treatment for an AUD.

Subjects were randomized into 20 weeks of BCT or 20 weeks of ICBT only. The authors found that there were no significant differences in attendance across conditions nor was there any difference post-treatment in percent days of heavy drinking (PDHD). However, for both groups at 6- and 12-month follow-up assessments, those in BCT had significantly fewer PDHD, and at 12-months, using growth curve modeling, both men and women in the BCT condition increased their heavy days of drinking at a significantly slower rate than those in ICBT only. Findings were similar on for couple functioning. Both men and women in the BCT condition reported better couple functioning at post-treatment, 6-month follow-up, and 12-month follow-up. Growth curve modeling showed faster improvements in relationship adjustment (DAS scores) during treatment and slower declines in relationships adjustment over the 12-months after treatment completion among BCT than ICBT participants.

Summary

In contrast to Key Question 1, there is more evidence to address the second key question, **what is the effectiveness of family involved interventions compared to alternative interventions in improving outcomes for adult patients with mental health conditions** *[i.e., how do family involved interventions compare to (a) any individually-oriented psychosocial intervention or (b) any alternative family involved intervention]?* The majority of studies addressing Key Question 2 are aimed at the three different time points in the trajectory of treatment: treatment initiation or engagement, attendance, and treatment response. As with the results, the discussion focuses on the evidence at these stages and then discusses some of the methodological considerations for this set of studies.

Initiation

The largest amount of evidence on treatment initiation came from the three studies that assessed CRAFT. While these studies varied in quality, their consistency suggests that CRAFT is efficacious at promoting treatment initiation for people with SUDs, but there is little evidence on whether that engagement is sustained or if that engagement leads to reduced patient symptoms. Evidence from O'Farrell and colleagues[64] also supports the finding that active family involved interventions improve patient engagement.

Attendance and Adherence

We found some evidence from five trials to suggest that family treatment improves treatment attendance in AUD and drug use disorder trials. Ten trials, however, did not show any differences in attendance by condition. The evidence, therefore, is inconsistent on whether family involved treatments improve session attendance. Likewise, there was conflicting evidence, based on two studies, on whether family treatment significantly improved medication adherence.

Effectiveness of Interventions on Treatment for AUD and Drug Use Disorder Symptoms

Although results from individual studies that assessed whether treatment that included families as active participants improved abstinence or reduced substance use behaviors were not consistent, results from pooled analyses showed that, across studies, family involved treatments, specifically BCT or BFT, resulted in a significantly higher proportion of days abstinent than ICBT. These differences were consistent and persistent across all time points, but the short-term effect appeared to be strongest. These same patterns were seen when data from AUD and drug use disorder trials were stratified. These findings are largely consistent with a recent prior review of BCT for SUDs which reported 'robust' findings that BCT was better than control conditions in reducing the frequency of use (d = 0.45), reducing the consequences of use (d = 0.50), and improving relationship satisfaction (d = 0.51).[123]Powers and colleagues[123] included non-US studies and child-focused studies of BCT.

However, when the only two studies not either conducted or first-authored by Dr. Fals-Stewart (both targeted at AUDs) were examined separately in pooled analyses, these patterns differed slightly. There were no differences between BCT and ICBT at post-treatment or long-term, but there were significant differences in the short-term. Because all of the drug use trials included were either first-authored by or used data collected by Dr. Fals-Stewart, we have no evidence, outside of his work, on trials that met our inclusion criteria, to compare BCT to ICBT for drug use disorders. Therefore, although there is compelling evidence to suggest that BCT is effective at improving PDA, especially for periods within 6 months of treatment completion, questions remain about its effectiveness immediately post-treatment and for long-term abstinence or harm reduction.

Effectiveness of Interventions on Treatment for Family Outcomes (Couple and Family Functioning)

Like findings on abstinence and reduction of drug or alcohol use behaviors, active family treatments for SUDs showed better short- and long-term improvements in couple functioning than individual treatments in pooled analyses, although for individual studies these differences were not always statistically significantly, especially at later time points (e.g., 12 months). Passive attention control treatments that included families were not significantly different from ICBT, but they were significantly different from BCT, with BCT showing significant improvements in couple functioning. Some evidence from three studies of variable quality (1 poor, 1 fair, and 1 good quality) suggests BCT also reduces intimate partner violence.

Effectiveness of Interventions on Relapse Prevention for AUDs and Drug Use Disorders

Our findings showed mixed results in treatments that added additional relapse prevention treatment to standard BCT, with one study[72] failing to show significant differences in AUD between those assigned to BCT and those assigned to BCT with relapse prevention and another study[4] demonstrating a significant increase in PDA for those assigned to BCT plus relapse prevention versus those in standard BCT at both short-term and long-term assessments. In the latter study, those with the most severe drinking and poorest couple functioning at baseline benefitted the most from BCT plus relapse prevention. The interaction between marital happiness and relapse was also considered in the former study, but this relationship was not significant. No studies addresses relapse for those in drug use disorder trials.

Sub-Groups of Interest

Veterans. Two studies of the 22 studies reviewed identified Veterans as participants. No direct comparisons between Veterans and non-Veteran samples were found among studies that met our inclusion criteria. Findings from the one trial we reviewed that provided substance use outcomes with Veterans[4, 65]demonstrated comparable or better rates of PDA from alcohol use (post-treatment: 98.0%; short-term follow-up: 87.6%; long-term follow-up: 82.7%) than average rates of PDA reported in the AUD trials included in our pooled analyses. However, without direct comparisons within trials between Veteran and non-Veteran samples and between BCT and ICBT, we can draw few conclusions on whether treatment response for Veterans differs from treatment response for non-Veterans.

Intimate Partners versus Other Family Members. While the data are limited, it appears that treatments involving family members, including those who are and are not intimate partners, are successful in increasing SUD treatment initiation among those with SUDs. Once in treatment, however, the data are mixed (one study supported BFT over ICBT or medication only,[68] another found non-significant differences between BFT and ICBT[77]). Only one study[82] limited participation to non-intimate partners. While subjects in the BFT arm were more likely to attend treatment than those in ICBT in this trial, there were no significant differences across conditions in PDA or PDHD across any time point.

Women. Pooled analyses showed little difference by gender in the overall effect of BCT compared to ICBT. One study by McCrady and colleagues,[75] however, found women with psychological comorbidities had significantly higher PDA with BCT than ICBT, those with poor relationship functioning at baseline responded better to BCT than ICBT, and those with the best relationship functioning at baseline had smaller differences over time in PDHD.

Bipolar Disorder

Overview

We identified 2 studies that addressed KQ2A, comparing family treatment to individual therapy.[91, 92] Three studies addressed KQ2B comparing a family therapy with a different family intervention.[89, 90, 93] Outcomes are presented in Appendix D, Tables 6 to 8.

Treatment Response: Symptoms

Comparisons with traditional individual-oriented therapies (KQ2A; 2 trials)

FFT. One study reporting symptoms compared FFT to alternative, empirically supported individual therapies (cognitive behavioral therapy or interpersonal and social rhythm therapy), with clinical status assessed at follow-up visits.[92] Based on DSM-IV criteria, the odds of being well in any given study month were greater for patients in any one of three intensive therapy groups (one of which was FFT) compared to the control condition, individually-oriented collaborative care. However, when the authors stratified the intensive therapy group by type of therapy, there was no difference between family-focused therapy and collaborative care. No significant differences between conditions were reported,[92] suggesting FFT may perform similarly to other empirically supported, intensive interventions in improving symptoms of bipolar disorder.

Relapse and recovery outcomes were reported in two studies comparing FFT to individual therapy. No significant differences in recovery or time to recovery were observed between FFT and either of two other intensive, individual therapy control groups (cognitive behavioral therapy or interpersonal and social rhythm therapy). Both the combined intensive therapy group and the FFT group alone (secondary analysis) were significantly better than individually-oriented collaborative care.[92] A second study found no difference in number of subjects with one or more relapses during one year of active treatment but 32% lower rates of relapse and 48% lower rates of hospitalization in the FFT group compared to the individually-focused treatment group during the year after treatment.[91]

Comparisons with alternative family therapies (KQ2B; 3 trials)

<u>*FFT.*</u> Another study reported symptoms when FFT was compared to another therapy with some family involvement. A significant treatment versus time interaction was observed for symptoms scores at both 12 and 24 months follow-up, indicating FFT results in greater improvement in symptoms than participants in a "crisis management" group (modeled after standard community care with 2 family psychoeducation sessions).[90, 96] There was also a significant difference between FFT and crisis management participants in the percentage of subjects who survived one year without relapse (71% vs. 47%) when study dropouts were excluded. Using the intent-to-treat sample, relapse at 24 months was significantly lower in the FFT group.[90, 96] Relapse rates at 24 months after randomization were 35% for FFT participants and 54% for crisis management participants. Patients in crisis management relapsed an average of 20 weeks sooner than FFT participants.

Relapse and family functioning interactions. This same trial found no main effect of family distress or a treatment by family distress interaction for relapse among patients randomized to FFT or crisis management.[90] Differences in percent relapsed were noted for participants with parental relatives (fewer relapses in participants from low expressed emotion parental homes compared to those from high expressed emotion parental homes) but not spousal relatives.[90]

<u>*FFT-HPI.*</u> Participants whose caregivers received FFT-HPI had significantly fewer symptoms of depression (5.6 points on the HAM-D; d = 0.67, medium effect) and mania (4.2 points on the YMRS; d = 0.34, small effect), indicating greater symptom relief, than patients whose caregivers received health education only.[93]

<u>*Problem Centered Systems Therapy for the Family (PCSTF)*</u>. Miller and colleagues (2004) failed to find differences in recovery between a general family therapy (PCSTF; 10 to 15 sessions focused on comprehensive assessment, problem identification, and task-oriented problem solving) and an alternative family therapy (disorder-specific multifamily groups [MFGs]).[89] The multifamily psychoeducational group therapy (6 sessions with 4 to 6 patients and their family members) focused on providing information about bipolar disorder, coping strategies for living with a family member with a mood disorder, and a forum to discuss differences in patients' and family members' perspectives on bipolar disorder. Among patients who recovered, the frequency of mood episode recurrence did not differ among the treatment groups but frequency of hospitalization was lower in the multifamily therapy group (5%) versus family therapy conducted with one family at a time (31%) or medication only (38%).[97]

Treatment Response: Family or Couple Functioning

Comparisons with traditional individual-oriented therapies (KQ2A; 1 trial)

<u>*FFT.*</u> Family or couple function was evaluated in one study. Significantly greater improvements in relationship functioning and satisfaction were found among subjects receiving intensive psychosocial treatment (family or individual) than those receiving individually-focused usual care.[95]

Comparisons with alternative family therapies (KQ2B). No trials.

Treatment Attendance and Medication Adherence

FFT

Attendance at therapy sessions was reported in two studies. FFT was not significantly different from multifamily therapy[89] or from other individually-oriented intense treatments.[92] A study of FFT compared to individual care reported no difference in medication adherence.[91] Family therapy (compared to crisis management with a limited family component)[90] resulted in greater medication adherence following treatment.

Summary

Two studies reported greater recovery at 12 months[92] or lower relapse at 24 months[91] based on symptom assessment in individuals who participated in family-focused therapy compared to individually oriented treatment (KQ2A). Rehospitalization was also lower in the family-focused therapy group.[91] In addition, the odds of being classified as "well" in any given month were greater for participants in any of 3 intensive therapies (including family-focused therapy) compared to individually-focused collaborative care.[92]

Two studies reported reduced symptom scores among patients whose family participated in family-focused therapy[90] or family-focused therapy with a health-promoting focus[93] versus an alternative family involved intervention (KQ2B). Lower relapse and longer relapse-free survival following family-focused therapy were also reported in one of the studies.[5] However, one study reported no difference in recovery at 28 months between family treatment delivered to individual families and multi-family therapy.[89] This study involved a shorter treatment interval (all treatment completed within 6 months vs. 9 months in the other two studies).

One study reported a significant difference between three intensive therapies (one of which was family-focused therapy) and individually-oriented collaborative care (KQ2A) in relationship functioning or satisfaction.[95] In two studies, problem-centered family therapy[89] and three intensive therapies (including family-focused therapy)[92] were not observed to improve treatment attendance compared to individually-focused collaborative care (KQ2A) [92] or multifamily therapy (KQ2B.)[89] Results for improvements in medication adherence were mixed with no difference in a study of family-focused therapy compared to individual therapy (KQ2A)[91] or family-focused therapy compared to crisis management with limited family involvement (KQ2B).[5]

Overall, although studies typically assessed symptoms and reported either the symptom scores or relapse/recovery based on symptom scores, few studies assessed other outcomes of interest including global functioning (2 studies), health care utilization (1 study), family outcomes (1 study), attendance (2 studies), or medication adherence (3 studies). No study reported quality of life or satisfaction with care.

Many of the studies reviewed above were cited in a systematic review of family psychosocial interventions for bipolar disorder completed by Justo et al.[124] All of the studies in their review were randomized or quasi-randomized trials that enrolled adults and involved psychoeducational interventions or psychotherapy. Overall, based on 5 studies reviewed by Justo and colleagues[124] that compared family interventions to no intervention, two of which met eligibility for our review,[89, 94] no added effect of the family intervention to medication only was observed. In three studies that compared one family intervention to another family intervention or individual therapy, all of which were included in our review,[89-91] results were inconsistent. Of the 7 studies in the Justo et al. review, 5 were conducted in the United States. Four of the five studies were eligible for inclusion in our review.[5, 89, 91, 94] The fifth study was published in 1990 and did not meet our eligibility criteria. As reported in the Cochrane review, that study found no significant clinical improvement when a family intervention was compared to no intervention.

Schizophrenia Spectrum Disorders
Overview

Four studies addressing KQ2 met our search criteria; one comparing a family intervention to individual oriented therapies (KQ2A) and three comparing two family involved therapies (KQ2B). Data are presented in Appendix D, Tables 10 to 12.

Comparisons with Traditional Individual-Oriented Therapies (KQ2A; 1 trial)

One trial examined differences between a two-year multiple family group (MFG) intervention and standard individual mental health care (case management and medication management) within outpatient mental health service clinics.[101-103] While the present review focuses on treatment comparisons at post-treatment and after treatment completion, the length of this intervention (2 years) increases the relevance of mid-treatment findings. At mid-treatment (1 year post-baseline), subjects in the MFG group showed significant improvement in negative symptoms as measured by MSANS (Modified Scale for the Assessment of Negative Symptoms),[101] with subjects in the MFG scoring, on average, one point better on a 25 point scale. At post-treatment, there were no statistical differences in hospitalization between the two groups. MFG subjects had statistically higher use of outpatient services that was attributable to greater time spent in the intervention for MFG participants.[103] At the one-year follow-up, differences between the MFG group and their standard care counterparts on overall psychiatric hospitalization rates were non-significant. However, hospitalization in state level facilities (which provide longer term care and include patients referred directly from the criminal justice system) was 12% lower (significant difference) for MFG subjects than for standard care subjects. No significant group differences were observed in outpatient service use at one year post-treatment.[103] Differences between groups on family functioning or by distressed and non-distressed families were not reported.

In another study of note (not reported in our tables), Herz and colleagues[125] studied the effectiveness of a program of relapse prevention (an early intervention treatment strategy with psychoeducation for patient and family, active monitoring of the subject for prodromal symptoms, weekly group therapy for the patient, and a biweekly multifamily group) to treatment as usual. Treatment as usual included individual supportive therapy and medication management biweekly for 15 to 30 minutes. Significant differences in relapse and rehospitalization rates were found, favoring the intervention. However, only 29% (12 of 41) of the relapse prevention patients' families actually attended family groups, and full results were not reported for those who attended family groups versus those who did not. Of note, only one patient from these twelve families relapsed; however, this number is too low to draw conclusions as to the significance of the family component of the relapse prevention program. Given the lack of clarity regarding which subjects actually received family involvement in their care and the outcomes of those who received family involved care, this study did not meet eligibility criteria for our review. We elected to present findings here given their relevance.

Comparisons with Alternative Family Therapies (KQ2B; 3 trials)

One trial compared Assertive Community Treatment (ACT), which includes a family education and engagement component, to ACT plus a biweekly multi-family group.[29] Number of hospital admissions, rates of annual rehospitalization, and subjects' symptoms decreased throughout the two year intervention for participants in both groups pre-treatment to post-treatment; however, there were no significant differences between the groups. Data were not reported by treatment group and therefore are not included in appendix tables. One reported area of differing outcomes by treatment group was in employment rates. Employment rate for subjects in the MFG was significantly higher between months four and twenty (of the two year intervention); however, differences were non-significant at the final reporting point (end of the twenty four month intervention). Family outcomes (family dissatisfaction with the subject, reported friction between the subject and others) improved significantly for both groups pre- and post-treatment, but direct comparisons between the two treatment groups were not reported.

The trial comparing Applied Family Management (AFM) to Supportive Family Management (SFM)[24, 104] showed no differences in the likelihood a subject would stabilize, and no significant interactions between family management and medication dosage. Rehospitalization and relapse outcomes were reported only for the 313 subjects who stabilized and only during the two years of treatment. There were no significant differences in rehospitalization, mean days to rehospitalization, time to psychotic relapse, or time to use of first rescue medication between the AFM and SFM groups overall.[24] Rehospitalization also did not significantly differ when comparing the two levels of family treatment within the three medication dosage groups. There were also no significant differences in social adjustment between the two treatment groups from baseline to post-treatment in social functioning, family relationships, or the romance/sexual factors of the social adjustment scale.[104] However, the more intensive AFM treatment was associated with significantly lower levels of rejecting attitudes by family members toward the subject (0.32 scale points at 1 year; 0.31 effect size; 1.03 scale points at 2 years; 0.30 effect size; $p < 0.01$) and significantly less family friction then the less intensive SFM intervention. However, authors note that given the non-significant differences on primary outcomes and small differences on family outcomes, differences across these treatment conditions may have limited clinical significance.

A third trial was comprised of 108 subjects with a dual diagnosis of active substance abuse or dependence and either schizophrenia, schizoaffective, or bipolar disorder.[99, 100] Patients and a family member received weekly psychoeducation in both groups, however the FPE (Family Psychoeducation) arm sessions were brief, lasting 2-3 months. In the Family Intervention for Dual Disorders (FIDD) arm, 20-30 sessions (over 18 months) were conducted and problem solving strategies and training in communication were added. Additionally, patients and family members in both groups were encouraged to attend multiple family support groups for up to 36 months. Engagement, defined as subjects participating in 2 or more sessions, was high for both groups (>80%) and not significantly different by group. Treatment exposure, defined as attending at least 3 sessions for the FIDD group or 6 educational sessions the FPE group, did not differ between groups. Attendance in the multiple family support groups was low for both conditions (15% for FIDD and 11% for FPE; difference non-significant); these groups were discontinued three years into the study. The FIDD group Brief Psychiatric Rating Scale rating was significantly higher than the FPE group over the three year follow up period; the effect was small for total score (0.17) but moderate for the psychosis subscale (0.32). Overall subject functioning, as measured by the Global Assessment Scale, was higher in the FIDD group (p = 0.08), over the three year follow up period. In the FIDD group, the BPRS psychosis symptom reduction was much stronger for women than for men. The more intensive FIDD subjects did not show significant improvement in alcohol or drug use or percent stable days compared to their FPE counterparts, but both groups improved significantly in these areas as compared to baseline. Social problem solving skills did not improve significantly for the FIDD group as compared to the FPE group, as was hypothesized. Outcomes on the <u>individual</u> functioning of family members, versus the family as a unit, and on how having a relationship with an individual with a mental illness affects the family member were collected; however, those outcomes are outside the scope of this review and thus are not reported here.

Results were not reported by relationship distress in trials comparing family involved therapies.

Summary and Discussion

Evidence synthesized in numerous prior reviews supports the efficacy of family interventions, typically psychoeducational family treatments, that include elements of education on the illness, family support, crisis intervention, and problem-solving skills training to improve relapse and rehospitalization rates outcomes for schizophrenia spectrum patients, compared to no intervention or medication only (KQ1).[126-130] Psychoeducational family treatments of at least 9 months, in combination with medication, have been previously recommended by existing treatment guidelines[127] with "good" evidence of leading to improved relapse rates among patients.[6, 126-128]

The Schizophrenia Patient Outcomes Research Team (PORT), funded in 1992 by the Agency for Health Care Policy and Research and the National Institute of Mental Health, issued psychosocial treatment recommendations in 1998, 2003, and 2009 which included recommendations for family based treatment. They recommend that patients with ongoing contact with their families, or who have "non-family" caregivers, should be offered psychosocial intervention that provides a combination of family education, family support, crisis intervention, and problem solving skills training,[127] regardless of level of a family's expressed emotion. Their initial recommendations were refined and expanded to include shorter interventions (less than nine months), in recognition that more complex and lengthy interventions are difficult to actually implement.[128, 129]

Research summarized in prior reviews has largely established that family psychoeducational treatments are superior to treatment as usual in reducing relapse rates.[131, 132] However, these interventions are not consistently superior to comprehensive and intensive patient-only interventions[132] and the effects of these interventions over long term follow-ups are mixed.[33, 130, 131, 133, 134] Recently a Cochrane review[126] also supported the above review findings but cautioned that these effects may be overestimated due to poor methodological quality. Also, as noted in the Cochrane review,[126] many previous schizophrenia studies were conducted in China and other countries, so the results may not be applicable to a US. Veteran population. Family interventions for schizophrenia which met our inclusion criteria (conducted in the US since 1996 and including patient outcomes), have not included a no treatment, waitlist, or medication only comparison condition. Therefore, we cannot contribute to the body of literature establishing the general efficacy of family treatments compared to waitlist or medication management only (KQ1). While there is an important clinical need to provide some form of psychosocial intervention to patients with serious mental illness, comparisons of relatively untested programs to equally rigorous comparators complicate efforts to demonstrate the initial efficacy of untested programs.

Our findings address how family interventions compare to individually oriented care (1 trial) or other family interventions (3 trials) and include a wider breadth of patient outcomes and more complex patients with either co-occurring problems (1 trial) or co-morbid substance use disorders (1 trial) than trials conducted prior to our review period. Additionally, to address an existing gap in the literature,[9, 130] one trial examined the efficacy of family involved treatments in improving patient outcomes for patients who are relatively stable (those who have not recently suffered a psychotic relapse or hospitalization)[101-103] by recruiting participants from a community mental health setting, regardless of recent relapse or hospitalization. Dyck and colleagues[101, 102] found an intervention including multiple family groups was superior to individually-oriented treatment at the mid-treatment time point (one year after randomization) in rates of negative symptoms and rates of hospitalization. At post-treatment and long term follow-up (1 year post), the only significant difference across conditions was in rates of state-level psychiatric facility hospitalizations.[103] State-level psychiatric hospitalizations are reserved for those patients with the most severe symptoms, thus this finding may suggest that family intervention is more beneficial than individual care for those with the most severe symptoms, consistent with earlier findings.[129] Additionally, these findings are consistent with prior work suggesting erosion of treatment effects can be found across conditions at long term follow-ups.[33, 131]

Three other trials each compared a less intensive to a more intensive family intervention.[24, 29, 99, 104] Few differences were found between conditions, although improvements in both groups as compared to baseline were noted for several outcomes. This is consistent with past reviews identifying that differences among intensive interventions and among alternative family interventions with different theoretical underpinnings are largely non-significant.[130, 132] The subjects in McFarlane and colleagues[29] Assertive Community Treatment trial all showed improvement over the two year intervention, but the addition of multiple family groups yielded only one significant additional benefit, employment rates during treatment. However, these differences were also non-significant at the 24 month end point.

Schooler et al.[24] found that the addition of in-home behavioral single family therapy to a larger family-oriented treatment package did not provide significant additional benefits in subjects' need for rescue medication, relapse delay, or hospitalization. Mueser et al.,[104] examining subjects in the same study, found the more intensive family intervention lead to significantly less family friction and better attitudes towards the patient than the family-oriented treatment package delivered in clinics, without in-home BFT. There were no differences in patient social functioning between groups. Outcome data was collected only for subjects who successfully stabilized and complied with treatment, eliminating the most severely ill patients (41% of the 528 randomized), who may stand to benefit more from the more intensive family treatment.

Mueser and colleagues' trial[99, 100] enrolled subjects dually diagnosed with both schizophrenia spectrum and substance use disorders, and they expanded the definition of family to include "any caring, but non-professional relationship," including clergy and friends as well as relatives. The longer, skills oriented intervention (FIDD) was associated with greater improvements in subject psychiatric functioning and symptoms than brief (2-3 month) family psychoeducation only treatment, but did not reduce substance use. The initial success in engaging subjects and their family members in both levels of treatment suggests acceptability of family intervention for dual diagnosis patients. However, the vast majority of families (over 80%) in both study arms did not participate in multi-family groups offered between the end of the psychoeducation and skills intervention and the final data collection point (three years after randomization). How to motivate families and patients to participate in program offerings post-treatment is an area that needs further research. None of the schizophrenia studies included in our review provided results comparing distressed to non-distressed families.

Posttraumatic Stress Disorder

Overview

One study that met our criteria addressed KQ2. Relevant to KQ2A, Glynn and colleagues compared an individually-oriented treatment (exposure therapy) to that same intervention followed by PTSD-specific behavioral family therapy. Findings are presented in Appendix D, Tables 14 to 16.

Comparisons with Traditional Individual-Oriented Therapies

Differences in symptom change and social adjustment were non-significant between those who participated in exposure therapy versus exposure therapy plus BFT.[8] Additionally, Glynn and colleagues[8] collapsed all those participating in BFT with those not participating in BFT. They found greater increases in social problem solving skills over the course of treatment among those participating in BFT than those who did not participate in BFT. However, those who participated in exposure therapy plus BFT were more likely to drop out of treatment than those who participation in exposure therapy alone.[8]

No studies compared different family involved therapies. Additionally, the role of family distress in predicting differential response across conditions was not examined.

Sexual Functioning Disorders

No studies compared family interventions to traditional individual-oriented therapies or to different family interventions.

Other Conditions

Depression

No studies that met our inclusion criteria included a comparison of family involved therapy and individual or alternative family involved therapy. However, we did identify two recent Cochrane reviews that explored the role of family members in the treatment of depression. Barbato and D'Avanzo[135] included randomized controlled trials or quasi-randomized controlled trials comparing marital therapy to other psychosocial and medication treatments or to non-active treatments.[135] The studies included heterosexual couples between the ages of 16 and 65 years with a depressed spouse (primary diagnosis by DSM-IV, International Classification of Diseases (ICD-10), or Research Diagnostic Criteria codes). Treatment was community or outpatient based. Eight trials were included; three of these were conducted in the United States (publication dates 1989-1992). The overall conclusion from the review was that there was no evidence that marital therapy was different than individual psychotherapy in terms of depressive symptoms (data from 6 studies with a total of 167 subjects) or persistence of depression (3 studies, 106 subjects) following treatment. Marital distress was lower following treatment in the marital therapy groups than in the individual therapy groups (5 studies, 137 subjects). There was no difference in the number of drop-outs (6 studies, 210 subjects). In distressed couples, there was no difference in depression outcomes (4 studies, 90 subjects) or drop-outs (4 studies, 109 subjects). Marital stress was significantly reduced (4 studies, 90 subjects). Two studies (60 subjects) that compared marital therapy to no or minimal therapy did report a reduction in depressive symptoms following treatment. The three studies from the United States, all of which compared marital therapy to individual therapy, found no difference in depressive symptoms. Two of the studies reported persistence of depression with no difference between treatment groups. The authors of the review noted small sample sizes, unclear sample representation, short follow-up periods (or assessment only at the end of treatment), and large number of drop-outs as methodological weaknesses of this literature.

The second review focused on family therapy for depression.[136] Randomized controlled trials and controlled clinical trials were included if the treatment involved 6 or more sessions of at least one hour duration and no group therapy with multiple families. Family therapy was compared to no intervention or an alternative intervention. Six studies were included in the review however two enrolled adolescents and one enrolled children. Of the three studies enrolling adults, two were conducted in the United States. In one study published in 1985, an inpatient family intervention (psychoeducation based) reduced symptoms, improved family attitude toward treatment, and improved global functioning compared to individual treatment. The results were significant only for the female patients. The second study is reviewed above.[89] Overall, the authors of the review concluded that there was insufficient evidence to assess the effectiveness of family therapy for treatment of depression. The use of psychological interventions with an evidence base was recommended.

Summary

Recent prior reviews have established that there is low[135] or insufficient[136] strength of evidence to assess whether family therapy is more effective than no treatment or waitlist in reducing symptoms of depression and increasing family functioning. An early review[9] included data from 3 studies published prior to our inclusion date. One study of behavioral marital therapy found no difference between behavioral marital therapy and individual cognitive therapy for improving depression symptoms in maritally distressed couples;[45] both interventions were superior to wait list control.[45] A second study included distressed and non-distressed couples.[44] In that study, behavioral marital therapy and individual cognitive therapy were comparable for maritally distressed couples. Cognitive therapy was superior for alleviating depression in non-maritally distressed couples. A similar result was reported in a study comparing interpersonal psychotherapy for depression (IPT) without family involvement to IPT delivered as a couple therapy (i.e., both the patient and his or her intimate partner participate in treatment sessions).[137] The study that was eligible for and included in our review enrolled mildly to moderately distressed couples and found brief couple therapy to be superior to waitlist for reducing symptoms and improving couple function.[114]

Eating Disorders

The same study that reported outcomes for KQ1 (group CBT with spouse vs. wait list control) included a comparator active treatment group (standard CBT).[115] Results (see Appendix D, Tables 22 to 24) were reported post-treatment and at 6 month follow-up. There were no significant differences between the two active CBT groups for binge abstinence or days binged (either by 7-day recall or the EDEQ.[116, 117] Depression scores (BDI[112]) decreased for both groups but did not differ between groups. There were no differences between active CBT groups on the Rosenberg Self-Esteem Score.[138] Couple functioning (Dyadic Adjustment Scale)[109] did not differ between CBT groups post-treatment or at follow-up, however, subjects in the CBT with spouse group reported being in better agreement with their spouses regarding a plan of action for binge eating (p = 0.04). Attendance at treatment sessions was comparable.

Summary

Patient or couple functioning outcomes for women in the group CBT for binge eating disorder with spouse involvement group did not differ from results for women in the standard CBT group with the exception of better agreement on a plan for managing binge eating.

Smoking Cessation

One study of partner-assisted therapy in conjunction with individual counseling met eligibility criteria.[118] The study was conducted at an Army Medical Center and enrolled 625 women who were pregnant and their intimate partners. Partner-assisted therapy with individual counseling was compared to individual counseling alone or to usual care. Outcomes were assessed at 28 weeks of pregnancy and at 2-, 6-, and 12-months postpartum. Results are presented in Appendix D, Tables 22 to 24. No differences were observed between groups for abstinence from smoking, time to relapse, or social support (including smoking-specific support, instrumental support, or emotional support).

Summary

Abstinence from smoking, time to relapse, and social support did not differ for pregnant women who participated in partner-assisted therapy with woman-only counseling, woman-only counseling, or usual care.

SUMMARY AND DISCUSSION

This evidence synthesis summarizes the efficacy of family involved psychosocial treatments in improving the outcomes of patients with mental health conditions in the US since 1995. Two key questions were identified. Our search yielded 51 articles (39 trials), including trials of family interventions for substance use disorders (22 trials), bipolar disorder (6 trials), schizophrenia and related disorders (4 trials), PTSD (2 trials), sexual functioning disorders (2 trials), depression (1 trial), binge eating disorder (1 trial), and nicotine dependence (1 trial).

Overall, this review represents a variety of studies examining family involved treatments for mental health conditions. Trials were highly heterogeneous in terms of intervention characteristics, size, population, and findings. In many cases, the family intervention was manualized and withdrawals from the trials were adequately described. Typically, well-validated outcome measures were employed, diagnoses were verified by structured clinical interviews, and exclusion/inclusion criteria were clearly described. However, few studies included a description of allocation concealment or blinding procedures and measures used to assess the same construct were highly variable across trials. Frequently, intent to treat analyses were either not described or not employed, assessments of treatment integrity were frequently not described, and for many studies, samples were small and analyses underpowered. Additionally, many studies were conducted on mostly white and male samples, who were under 40 years old, and in all but two trials, Veteran status among participants was not reported. While post-treatment symptom severity was frequently reported, many of our other outcomes of interest were not. Most notable was the frequent absence of assessments of global family/couple adjustment, communication, conflict, observational family/couple interactions, intimate partner violence, adherence, attendance, and satisfaction with care. The substance use literature posed the largest exception to this, with studies frequently examining global family/couple adjustment, adherence, attendance, and satisfaction with care. This likely reflects the more advanced stage of development of this literature.

The majority of studies fell into either Baucom and colleague's[9] disorder specific couple/family treatment and/or partner-assisted treatment categories. The purposes of family involvement also varied and included, but were not limited to, engaging patients in care, family members acting as out-of-session coaches, psychoeducation to improve family's support for patients, and addressing family conflict that could exacerbate symptoms.

SUMMARY OF EVIDENCE BY KEY QUESTION

Key Question #1. What is the efficacy of family involved interventions in improving outcomes for adult patients with mental health conditions [i.e., how do family involved psychosocial treatments compare to no psychosocial treatment: (a) waitlist/no treatment or (b) medication management only]?

The level of development of the evidence for family involved treatments varied greatly across conditions. Consequently, family treatments for some conditions had a number of efficacy trials prior to our search timeframe (i.e., schizophrenia and substance use disorder). For these conditions, the trials reviewed were more applicable to KQ2. See Table 1 for a review of the efficacy status of family treatments for mental health conditions prior to our review.

Substance Use Disorders

One trial[64] found that among patients completing an inpatient alcohol detoxification program, a single family session and single family follow-up to help plan for continuing care (partner-assisted treatment[9]) did not result in significantly improved percent days abstinent post-intervention or greater attendance to continuing care. However, 92% of those receiving the family intervention were more likely to enter a continuing care program, a 30% improvement over patients hospitalized for substance use detoxification whose families did not participate in their aftercare planning.

Bipolar Disorder

Two trials compared a family intervention to a drug-only treatment. In one trial medication management alone was compared to medication management plus either Problem Centered Systems Therapy of the Family (PCSTF; a general family therapy[9]) or psychoeducational multifamily groups (a disorder specific family intervention[9]). There were no differences in symptoms between either family involved treatments or medication management alone.[89, 97, 98] However, compared to medication management only, patients from distressed families reported significantly lower rates of depressive episodes (psychoeducational multifamily groups: 1.4 fewer episodes per year, d = 1.0; PCSTF: 0.9 fewer episodes, d = 0.70), shorter duration of depressive episodes (psychoeducational multifamily groups: 14% less time; d = 0.82), and fewer mood episodes (psychoeducational multifamily groups: 1.7 fewer episodes, yearly, d = 0.82), suggesting a family intervention specific to bipolar disorder or a general family therapy could provide improved treatment response for patients with bipolar disorder in distressed families. In the other trial, while those assigned to psychoeducational marital therapy (a disorder specific couple intervention) did not report greater symptom relief than those assigned to medication management only, patients in marital therapy did report better global functioning (7 points on the 100 point GAS) and medication adherence (0.53 points on a 6 point scale) than those assigned to medication management only.[94] In both cases, family functioning outcomes were not reported.

Schizophrenia

No trials.

PTSD

One trial demonstrated exposure plus Behavioral Family Therapy (a disorder specific family therapy[9]) resulted in better PTSD outcomes than waitlist;[8] however these differences eroded at follow-up and drop out was worse among those in the family treatment condition. Another trial demonstrated significantly better engagement in treatment for the patients (Bosnian refugees) of those who participated in family support groups (CAFES; a trauma-specific family therapy), than waitlist.[105] Specifically, patients' whose family members participated in CAFES attended 4 more mental health visits than waitlist controls.

Sexual Functioning

One trial[106] found subjects assigned to sex therapy plus medication reported greater satisfaction with treatment than those assigned to medication alone (disorder specific couple treatment).[9, 106] Differences between conditions on erectile functioning up to two months after treatment were not significant. A second trial found no significant difference between those assigned to four weeks of cognitive-behavior sex therapy plus medication versus those assigned to medication alone after 4 weeks of treatment. Further descriptive statistics on differences between the two groups were provided at this post-treatment assessment but further formal testing was not provided.

Other Conditions Examined in Single Trials

One small trial of brief couple therapy for depression (n = 35; disorder specific couple treatment) found that couple therapy led to significantly improved depression symptoms and marital satisfaction. On continuous measures, scores on the BDI-II (d = 0.54), HAM-D (d = 0.72), and DAS (d = 0.43) were each significantly improved for participants in couple therapy compared to waitlist controls.[114] A trial of group CBT for binge eating disorder found that CBT with or without spouse involvement resulted in better symptom improvement than waitlist.[115]

Key Question #2. What is the effectiveness of family involved interventions compared to alternative interventions in improving outcomes for adult patients with mental health conditions [i.e., how do family involved interventions compare to (a) any individually-oriented psychosocial intervention or (b) any alternative family involved intervention]?

Substance Use Disorders

Twenty-one of 22 trials addressed KQ2. Fifteen trials compared family treatment to individually-oriented treatment as usual or manualized individual behavior therapy (13 of these trials examined BCT or BFT for an alcohol or substance use disorder; 2 trials examined alternative methods of family involvement in care) and 6 trials compared a family treatment to an alternative family involved treatment (3 trials examined CRAFT, a disorder-specific and partner-assisted treatment; 3 examined BCT or BFT). Findings are summarized by intervention below.

Behavioral Couple Therapy or Behavioral Family Therapy (disorder specific couple therapy[9])

Effects on substance use. BCT participants used substances for 1.2 fewer days per month (14.6 per year) at post-treatment, 3.3 days per month (40 per year) at 6 months, and 3.6 days per month (44 per year) for 12 month follow-ups. This same general pattern of results was found for studies addressing drug use only, alcohol use only, drug use disorders among men, and drug use disorders among women.

Effects on relationship adjustment. Better relationship adjustment following treatment was found among those assigned to BCT than ICBT, with 12.5% higher scores on the DAS, on average, among those who participated in BCT, one year after treatment.

Therapy with non-intimate partners (BFT). Findings are mixed for differences between ICBT and BFT, a version of BCT including non-intimate partners, with one trial finding no differences in substance use between BFT and individual treatment and a second trial finding significantly lower rates of substance use among those in BFT than those in individual treatment at 18 months after treatment (13.2% fewer days abstinence). However, these differences eroded at 30 month follow-ups.

Brief BCT. Two trials examined both a brief version of BCT and standard BCT for substance use disorders and found both BCT and brief BCT led to significant differences in PDA compared to ICBT, but few differences were found between the standard and brief versions of BCT.

BCT with relapse prevention. Two trials added a relapse prevention intervention to BCT (2 trials[4, 72, 86, 87]) with one trial finding no differences between conditions[72, 86, 87] and the other finding greater reductions in substance use, with 13.2% fewer days of use 18 months after treatment.[4] These differences eroded and were non-significant at the 30 month follow-up. In this trial, the benefits of BCT with relapse prevention were strongest for those in the most distressed relationships and with the most severe drinking behavior.[4]

Same sex couples. One trial compared BCT to ICBT with same sex couples, finding fewer percent days heavy drinking among BCT participants at long term follow-ups and significantly slower rates of erosion in treatment effects among BCT participants (i.e., BCT participants were slower to increase their rates of heavy drinking than ICBT patients after treatment).

Veterans. Two studies examined Veterans with alcohol use disorders.[4, 65] One found no difference between BCT and a general couple therapy on sexual satisfaction.[65] Rates of substance use after treatment were not reported. The second compared BCT to BCT with relapse prevention, discussed above.[4] Veterans participating in BCT[4] demonstrated comparable or better rates of PDA from alcohol use (post-treatment: 98.0%; short-term follow-up: 87.6%; long-term follow-up: 82.7%) than average rates of PDA reported in the AUD trials included in our pooled analyses. However, direct comparisons within trials between Veteran and non-Veteran have yet to be conducted, and research has yet to evaluate BCT compared to individual therapy among Veteran samples.

CRAFT (disorder-specific and partner-assisted treatment[9])

Across 3 trials[80, 81, 83] CRAFT was found to be superior to alternative family treatments in improving patients' initiation of substance use treatment 30-48%. Trials did not provide data on differences in overall rates of session attendance or substance use.

Alternatives to BCT and CRAFT

BCT versus non-disorder specific couple therapy. Two trials compared BCT to an alternative non-disorder specific couple treatment[65, 73] finding no differences between the couple interventions on substance use[73] or relationship functioning.[65, 73]

Adding additional treatment components to BCT. One trial added parenting skills training to BCT[71] and a second added attendance to AA and Al-Anon.[72, 86, 87] Both trials found no differences in symptoms or couple functioning between BCT with additional treatment components versus standard BCT.

Reciprocal relationship counseling. Carroll[77] found that the combination of reciprocal relationship counseling (disorder specific intervention[9]), contingency management, and naltrexone use was superior to contingency management plus naltrexone only in family functioning, but not in percent days abstinent or days in treatment.

Motivational and psychoeducational treatment with couple counseling for heroin users with pregnant partners. Jones and colleagues[70] found that subjects in a motivational and psychoeducational intervention that included couple therapy for male heroin users with pregnant intimate partners, actually had <u>higher</u> heroin use at short-term follow up, compared to an individual only counselor-led drug treatment support group.

Bipolar Disorder

Five RCTs provided data relevant to KQ2.

Family-Focused Therapy (FFT; 4 trials; disorder specific family treatment[9])

- FFT or an adapted version of FFT (FFT-HPI[93]) led to better symptom response than either individually-oriented care (1 trial[91]) or alternative family involved interventions (2 trials[90, 93]).

  - ☐ FFT leads to lower rates of relapse than crisis management with limited family involvement, 24 months after randomization (35% relapse versus 54%). Patients in crisis management relapsed an average of 20 weeks sooner than those in FFT.[5, 90]

  - ☐ FFT leads lower rates of relapse (28% versus 60%) and lower rates of hospitalization (12% versus 60%) than individual therapy one year after the end of active treatment.[91]

  - ☐ No significant differences were found between FFT and individual therapy on medication adherence.[91]

  - ☐ FFT-HPI leads to fewer manic (4.2 points on the YMRS; d = 0.34; small effect) and depression symptoms (5.6 points on the HAM-D; d = 0.67; medium effect) among bipolar patients than health education provided to families via DVDs.[93]

- One trial[92] found no significant differences in symptoms of bipolar disorder or family functioning between FFT and either cognitive behavioral therapy or interpersonal and social rhythm therapy, suggesting FFT may perform similarly to other empirically supported, highly intensive interventions in improving symptoms of bipolar disorder.

- Mixed findings limit conclusions that can be drawn about the role of FFT in session attendance or medication adherence.

Disorder Specific versus General Family Therapy (1 trial[89, 97, 98])

The difference in rates of recovery between general family therapy and disorder specific family therapy, delivered in multiple family groups, were non-significant.

Schizophrenia

Three trials addressed KQ2 (1 trial for KQ1 and 3 for KQ2 due to greater than 2 comparison conditions).

Multiple Family Groups (MFG; 1 trial)[101-103]

- One trial compared MFGs (disorder specific family therapy[9]), an interventions focused on psychoeducation, family functioning, and social support, to individually oriented psychosocial intervention. Results indicated that, at the one year point of a two year intervention, MFGs improved negative symptoms of schizophrenia (e.g., blunted affect, alogia, anhedonia, inattention, avolition) an average of one point on a 25 point scale and led to 12% lower rates of hospitalization at state level psychiatric hospitals than individual treatment.

- Differences in rates of hospitalization overall or at non-state level facilities, or use of crisis care, were non-significant at post-treatment and one year after treatment.

Assertive Community Treatment (ACT) With and Without a Biweekly Multi-Family Group (1 trial[29])

- No significant differences were found between groups on hospital admissions, symptoms, or family outcomes.

- Employment rates for ACT and multifamily groups were significantly different during treatment but non-significant at the final follow-up.

Applied Family Management (AFT; 1 trial[104])

- Non-significant differences were found between intensive and less intensive family interventions in symptoms or rates of hospitalization. Authors note group differences may have limited clinical significance.[104]

- A more intensive family therapy (AFM) improved family functioning (patient rejection scale) by 0.32 scale points at 1 year (medium effect size, 0.31) and 1.03 scale points (medium effect size, 0.30 effect size) at 2 year follow-up, over less intensive family interventions.

Family Intervention for Dual Disorders (1 trial; disorder specific family treatment9)

- Subjects with a comorbid substance use disorder and serious mental illness (e.g., schizophrenia, bipolar disorder) demonstrated greater improvements in psychiatric symptoms (BPRS psychosis, medium effect size, 0.32; BPRS total, small effect size, 0.17) when assigned to a longer term (9-18 months) psychoeducational family program than a brief (2-3 month) family intervention.[100]
- Differences in substance use and global functioning across conditions were non-significant

PTSD

One trial found no significant differences in PTSD outcomes between exposure therapy with Behavioral Family Therapy (disorder specific family intervention[9]) versus exposure therapy only,[8] however the family involved arm resulted in poorer rates of dropout than exposure alone.

Sexual Functioning

No trials.

Other Conditions Examined In Single Trials

There were no differences between family involved interventions and individually-oriented treatments in one trial examining smoking cessation in pregnant women[118] and a second examining binge eating disorder, with the exception of greater agreement between spouses regarding a plan of action for binge eating.[115]

EFFICACY

In Table 16 below, we summarize the efficacy status[23] and strength of evidence[62] for outcomes of interest (i.e., symptoms, family/couple functioning, and, in some cases, treatment engagement) for those family treatments demonstrating benefits over their comparators that met our review criteria. In three cases, studies demonstrated an individually-oriented, disorder specific intervention plus a family intervention led to greater improvements than waitlist/drug only conditions, but the combined treatment did not demonstrate significant gains over the individually-oriented treatment alone in the same trial.[8, 77, 115] Consequently, these trials are not included in the table below. These findings represent only studies performed in the US in the last 15 years that report on patient outcomes. Studies finding no significant differences between the treatment and the comparator at post-treatment or follow-up assessments on our outcomes of interest are not included as 'possibly efficacious studies' and, consequently, not incorporated.

STRENGTH OF EVIDENCE

In addition to identifying studies that have demonstrated efficacy or are possibly efficacious, we rated the confidence with which we draw these conclusions for the outcomes of interest (i.e., the 'strength of the evidence that underlies conclusions,' p. 513, Owens et al.[62]). Strength of evidence was considered by mental health condition, given the wide variety of interventions, techniques, and treatment targets of these interventions. In general, with the exception of behavioral couple therapy for SUDs, CRAFT for increasing treatment initiation among patients with SUDs, and Family Focused Therapy (FFT) for bipolar disorder, each intervention was typically examined in one or two trials. Additionally, the FFT studies contained highly diverse sets of comparison conditions and findings were largely mixed, limiting our confidence in the strength of evidence across these trials.

Several of the individual trials were of good or fair quality (low or medium risk of bias) but with a single, often small trial of a particular intervention for a particular outcome and imprecise estimates of effect, we have low confidence that the available evidence for the interventions examined in single trials reflect the true effect. As such, the strength of evidence for any given intervention, with the exception of BCT for drug use disorders and CRAFT for increasing treatment initiation among those with an SUD, is generally low. Specific ratings for treatments deemed efficacious or possibly efficacious are presented in Table 16. *Importantly, our strength of evidence ratings are based solely on the results of our search, which included only US studies of family involved psychosocial treatments for mental health conditions since 1995 that included patient outcomes. Also, this Table should be considered in tandem with Table 1, which identifies those interventions established as efficacious prior to our review, including behavioral family therapy and supportive family therapy for schizophrenia.*[6, 9]

Table 16. Family Interventions since 1996 that Improve Outcomes for US Patients with Mental Health Conditions

MH Condition	Intervention	Comparator	Outcome	Efficacy Status	Strength of Evidence
Alcohol Use Disorders	Behavioral Couple Therapy	Individual Behavioral Therapy	1) Substance Use	1	Moderate[a]
			2) Relationship Adjustment	1	Moderate[a]
			3) Intimate Partner Violence	3	Low
			4) Attendance	3	Low
	Brief family intervention to promote continuing care[64]	Treatment-as-usual	1) Substance Use	ND	Low
			2) Treatment Initiation	3	Low
	Behavioral Couple Therapy + relapse prevention[64]	Behavioral Couple Therapy	1) Substance Use	3	Low
			2) Relationship Adjustment	ND	Low
	Behavioral Family Treatment[82]	Individual Behavioral Therapy	1) Substance Use	3	Low
			2) Family Functioning	ND	Low
	CRAFT[81]	Alternative Family Treatments	1) Substance Use	ND	Low
			2) Family Functioning	ND	Low
			3) Treatment Initiation	3	Low
Drug Use Disorders	Behavioral Couple Therapy	Individual Behavioral Therapy	1) Substance Use	1	Moderate[a]
			2) Relationship Adjustment	1	Moderate[a]
			3) Intimate Partner Violence	3	Low
			4) Attendance	1	Low[b]
	Behavioral Family Treatment[68, 82]	Individual Behavioral Therapy	1) Substance Use	3	Low
			2) Family Functioning	3	Low
	CRAFT[80, 83]	Al-Anon/Nar-Anon	1) Substance Use	ND	Moderate
			2) Family Functioning	ND	Low
			3) Treatment Initiation	1	Moderate
Bipolar	Family-Focused Treatment-Health Promoting Intervention[93]	Health information DVDs reviewed by caregivers	1) Symptoms	3	Low
	Family-Focused Treatment	Crisis management with two in-home family psychoeducation sessions[5, 90]	1) Symptoms	3	Low
			2) Medication Adherence	3	Low
		Problem-focused, psychoeducational Individual therapy[91]	1) Symptoms	3	Low
			2) Medication Adherence	ND	Low
		Cognitive behavior therapy[92, 95]	1) Symptoms	ND	Low
		Interpersonal and social rhythm therapy[92, 95]	1) Symptoms	ND	Low
	Marital intervention + medication[94]	Medication only	1) Symptoms	ND	Low
			2) Global Functioning	4	Low
			3) Medication Adherence	4	Low

MH Condition	Intervention	Comparator	Outcome	Efficacy Status	Strength of Evidence
Schizophrenia	Multiple Family Groups[101-103]	Standard, Individually-oriented care	1) Symptoms	ND	Low
			2) Any Hospitalization	ND	Low
			3) State Hospitalization	3	Low
			4) MH Care Utilization	ND	Low
	Family intervention + in home behavioral family therapy (Applied Family Management[24, 104]	Family intervention	1) Symptoms	ND	Low
			2) Family Functioning	ND	Low
			3) Patient Rejection by Family	3	Low
			4) MH Care Utilization	ND	Low
			5) Attendance	ND	Low
Schizophrenia & Substance Use Disorder	Psychoeducation + skills oriented training (Family Intervention for Dual Disorder[99, 100]	Short term psychoeducation	1) Schizophrenia Symptoms	3	Low
			2) Substance Use	ND	Low
			3) Global Functioning	3	Low
			4) Medication Adherence	ND	Low
PTSD	Coffee and Family Education and Support[105]	Waitlist	1) Number of MH Visits	4	Low
Depression	Brief problem-focused couple therapy[114]	Waitlist	1) Symptoms	4	Low
			2) Relationship Adjustment	4	Low

Efficacy Status:
1 = Efficacious & Specific = superior to placebo, nonspecific, or alternative intervention in at least two studies conducted by independent research teams.
2 = Efficacious; superior to waitlist in RCTs conducted by two independent research teams.
3 = *Possibly* Efficacious & Specific; criteria met for efficacious and specific from a single study.
4 = *Possibly* Efficacious; criteria met for efficacious from a single study (Baucom, 1998;[9] Chambless & Hollon,1998[23])
ND = No significant differences found; MH = Mental health

Strength of Evidence:
High = High confidence evidence reflects true effect. The effect and confidence in the estimate of effect is unlikely to change with further research.
Moderate = moderate confidence that evidence reflects true effect. The effect and confidence of the effect may change with further research.
Low = Low confidence evidence reflects true effect. The effect and confidence of the effect will likely change with further research.[62]

[a]Seven of the nine trials comparing these conditions were written by or based on data collected by Dr. Fals-Stewart. See Substance Use Disorders Results for KQ2 for discussion.
[b]Several studies also found non-significant differences, leading to low strength of evidence.

CONCLUSIONS

Nearly half of the trials we located were examinations of family involved treatments for substance use disorders, typically BCT or BFT for substance use disorders (disorder specific couple or family therapy[9]). While findings were not without contradiction, behavioral couple therapy is superior to individual behavior therapy for improving substance use and relationship distress. CRAFT[81, 83] also increases the rates with which patients with substance use disorders initiate substance use treatment. Mixed findings indicate relapse prevention added to behavioral couple therapy may improve outcomes, especially among those with the most severe substance use and relationship distress. Finally, unlike other mental health conditions, two trials were conducted with Veterans,[4, 65] but only one trial reported substance use outcomes and compared BCT to BCT with relapse prevention (O'Farrell, 1998a), making it difficult to draw conclusions about whether Veteran samples achieve the same benefits from BCT as other samples. More research is clearly needed examining the efficacy of family involved treatments with Veteran samples.

Findings for bipolar disorder were also mixed, with single trials demonstrating family therapy improves symptoms over medication management alone, particularly for those in distressed families, and FFT improves symptoms over alternative treatment approaches in two trials, but performs similarly to other empirically supported, individually-oriented interventions in another trial. Specifically, 1) FFT or an adapted version of FFT (FFT-HPI[93]) led to greater symptom improvements than either an individually-oriented treatment (1 trial[91]) or alternative family involved interventions (2 trials[90, 93]), 2) FFT performed similarly to other empirically supported, highly intensive, individually-oriented interventions in improving symptoms of bipolar disorder,[92] 3) for patients in distressed families, improved symptoms of depression were found for those in either a disorder specific multifamily group or general family therapy than medication management alone,[98] and 4) marital psychoeducational therapy led to greater improvements in global functioning and medication adherence, but not in symptoms, than medication management alone.

Work conducted prior to the time frame of our review has established the efficacy of behavioral family therapy and supportive family therapy for schizophrenia.[9] Given the wealth of data prior to 1996 supporting these interventions for schizophrenia, we were surprised to find only 4 US trials since that time. These trials expanded upon the work conducted in prior studies by including complex cases (i.e., multiple diagnoses or problems), but provided limited additional clarity regarding which family treatments enhance patient outcomes or if family treatments improve outcomes outside of relapse/rehospitalization rates. As noted in previous reviews,[9] schizophrenia and bipolar disorders are chronic, lifelong illnesses. Consequently, appropriate outcomes include lengthening time to relapse, improving quality of life, and enhancing family functioning, rather than success in eliminating or 'curing' symptoms. Among our outcomes of interest, one trial found rates of state-hospitalization were lower among those in multiple family psychoeducational groups than those in a shorter individually-oriented intervention of psychoeducation only.[103] A second trial found no differences on our outcomes of interest at final follow-ups for those participating in Assertive Community Training with or without a biweekly multiple family group.[29] A third trial found family therapy with an in home behavioral family therapy component resulted in less patient rejection by families than the same intervention without in-home behavioral family therapy. Differences on symptoms and rates of hospitalization were non-significant. A final trial demonstrated greater improvements in symptoms of serious mental illness and functioning, but not lower substance use, among dually diagnosed patients (serious mental illness and SUDs) assigned to a 9-18 month psychoeducational family program versus a brief (2-3 month) family intervention. However, problems with recruitment and retention of these complex patients raises concerns about the feasibility of family treatment for this group, especially long-term interventions.[100] Additional evidence from non-US trials exists supporting family treatments for schizophrenia for the prevention or delay of relapse over the past 15 years and was not included in the present review. The applicability of results to US Veterans and even US patients from studies outside the United States, particularly in China, is limited. A recent, more inclusive review of family treatments for schizophrenia concluded the quality of reporting in most these studies was poor.[126]

Family treatments for a number of additional mental health conditions were examined in one or two trials, including PTSD (2 trials), erectile dysfunction (2 trials), depression (1 trial), binge eating disorder (1 trial), and smoking cessation (1 trial). A family support group to encourage treatment engagement among Bosnian refugees with PTSD found greater rates of engagement than waitlist only participants (one trial). Additionally, support was found for brief couple therapy for depression over waitlist in improving depression and couple functioning. Results from the remaining trials included largely non-significant differences between family treatments and either individual treatment (PTSD, binge eating, smoking) or, for erectile dysfunction, medication management.

Overall, the literature indicated family involved treatments for mental health conditions were as effective as or more effective than individually-oriented psychotherapies, with two exceptions. The addition of approximately 23 weeks of disorder-specific behavioral family therapy after 9 weeks (18 sessions) of exposure therapy for PTSD lead to greater rates of treatment dropout than exposure therapy alone or waitlist.[8] Additionally, male opiod users with pregnant female partners who participated in a combination of motivational enhancement, case management, contingency management, and psychoeducational couple therapy reported greater heroin use at short-term follow-ups than patients participating in usual care. Outside of these two trials, findings either favored family involvement or demonstrated no significant differences between family interventions and comparator conditions, even when comparators were robust, active individually-oriented interventions. However, outside of the SUD literature, the number of trials testing the same intervention with the same or similar comparators was limited, leading to low confidence in the consistency of these conclusions. Additionally, many studies did not evaluate family and couple functioning after treatment, treatment adherence, or satisfaction with care. Additionally, most studies did not report Veteran status of their participants. Consequently, while the present study sought to optimize the relevance of this review to Veterans by examining only US studies, the generalizability of findings from these trials to Veterans' samples is largely unknown.

LIMITATIONS

There were several important limitations to this review. First, in order to focus on recent, high quality studies, most applicable to Veterans, our review was limited to randomized controlled trials conducted over the last 15 years. As discussed above, some family interventions were established as efficacious prior to this time frame, limiting the need for, and consequently, volume of studies addressing KQ1. Secondly, this review was also limited to studies conducted in the US only. The efficacy of family interventions has been established in many studies internationally (i.e. in China for family treatments for serious mental illness), however, their applicability to the US Veteran population or US healthcare system is not known.[129] Third, developing and advancing a psychosocial intervention such that it is appropriate for testing in an RCT is a major task requiring years of work and even further complicated by the need to recruit both patients and their families for participation. Consequently, there are numerous family involved interventions not included in our review that are in various stages of development or are currently under evaluation in RCTs (e.g., Couple therapies for PTSD,[139] Family Member Provider Outreach Program,[140] Coaching into Care,[141] REACH[142]). While our focus on RCTs is warranted, given the VA's need for direction on which family interventions have established an evidence base, exclusions of these interventions under development is a potential limitation. Fourth, we elected to organize our findings by mental health condition, consistent with the organization of the DSM-IV. However, alternative methods of presenting findings exist. Findings could be presented comparing 'serious mental illness' (i.e., discussing schizophrenia and bipolar trials together) to other forms of mental illness or by type of intervention (family versus couple; disorder specific versus general family therapies; interventions using similar approaches, such as psychoeducational interventions). Conclusions using these alternative approaches to synthesizing findings would likely differ from those reached in this review.

Finally, interventions specifically targeting caregiver outcomes are important. However, given the VA's traditional focus on Veteran outcomes, our review included only studies which assessed participants' outcomes (including family and couple functioning). Interventions that solely seek to improve the distress and burden experienced by family members of those with mental illness are were not reviewed, and rates of improvement in the personal distress experienced by family members or caregivers were not included when reported in the trials reviewed. Our findings cannot speak to the efficacy of family interventions for mental health conditions in improving the functioning of patient's family members and caregivers.

RECOMMENDATIONS FOR FUTURE RESEARCH

There are a number of important gaps in our findings that highlight the need for future work. As discussed above, further work is needed to integrate our findings on patient outcomes with research examining how family/couple interventions effect outcomes for spouses and other family members (i.e., caregiver burden, distress, anxiety, etc). For substance use disorders, further work is needed establishing that patients' whose families participate in CRAFT have better reductions in substance use and better longer-term retention in treatment than those assigned to other interventions. Additionally, comparisons between BCT and other family involved interventions are warranted. Finally, a large number of the BCT trials reviewed were conducted within a single lab (i.e., Dr. Fals-Stewart) and further work outside of this laboratory is indicated.

A few trials found family interventions were most effective (i.e., resulted lower rates of symptoms) than comparison conditions for patients in distressed families and/or with more severe baseline symptoms (i.e., BCT with relapse prevention and family therapy for bipolar disorder). Family distress by condition interactions have also been found in studies of depression conducted prior to our review, suggesting that individuals benefit more from individual than marital therapy when in non-distressed relationships.[44, 137] If replicated, these findings could have important implications to personalizing treatment for those with greater family distress and/or more severe symptoms of mental illness. Future work should continue to test for these interactions.

With the exception of two interventions, BCT for substance use and CRAFT for the initiation of substance use treatment, in the past fifteen years, very few family treatments for improving adult mental health conditions have been investigated in more than one rigorous RCT in the US. Generally, the literature is in need of this work. Future trials are needed examining CRAFT,

BCT, and Family-Focused Therapy specifically in Veteran samples. Additionally, further work is needed to continue to establish the efficacy of interventions highlighted in Table 15 as possibly efficacious as they have demonstrated some significant improvements in patient functioning over comparison conditions in at least one trial (rated 3 or 4 on the status of their efficacy). This includes further trials of relapse prevention in addition to BCT, CRAFT for alcohol use disorders, brief BCT for substance use disorders, BFT (with non-intimate partners) for substance use disorders, family involvement to increase treatment initiation among patients hospitalized for substance use detoxification, Family-Focused Treatment-Health Promoting Intervention for bipolar disorder, Family Focused Treatment for bipolar disorder, marital therapy for bipolar disorder, in home behavioral family therapy as an addition to family treatments for schizophrenia, combined treatments for co-occurring schizophrenia and substance use disorders (Family Intervention for Dual Disorder), and support groups to promote treatment use among patients with PTSD (CAFES). Such trials are needed that use large samples, longer-term follow-ups, high quality methodologies, evaluate both patient and family outcomes, compare outcomes by 'type' of family member included (e.g., spouse, parent, sibling), and use standardized symptom measures that can facilitate comparisons across trials.

Evaluating applications of these interventions to patients with comorbid conditions (e.g., substance use and serious mental illness), non-white samples, older patients (i.e., over 65), and Veteran groups is warranted. Additionally, alternative types of family constellations (i.e., close friends, same sex couples) have received little attention among existing RCTs. For Veterans, preferences for which family members to include (i.e., intimate partners versus other family members), how these preferences vary by era (i.e., recently returning Veterans versus Vietnam/Korean War Veterans eras), and the availability and "type" of family members interested in participating (i.e., intimate partners versus other family members) is important to inform policy decisions, especially considering that current eligibility criteria for VA family-related services does not extend to close friends or intimate partners who do not reside with the Veteran. Additionally, research is needed evaluating methods of engaging families in care. This was demonstrating in a study of schizophrenia finding that 80% of families did not participate in optional follow up family group sessions.[99, 100] Additionally, trials of family interventions for several mental health conditions were notably limited or absent from the published literature in the US in the past 15 years, including studies of family treatments for depression, PTSD and other anxiety disorders, personality disorders, eating disorders, and sexual functioning disorders, warranting further work with these conditions.

Given the intent of the ESP is to provide an objective, non-biased approach to the review topic, providing our own cost-benefit analysis of interventions is beyond scope of this review. Additionally, this information was largely absent from RCTs reviewed. Consequently, future research is needed evaluating the costs and benefits of effective interventions. This work could further consider multifamily versus single family interventions for schizophrenia, intensive versus less intensive interventions for serious mental illness, and brief versus standard length interventions for substance use and other disorders (e.g., standard BCT versus brief BCT).

Finally, with the exception of a few studies within the schizophrenia literature, limited attention was paid among studies reviewed to interventions for patients with multiple diagnoses, conditions, or problems. Future research should work to identify efficacious family treatments for patients with commonly co-occurring conditions important to VA populations, such as PTSD and substance use disorders, serious mental illness and substance use disorders, comorbid personality disorders among patients seeking treatment for an Axis I condition. Patients were not excluded from trials due to diagnosis of a personality disorder, but findings were typically not stratified by other co-morbid conditions, preventing comparisons of treatment response by co-morbid conditions. Additionally, in the substance use literature, couples and families in which both the patient and the family member have a substance use disorder are typically excluded from trials. However, in practice, dual SUD couples and family members are not uncommon. Further work is also needed to identify evidence based practices and approaches to family involvement for patients with co-occurring intimate partner violence, suicidality, self-injury, or/ or traumatic brain injury.

REFERENCES

1. Milliken CS, Auchterlonie JL, Hoge CW. Longitudinal assessment of mental health problems among active and reserve component soldiers returning from the Iraq war. *JAMA*. 2007 Nov 14;298(18):2141-8.

2. Meis LA, Erbes CR, Polusny MA, et al. Intimate relationships among returning soldiers: the mediating and moderating roles of negative emotionality, PTSD symptoms, and alcohol problems. *J Trauma Stress*. 2010 Oct;23(5):564-72.

3. Bodenmann G, Plancherel B, Beach SR, et al. Effects of coping-oriented couples therapy on depression: a randomized clinical trial. *J Consult Clin Psychol*. 2008 Dec;76(6):944-54.

4. O'Farrell TJ, Choquette KA, Cutter HS. Couples relapse prevention sessions after behavioral marital therapy for male alcoholics: outcomes during the three years after starting treatment. *J Stud Alcohol*. 1998 Jul;59(4):357-70.

5. Miklowitz DJ, George EL, Richards JA, et al. A randomized study of family-focused psychoeducation and pharmacotherapy in the outpatient management of bipolar disorder. *Arch Gen Psychiatry*. 2003 Sep;60(9):904-12.

6. Dixon LB, Lehman AF. Family interventions for schizophrenia. *Schizophr Bull*. 1995;21(4):631-43.

7. Bryne M, Carr A, Clark M. The efficacy of couples-based interventions for panic disorder with agoraphobia. *J Fam Ther*. 2004;26:105-25.

8. Glynn SM, Eth S, Randolph ET, et al. A test of behavioral family therapy to augment exposure for combat-related posttraumatic stress disorder. *J Consult Clin Psychol*. 1999 Apr;67(2):243-51.

9. Baucom DH, Shoham V, Mueser KT, et al. Empirically supported couple and family interventions for marital distress and adult mental health problems. *J Consult Clin Psychol*. 1998 Feb;66(1):53-88.

10. DiMatteo MR. Social support and patient adherence to medical treatment: a meta-analysis. *Health Psychol*. 2004 Mar;23(2):207-18.

11. Sellwood W, Tarrier N, Quinn J, et al. The family and compliance in schizophrenia: the influence of clinical variables, relatives' knowledge and expressed emotion. *Psychol Med*. 2003 Jan;33(1):91-6.

12. Butzlaff RL, Hooley JM. Expressed emotion and psychiatric relapse: a meta-analysis. *Arch Gen Psych*. 1998 Jun;55(6):547-52.

13. Miklowitz DJ, Goldstein MJ, Nuechterlein KH, et al. Family factors and the course of bipolar affective disorder. *Arch Gen Psych*. 1988 Mar;45(3):225-31.

14. Hooley JM, Gotlib, I.H. A diathesis-stress conceptualization of expressed emotion and clinical outcome. *Appl Prev Psychol*. 2000;9:131-51.

15. Tarrier N, Sommerfield C, Pilgrim H. Relatives' expressed emotion (EE) and PTSD treatment outcome. *Psychol Med.* 1999 Jul;29(4):801-11.

16. Miklowitz DJ. The role of family systems in severe and recurrent psychiatric disorders: a developmental psychopathology view. *Dev Psychopathol.* 2004 Summer;16(3):667-88.

17. Wendel JS, Miklowitz DJ, Richards JA, et al. Expressed emotion and attributions in the relatives of bipolar patients: an analysis of problem-solving interactions. *J Abnorm Psychol.* 2000 Nov;109(4):792-6.

18. Monson CM, Taft CT, Fredman SJ. Military-related PTSD and intimate relationships: from description to theory-driven research and intervention development. *Clin Psychol Rev.* 2009 Dec;29(8):707-14.

19. Epstein EE, McCrady BS. Behavioral couples treatment of alcohol and drug use disorders: current status and innovations. *Clin Psychol Rev.* 1998 Sep;18(6):689-711.

20. Smith JE, Meyers, R.J. Motivating substance abusers to enter treatment: Working with family members. New York: Guilford Press; 2005.

21. Monson CM, Fredman, S.J., Dekel, R.D. Posttraumatic stress disorder in an interpersonal context. In: J.G. B, ed Interpersonal Processes in the Anxiety Disorders: Implications for Understanding Psychopathology and Treatment. 2010:179-208.

22. Lutz ME. Sobering decisions: Are there gender differences? *Alcohol Treat Q.* 1991;8:51-64.

23. Chambless DL, Hollon SD. Defining empirically supported therapies. *J Consult Clin Psychol.* 1998 Feb;66(1):7-18.

24. Schooler NR, Keith SJ, Severe JB, et al. Relapse and rehospitalization during maintenance treatment of schizophrenia. The effects of dose reduction and family treatment. *Arch Gen Psych.* 1997 May;54(5):453-63.

25. Falloon IR, Boyd, J.L., McGill, C.W. Family care of schizophrenia: A problem solving approach to the treatment of mental illness. New York: Guilford Press; 1984.

26. Tarrier N, Barrowclough C, Vaughn C, et al. Community management of schizophrenia. A two-year follow-up of a behavioural intervention with families. *Br J Psychiatry.* 1989 May;154:625-8.

27. Xiong W, Phillips, M.R., Hu, X. Family-based intervention for shizophrenic patients in China. A randomised controlled trial. *Br J Psychiatry.* 1994;165(2):239-47.

28. Randolph ET, Glynn, S.M., Eth, S., Paz, G.G., Leong, G.B., Shaner, A.L. Family therapy for schizophrenia: Two year outcome. Annual Meeting of the American Psychiatric Association; 1995 May, 1995; Miami, Florida.

29. McFarlane WR, Dushay RA, Stastny P, et al. A comparison of two levels of family-aided assertive community treatment. *Psychiatric Services.* 1996 Jul;47(7):744-50.

30.   Leff J, Vaughn, C. Expressed emotion in families: Its significance for mental illness. New York: Guilford Press; 1985.

31.   Zhang M, Wang M, Li J, et al. Randomised-control trial of family intervention for 78 first-episode male schizophrenic patients. An 18-month study in Suzhou, Jiangsu. *Br J Psychiatry Suppl.* 1994 Aug(24):96-102.

32.   McFarlane WR, Lukens E, Link B, et al. Multiple-family groups and psychoeducation in the treatment of schizophrenia. *Arch Gen Psych.* 1995 Aug;52(8):679-87.

33.   Hogarty GE, Anderson CM, Reiss DJ, et al. Family psychoeducation, social skills training, and maintenance chemotherapy in the aftercare treatment of schizophrenia. II. Two-year effects of a controlled study on relapse and adjustment. Environmental-Personal Indicators in the Course of Schizophrenia (EPICS) Research Group. *Arch Gen Psych.* 1991 Apr;48(4):340-7.

34.   Sisson RW, Azrin NH. Family-member involvement to initiate and promote treatment of problem drinkers. *J Behav Ther Exp Psychiatry.* 1986 Mar;17(1):15-21.

35.   Hunt GM, Azrin NH. A community-reinforcement approach to alcoholism. *Behav Res Ther.* 1973 Feb;11(1):91-104.

36.   Azrin NH. Improvements in the community-reinforcement approach to alcoholism. *Behav Res Ther.* 1976;14(5):339-48.

37.   O'Farrell TJ, Cutter, H.S.G., Floyd, F.J. Evaluating behavioral marital therapy for male alcoholics: Effects on marital adjustment and communication from before to after treatment. *Behav Ther.* 1985;16:147-67.

38.   O'Farrell TJ. A behavioral marital therapy couples' group program for alcoholics and their spouses. In: O'Farrell TJ, ed Treating alcohol problems: Marital and family interventions. New York: Guilford Press; 1993:170-209.

39.   Riley AJ, Riley EJ. A controlled study to evaluate directed masturbation in the management of primary orgasmic failure in women. *Br J Psychiatry.* 1978 Nov;133:404-9.

40.   Ersner-Hershfield R, Kopel S. Group treatment of preorgasmic women: evaluation of partner involvement and spacing of sessions. *J Consult Clin Psychol.* 1979 Aug;47(4):750-9.

41.   Everaerd W, Dekker J. A comparison of sex therapy and communication therapy: couples complaining of orgasmic dysfunction. *J Sex Marital Ther.* 1981 Winter;7(4):278-89.

42.   Zimmer D. Does marital therapy enhance the effectiveness of treatment for sexual dysfunction? *J Sex Marital Ther.* 1987 Fall;13(3):193-209.

43.   Hurlbert DF. A comparative study using orgasm consistency training in the treatment of women reporting hypoactive sexual desire. *J Sex Marital Ther.* 1993 Spring;19(1):41-55.

44.   Jacobson NS, Dobson K, Fruzzetti AE, et al. Marital therapy as a treatment for depression. *J Consult Clin Psychol.* 1991 Aug;59(4):547-57.

45.   O'Leary KD, Beach SR. Marital therapy: a viable treatment for depression and marital discord. *Am J Psychiatry.* 1990 Feb;147(2):183-6.

46.   Mehta M. A comparative study of family-based and patient-based behavioural management in obsessive-compulsive disorder. *Br J Psychiatry.* 1990 Jul;157:133-5.

47.   Emmelkamp PM, de Lange I. Spouse involvement in the treatment of obsessive-compulsive patients. *Behav Res Ther.* 1983;21(4):341-6.

48.   Emmelkamp PM, de Haan E, Hoogduin CA. Marital adjustment and obsessive-compulsive disorder. *Br J Psychiatry.* 1990 Jan;156:55-60.

49.   Cobb JP, Mathews AM, Childs-Clarke A, et al. The spouse as co-therapist in the treatment of agoraphobia. *Br J Psychiatry.* 1984 Mar;144:282-7.

50.   Emmelkamp PM, van Dyck R, Bitter M, et al. Spouse-aided therapy with agoraphobics. *Br J Psychiatry.* 1992 Jan;160:51-6.

51.   Hand I, Angenendt, J., Fischer, M., Wilke, C. Exposure in-vivo with panic management for agoraphobia: Treatment rationale and long-term outcome. In: Hand I, Wittchen, H-U, ed Panic and phobias: Empirical evidence of theoretical models and long-term effects of behavioral treatments. Berlin: Springer-Verlag; 1986:104-27.

52.   Jannoun L, Munby, M., Catalan, J., Gelder, M. A home-based program for agoraphobia. *Behav Ther.* 1980;11:294-305.

53.   Oatley K, Hodgson D. Influence of husbands on the outcome of their agoraphobic wives' therapy. *Br J Psychiatry.* 1987 Mar;150:380-6.

54.   Barlow DH, O'Brien, G.T., Last, C.G. Couples treatment of agoraphobia. *Behav Ther.* 1984;15:41-58.

55.   Arnow BA, Taylor, C.B., Agras, W.S., Telch, M.J. Enhancing agoraphobia treatment outcomes by changing couple communication patterns. *Behav Ther.* 1985;16:452-67.

56.   Chambless DL, Ollendick TH. Empirically supported psychological interventions: controversies and evidence. *Annu Rev Psychol.* 2001;52:685-716.

57.   Nathan PE, Gorman, J.M. A Guide to Treaments That Work. New York: Oxford University Press; 1998.

58.   Kendall PC. Empirically supported psychological therapies. *J Consult Clin Psychol.* 1998 Feb;66(1):3-6.

59.   Association AP. Diagnostic and Statistical Manual, Third Edition DSM-III. Third ed; 1994.

60.   Association AP. Diagnostic and Statistical Manual, Fourth Edition, DSM-IV-TR. Fourth ed; 2000.

61.   Cochrane Handbook for Systematic Reviews of Interventions. In: Higgins JPT, Green S, eds. Version 5.1.0 (updated March 2011) ed: The Cochrane Collaboration; 2011.

62.   Owens DK, Lohr KN, Atkins D, et al. AHRQ series paper 5: grading the strength of a body of evidence when comparing medical interventions--agency for healthcare research and quality and the effective health-care program. *J Clin Epidemiol.* 2010 May;63(5):513-23.

63.   Kelley ML, Fals-Stewart W. Couples- versus individual-based therapy for alcohol and drug abuse: effects on children's psychosocial functioning. *J Consult Clin Psychol.* 2002 Apr;70(2):417-27.

64.   O'Farrell TJ, Murphy M, Alter J, et al. Brief family treatment intervention to promote continuing care among alcohol-dependent patients in inpatient detoxification: a randomized pilot study. *J Sub Abuse Treat.* 2008 Apr;34(3):363-9.

65.   O'Farrell TJ, Kleinke CL, Cutter HS. Sexual adjustment of male alcoholics: changes from before to after receiving alcoholism counseling with and without marital therapy. *Addict Behav.* 1998 May-Jun;23(3):419-25.

66.   Fals-Stewart W, Birchler GR, O'Farrell TJ. Behavioral couples therapy for male substance-abusing patients: effects on relationship adjustment and drug-using behavior. *J Consult Clin Psychol.* 1996 Oct;64(5):959-72.

67.   Fals-Stewart W, O'Farrell TJ, Birchler GR. Behavioral couples therapy for male methadone maintenance patients: effects on drug-using behavior and relationship adjustment. *Behav Ther.* 2001;32:391-411.

68.   Fals-Stewart W, O'Farrell TJ. Behavioral family counseling and naltrexone for male opioid-dependent patients. J *J Consult Clin Psychol.* 2003 Jun;71(3):432-42.

69.   Fals-Stewart W, Klostermann K, Yates BT, et al. Brief relationship therapy for alcoholism: a randomized clinical trial examining clinical efficacy and cost-effectiveness. *Psychol Addict Behav.* 2005 Dec;19(4):363-71.

70.   Jones HE, Tuten M, O'Grady KE. Treating the partners of opioid-dependent pregnant patients: feasibility and efficacy. *Am J Drug Alcohol Abuse.* 2011 May;37(3):170-8.

71.   Lam WK, Fals-Stewart W, Kelley ML. Parent training with behavioral couples therapy for fathers' alcohol abuse: effects on substance use, parental relationship, parenting, and CPS involvement. *Child Maltreat.* 2009 Aug;14(3):243-54.

72.   McCrady BS, Epstein EE, Hirsch LS. Issues in the implementation of a randomized clinical trial that includes Alcoholics Anonymous: studying AA-related behaviors during treatment. *J Stud Alcohol.* 1996 Nov;57(6):604-12.

73.   Walitzer KS, Dermen KH. Alcohol-focused spouse involvement and behavioral couples therapy: evaluation of enhancements to drinking reduction treatment for male problem drinkers. *J Consult Clin Psychol.* 2004 Dec;72(6):944-55.

74.   Fals-Stewart W, Birchler GR, Kelley ML. Learning sobriety together: A randomized clinical trial examining behavioral couples therapy with alcoholic female patients. *J Consult Clin Psychol.* 2006 Jun;74(3):579-91.

75.   McCrady BS, Epstein EE, Cook S, et al. A randomized trial of individual and couple behavioral alcohol treatment for women. *J Consult Clin Psychol.* 2009 Apr;77(2):243-56.

76.   Winters J, Fals-Stewart W, O'Farrell TJ, et al. Behavioral couples therapy for female substance-abusing patients: effects on substance use and relationship adjustment. *J Consult Clin Psychol.* 2002 Apr;70(2):344-55.

77.   Carroll KM, Ball SA, Nich C, et al. Targeting behavioral therapies to enhance naltrexone treatment of opioid dependence: efficacy of contingency management and significant other involvement. *Arch Gen Psychiatry.* 2001 Aug;58(8):755-61.

78.   Fals-Stewart W, Lam WK. Brief behavioral couples therapy for drug abuse: A randomized clinical trial examining clinical efficacy and cost-effectiveness. *Fam Syst Health.* 2008;26(4):377-92.

79.   Fals-Stewart W, O'Farrell TJ, Lam WKK. Behavioral couple therapy for gay and lesbian couples with alcohol use disorders. *J Subst Abuse Treat.* 2009 Dec;37(4):379-87.

80.   Kirby KC, Marlowe DB, Festinger DS, et al. Community reinforcement training for family and significant others of drug abusers: a unilateral intervention to increase treatment entry of drug users. *Drug Alcohol Depend.* 1999 Aug 2;56(1):85-96.

81.   Miller WR, Meyers RJ, Tonigan JS. Engaging the unmotivated in treatment for alcohol problems: a comparison of three strategies for intervention through family members. *J Consult Clin Psychol.* 1999 Oct;67(5):688-97.

82.   O'Farrell TJ, Murphy M, Alter J, et al. Behavioral family counseling for substance abuse: a treatment development pilot study. *Addict Behav.* 2010 Jan;35(1):1-6.

83.   Meyers RJ, Miller WR, Smith JE, et al. A randomized trial of two methods for engaging treatment-refusing drug users through concerned significant others. *J Consult Clin Psychol.* 2002 Oct;70(5):1182-5.

84.   Fals-Stewart W, O'Farrell TJ, Feehan M, et al. Behavioral couples therapy versus individual-based treatment for male substance-abusing patients. An evaluation of significant individual change and comparison of improvement rates. *J Substance Abuse Treat.* 2000 Apr;18(3):249-54.

85.   Fals-Stewart W, Kashdan TB, O'Farrell TJ, et al. Behavioral couples therapy for drug-abusing patients: effects on partner violence. *J Substance Abuse Treat.* 2002 Mar;22(2):87-96.

86.   McCrady BS, Epstein EE, Hirsch LS. Maintaining change after conjoint behavioral alcohol treatment for men: outcomes at 6 months. *Addiction.* 1999 Sep;94(9):1381-96.

87.   McCrady BS, Epstein EE, Kahler CW. Alcoholics anonymous and relapse prevention as maintenance strategies after conjoint behavioral alcohol treatment for men: 18-month outcomes. *J Consult Clin Psychol.* 2004 Oct;72(5):870-8.

88.   Sobell LC SM. Timeline followback user's guide. A calendar method for assessing alcohol and drug use. Toronto: Addiction Research Foundation; 1996.

89.   Miller IW, Solomon DA, Ryan CE, et al. Does adjunctive family therapy enhance recovery from bipolar I mood episodes? *J Affect Disord.* 2004 Nov 1;82(3):431-6.

90.   Miklowitz DJ, Simoneau TL, George EL, et al. Family-focused treatment of bipolar disorder: 1-year effects of a psychoeducational program in conjunction with pharmacotherapy. *Biol Psychiatry.* 2000 Sep 15;48(6):582-92.

91.   Rea MM, Tompson MC, Miklowitz DJ, et al. Family-focused treatment versus individual treatment for bipolar disorder: results of a randomized clinical trial. *J Consult Clin Psychol.* 2003 Jun;71(3):482-92.

92.   Miklowitz DJ, Otto MW, Frank E, et al. Psychosocial treatments for bipolar depression: a 1-year randomized trial from the Systematic Treatment Enhancement Program. *Arch Gen Psych.* 2007 Apr;64(4):419-26.

93.   Perlick DA, Miklowitz DJ, Lopez N, et al. Family-focused treatment for caregivers of patients with bipolar disorder. *Bipolar Disord.* 2010 Sep;12(6):627-37.

94.   Clarkin JF, Carpenter D, Hull J, et al. Effects of psychoeducational intervention for married patients with bipolar disorder and their spouses. *Psych Services.* 1998 Apr;49(4):531-3.

95.   Miklowitz DJ, Otto MW, Frank E, et al. Intensive psychosocial intervention enhances functioning in patients with bipolar depression: results from a 9-month randomized controlled trial. *Am Journal Psych.* 2007 Sep;164(9):1340-7.

96.   Miklowitz DJ, Thomson, M.C. Family variables and interventions in schizophrenia. In: Sholevar GP, Schwoeri, L.D. , ed Textbook of marital and family therapy. Washington D.C.: American Psychiatric Publishing, Inc.; 2003.

97.   Solomon DA, Keitner GI, Ryan CE, et al. Preventing recurrence of bipolar I mood episodes and hospitalizations: family psychotherapy plus pharmacotherapy versus pharmacotherapy alone. *Bipolar Disord.* 2008 Nov;10(7):798-805.

98.   Miller IW, Keitner GI, Ryan CE, et al. Family treatment for bipolar disorder: family impairment by treatment interactions. *J Clin Psych.* 2008 May;69(5):732-40.

99.   Mueser KT, Glynn SM, Cather C, et al. Family intervention for co-occurring substance use and severe psychiatric disorders: participant characteristics and correlates of initial engagement and more extended exposure in a randomized controlled trial. *Addict Behav.* 2009 Oct;34(10):867-77.

100. Mueser KT, Glynn SM, Cather C, et al. A randomized controlled trial of family intervention for co-occurring substance use and severe psychiatric disorders. *Schizophr Bull*. 2012; In Press.

101. Dyck DG, Short RA, Hendryx MS, et al. Management of negative symptoms among patients with schizophrenia attending multiple-family groups. *Psychiatr Serv*. 2000 Apr;51(4):513-9.

102. Dyck DG, Hendryx MS, Short RA, et al. Service use among patients with schizophrenia in psychoeducational multiple-family group treatment. *Psychiatr Serv*. 2002 Jun;53(6):749-54.

103. McDonell MG, Short RA, Hazel NA, et al. Multiple-family group treatment of outpatients with schizophrenia: impact on service utilization. *Fam Process*. 2006 Sep;45(3):359-73.

104. Mueser KT, Sengupta A, Schooler NR, et al. Family treatment and medication dosage reduction in schizophrenia: effects on patient social functioning, family attitudes, and burden. *J Consult Clin Psychol*. 2001 Feb;69(1):3-12.

105. Weine S, Kulauzovic Y, Klebic A, et al. Evaluating a multiple-family group access intervention for refugees with PTSD. *J Marital Fam Ther*. 2008 Apr;34(2):149-64.

106. Aubin S, Heiman JR, Berger RE, et al. Comparing Sildenafil alone vs. Sildenafil plus brief couple sex therapy on erectile dysfunction and couples' sexual and marital quality of life: a pilot study. *J Sex Marital Ther*. 2009;35(2):122-43.

107. Banner LL, Anderson RU. Integrated sildenafil and cognitive-behavior sex therapy for psychogenic erectile dysfunction: a pilot study. *J Sex Med*. 2007 Jul;4(4 Pt 2):1117-25.

108. Rosen RC, Riley A, Wagner G, et al. The international index of erectile function (IIEF): a multidimensional scale for assessment of erectile dysfunction. *Urology*. 1997 Jun;49(6):822-30.

109. Spanier GB. Effects of behavioral marital therapy: a meta-analysis of randomized controlled trials. *J Consult Clin Psychol*. 1976;38:15-28.

110. Schaefer MT, Olson, D.H. Assessing intimacy: the pair inventory. *J Marital Fam Ther*. 1980;7:47-60.

111. Althof SE, Corty EW, Levine SB, et al. EDITS: development of questionnaires for evaluating satisfaction with treatments for erectile dysfunction. *Urology*. 1999 Apr;53(4):793-9.

112. Beck AT, Ward CH, Mendelson M, et al. An inventory for measuring depression. *Arch Gen Psych*. 1961 Jun;4:561-71.

113. Beck AT, Epstein N, Brown G, et al. An inventory for measuring clinical anxiety: psychometric properties. *J Consult Clin Psychol*. 1988 Dec;56(6):893-7.

114.   Cohen S, O'Leary KD, Foran H. A randomized clinical trial of a brief, problem-focused couple therapy for depression. *Behav Ther.* 2010 Dec;41(4):433-46.

115.   Gorin AA, Le Grange D, Stone AA. Effectiveness of spouse involvement in cognitive behavioral therapy for binge eating disorder. *Intern J Eat Disord.* 2003 May;33(4):421-33.

116.   Fairburn CG, Beglin SJ. The evaluation of a new instrument for detecting eating disorders in community samples. Oxford University; 1991.

117.   Fairburn CG, Beglin SJ. Assessment of eating disorders: interview or self-report questionnaire? *Intern J Eat Disord.* 1994 Dec;16(4):363-70.

118.   McBride CM, Baucom DH, Peterson BL, et al. Prenatal and postpartum smoking abstinence a partner-assisted approach. *Am J of Prevent Med.* 2004 Oct;27(3):232-8.

119.   Miller IW, Bishop S, Norman WH, et al. The Modified Hamilton Rating Scale for Depression: reliability and validity. *Psychiatry Res.* 1985 Feb;14(2):131-42.

120.   Beck AT, Steer RA, Brown GK. Beck Depression Inventory - Manual 2nd ed. San Antonio, TX: The Psychological Corporation; 1996.

121.   Christensen A, Atkins DC, Berns S, et al. Traditional versus integrative behavioral couple therapy for significantly and chronically distressed married couples. *J Consult Clin Psychol.* 2004 Apr;72(2):176-91.

122.   Fals-Stewart Felony Complaint. http://www.ag.ny.gov/media_center/2010/feb/feb16a_10.html OR http://www.wivb.com/dpp/search/Fals-Stewart-felony-complaint. Accessed on January 2012.

123.   Powers MB, Vedel E, Emmelkamp PM. Behavioral couples therapy (BCT) for alcohol and drug use disorders: a meta-analysis. *Clin Psychol Rev.* 2008 Jul;28(6):952-62.

124.   Justo LP, Soares BG, Calil HM. Family interventions for bipolar disorder. Cochrane Database Syst Rev. 2007(4):CD005167.

125.   Herz MI, Lamberti JS, Mintz J, et al. A program for relapse prevention in schizophrenia: a controlled study. *Arch Gen Psych.* 2000 Mar;57(3):277-83.

126.   Pharoah F, Mari J, Rathbone J, et al. Family intervention for schizophrenia. Cochrane Database Syst Rev. 2010(12):CD000088.

127.   Lehman AF, Steinwachs DM. Translating research into practice: the Schizophrenia Patient Outcomes Research Team (PORT) treatment recommendations. *Schizophr Bull.* 1998;24(1):1-10.

128.   Lehman AF, Kreyenbuhl J, Buchanan RW, et al. The Schizophrenia Patient Outcomes Research Team (PORT): updated treatment recommendations 2003. *Schizophr Bull.* 2004;30(2):193-217.

129. Dixon LB, Dickerson F, Bellack AS, et al. The 2009 schizophrenia PORT psychosocial treatment recommendations and summary statements. *Schizophr Bull.* 2010 Jan;36(1):48-70.

130. Glynn SM, Cohen AN, Niv N. New challenges in family interventions for schizophrenia. *Expert Rev Neurother.* 2007 Jan;7(1):33-43.

131. Pilling S, Bebbington P, Kuipers E, et al. Psychological treatments in schizophrenia: I. Meta-analysis of family intervention and cognitive behaviour therapy. *Psychol Med.* 2002 Jul;32(5):763-82.

132. Pitschel-Walz G, Leucht S, Bauml J, et al. The effect of family interventions on relapse and rehospitalization in schizophrenia--a meta-analysis. *Schizophr Bull.* 2001;27(1):73-92.

133. Hornung WP, Feldmann R, Klingberg S, et al. Long-term effects of a psychoeducational psychotherapeutic intervention for schizophrenic outpatients and their key-persons--results of a five-year follow-up. *Eur Arch Psychiatry Clin Neurosci.* 1999;249(3):162-7.

134. Tarrier N, Barrowclough C, Porceddu K, et al. The Salford Family Intervention Project: relapse rates of schizophrenia at five and eight years. *Br J Psychiatry.* 1994 Dec;165(6):829-32.

135. Barbato A, D'Avanzo B. Marital therapy for depression. Cochrane Database Syst Rev. 2006(2):CD004188.

136. Henken HT, Huibers MJ, Churchill R, et al. Family therapy for depression. Cochrane Database Syst Rev. 2007(3):CD006728.

137. Foley SH, Rounsaville BJ, Weissman MM, et al. Individual versus conjoint interpersonal therapy for depressed patients with marital disputes. *Int J Family Psychiatry.* 1989;10:29-42.

138. Rosenberg M. Society and the adolescent self-image. Princeton, NJ: Princeton University Press; 1965.

139. Monson CM, Fredman SJ, Adair KC, et al. Cognitive-behavioral conjoint therapy for PTSD: pilot results from a community sample. *J Trauma Stress.* 2011 Feb;24(1):97-101.

140. Glynn SM, Dixon LB, Cohen A, et al. The Family Member Provider Outreach program. Psychiatric Services. 2008 Aug;59(8):934.

141. Sayers SL. Coaching into care: a pilot program to enhance outreach to military Veterans and their family members. VA Mental Health Annual Conference; 2011 August 23; Baltimore, Maryland.

142. Sherman MD, Fischer, E.P., Sorocco, K., McFarlane, W.R. Adapting the Multifamily Group Model to the Veterans Affairs system: The REACH Program. Research and Practice. 2009;40:593-600.

APPENDIX A. SEARCH STRATEGIES

Database: Ovid MEDLINE(R)
Search Strategy:
----

1   exp family/
2   couples.mp.
3   exp home nursing/
4   (grandparent: or grandmother: or grandfather:).mp.
5   exp legal guardians/
6   or/1-5
7   couples therapy/ or family therapy/ or marital therapy/
8   6 or 7
9   exp Infertility/ or exp Infertility, Male/ or exp Infertility, Female/ or exp Fertilization in Vitro/ or exp Reproductive Techniques, Assisted/ or exp Insemination, Artificial/
10   8 not 9
11   limit 10 to (english language and yr="1980 -Current")
12   limit 11 to ("newborn infant (birth to 1 month)" or "infant (1 to 23 months)" or "preschool child (2 to 5 years)" or "child (6 to 12 years)")
13   11 not 12
14   limit 13 to meta analysis
15   (systematic adj review:).mp.
16   13 and 15
17   14 or 16
18   limit 13 to randomized controlled trial

Database: PsycINFO
Search Strategy:
----

1   exp family/ or exp family members/ or exp spouses/ or exp couples/
2   exp caregivers/ or exp stepparents/ or exp siblings/ or caretaker:.mp.
3   exp grandparents/ or legal guardian:.mp.
4   or/1-3
5   couples therapy/ or family therapy/ or marital therapy/
6   4 or 5
7   exp Infertility/ or exp Reproductive Technology/
8   6 not 7
9   limit 8 to (english language and yr="1980 -Current")
10   limit 9 to 100 childhood <birth to age 12 yrs>
11   9 not 10
12   meta analysis/ or (systematic adj review:).mp.
13   11 and 12
14   (randomized or rct).mp.
15   11 and 14

APPENDIX B. CRITERIA USED IN QUALITY ASSESSMENT[62]

Risk of bias	Internal validity: study design and the quality of individual studies included in the review. Study design limitations may bias the estimates of treatment effect (such as lack of allocation concealment, or lack of blinding). Other areas for potential bias include stopping early for benefit and selective outcome reporting.
Consistency	The effect sizes from the included studies are similar and have the same direction of effect (positive or negative).
Directness	Interventions are directly related to health outcomes. For CERs, head-to-head comparisons are made. Indirectness is suspected if surrogate or intermediate outcomes are used instead of health outcomes. For CERs, indirectness is also suspected if more than one body of evidence is needed to link interventions, ad in the das with placebo controlled trials. Directness also includes applicability and relevance of the included studies to the VA population or to specific subpopulations within the VA. Applicability may also include settings (e.g., primary care vs. specialty care) and physician experience.
Precision	The degree of certainty surrounding an estimate of effect for each outcome of interest. Uncertainty of effect does not allow for a clinically useful conclusion, and is unable to rule out an important benefit or harm.
Risk of publication bias	Publication bias can result in an overestimate of effect. Publication bias is suspected if evidence is derived from a small number of commercially funded trials with small sample sizes and a small number of event.

APPENDIX C. PEER REVIEW COMMENTS/AUTHOR RESPONSES

REVIEWER COMMENT	RESPONSE
1. Are the objectives, scope, and methods for this review clearly described?	
Yes. On page 9 Introduction PL 110-387 signed in Oct 2008 added Marriage and Family Counseling and dropped the contingency on non-service connected Veterans. The May 2010 PL just added primary caregivers to eligible individuals	We have revised this part of the introduction to clarify that PL 110-387 expanded coverage and that PL 111 added primary caregivers to eligible folks.
Yes	
No. There is a good measure of ambiguity about the goals and scope of this review. This ambiguity is generated from the following factors: 1) The background of the review highlights the legislation that expands the services to family members (the 2010 Caregiver legislation, but also applies to 2008 legislation that provides for marriage counseling as a VA service). I believe it was fair to say that the primary impetus for this legislation was the national pressure on VA to provide expanded services to family members, in reference to greater mental health needs of family members, and the impact that both medical and mental health issues of Veterans have on families. The focus of the review, however, is on the treatment of individual disorders, and not on outcomes of family members as individuals or the marital/family unit. This may create a disconnect in the reader's mind about the rationale for the review. The rationale for the change in services, however, does include that family members constitute important members of the treatment team. This is a key part to the rationale that a review is needed to examine the evidence that family member involvement does improve outcomes. A more nuanced and spelled out rationale would help set the reader's expectations a bit better. 2) The definitions of different types treatments defined by Baucom et al. were described as part of the background, but no systematic differentiations regarding these classifications of how family members are involved in treatment were made in this review (only brief occasional mentions). Thus, the review is not really a proper follow-up to Baucom et al. One consequence of this is that the review did not place marital distress or family dysfunction as clinical syndromes, unlike Baucom et al., where the authors treated those outcomes as treatable entities in and of themselves. This would be expected given the background/introduction of the review. Although the Limitations section discuss this point, it should be highlighted in the beginning of the review 3) There was very little emphasis was made on relationship distress as a moderator in the review, with only a mention in the sections on couples therapy interventions for ED and also for depression. This is potentially highly relevant in that findings in the pre-1995 period of time prior was that couples therapy for depression may not be effective, and perhaps ill-advised in couples who do not consider themselves maritally distressed, only with a partner with depression. This finding may be relevant for other disorders, and although few studies have addressed the issue in their designs, it should be part of the dialogue from the beginning of the review and part of the discussion and recommendations for future research. 4) Behavioral Couples Therapy (BCT) versions as treatments for substance abuse and alcohol use disorders were referenced often in the review with no qualifier that these are variants of BCT specifically designed to treat these disorders, except in the more detailed descriptions of the Appendices (which may not get read by many readers). They include procedures never used in standard BCT or expanded Integrative Behavioral Couples Therapy (IBCT) designed to treat marital distress. IBCT being disseminated throughout VA currently would very likely not be effective for substance abuse or alcohol use disorders. This ambiguity could be very misleading to readers unfamiliar with the literature.	1) We have clarified in the introduction the rationale for the review. 2) We have clarified the scope of the review in the introduction and highlighted the review is not intended as a strict update to Baucom and colleagues' review. 3) We agree this is an important issue. We have highlighted throughout the results section when this information is available and included a discussion of findings relevant to this question in the discussion. 4) Thank you for your suggestion. We have clarified this in the results section for substance use disorders and refer to BCT as a 'disorder specific couple/family treatment' in additional places for clarity.
Yes. All methods are clearly described. Methodology is rigorous and effectively implemented. Outcomes of interest were well selected and decisions to include and exclude studies seem sensible given the intent to extrapolate findings to U.S. Veteran populations.	Thank you.
Yes. Objectives, scope and methods are clearly articulated and findings are clearly summarized in multiple formats. Tables which include main findings are particularly facilitative (e.g., Table 8).	Thank you.

REVIEWER COMMENT	RESPONSE
Yes	
Yes	
2. Is there any indication of bias in our synthesis of the evidence?	
No	
No	
No	
No. There is no indication of bias.	
No	
Although I understand ESP's rationale, I believe that given the undeveloped nature of this literature, limiting the review only to RCTs may have been overly limiting to understand the relevant clinical issues, trends, or promising practices.	We certainly agree with the need to disseminate information on those promising interventions underdevelopment that are currently or soon to be subjected to more rigorous RCTs to evaluate their efficacy. Given the size of this review as it currently stands, limited to RCTs, it was beyond the scope of the project to expand our search to other study designs (e.g., open trials; quasi-experiments). We have added this to the limitation section.
3. Are there any published or unpublished studies that we may have overlooked?	
Please refer to reviews by Shirley Glynn and Lisa Dixon	These reviews have both been integrated into the discussion section specific to findings for schizophrenia.
No	
No	
No. I am not aware of studies that have been overlooked.	
No. Review appears extensive and literature search process is clearly displayed in Figure 2.	Thank you.
I was surprised to see that none of Candice Monson's work on couples therapy for PTSD was included. I don't have the studies in front of me, so it may be that is because they were not RCTs. If so, see my comment above.	You are correct. Dr. Monson's currently published work did not meet our inclusion criteria (i.e., currently she has no published RCTs). We referenced this work in our limitations.
4. Please write any additional suggestions or comments below. If applicable, please indicate the page and line numbers from the draft report.	
Page 5 and 62 Recommendation for Future Research – PL lists eligible individuals for family services and that does not include close friends or intimate partner unless they are residing with the Veteran. Page 5 and 62 Family Services and Caregiver Services are administered from two different Program Offices and are conceptualized as different – perhaps introducing caregivers brings in a different topic?	We have revised the introduction to better describe the two laws that have expanded services. In this explanation we also describe that PL 111-163 is only for a select group of family members. We have also highlighted the issue of who is eligible for these services in the discussion.
Overall, the review was comprehensive and inclusive, providing a critical snapshot of the state of the evidence for family-involved psychosocial treatments for mental health conditions of relevance to Veterans.	Thank you.

REVIEWER COMMENT	RESPONSE
There was very little integration of the findings of this review with the findings from Baucom et al. (1998). Combining the findings from this review with the previous is important since many interventions showing strong evidence of effectiveness (e.g., Family Psychoeducation for schizophrenia spectrum disorders), have not been as extensively examined in the period from 1995 forward. As stated above, this review did not continue with the classification of types of family involvement, which significantly weakens our understanding of the actual interventions being examined.	We have taken better care to highlight the specific interventions that are reviewed and which category of intervention they fall under throughout the document (results and discussion section).
There was only a brief final mention in the recommendations of comorbidity as a factor examined in very few of the studies. This issue should be mentioned earlier and in greater detail since comorbidity is the norm for Veterans and indeed many older adults, Veterans or not. This recommendation should be front and center.	We have included a more explicit review of the types of co-occurring problems that were inclusion and exclusion criteria in the trials reviewed. We have also expanded the discussion of this issue in our future research section.
The term "slower rate of relapse" was used consistently in the section on family involved treatments of substance and alcohol abuse. I believe the authors mean "lower rate of relapse" since most or all of the findings are rates at various endpoints and do not describe a slope or growth curve of relapse across time.	Following the review of this draft, we conducted pooled analyses of the BCT studies which allowed us to draw more definitive conclusions about the efficacy of BCT compared to individual treatment. See results section.
On page 10, the authors state "Most prior reviews have focused on specific conditions (i.e., depression or substance use disorders), limiting the ability of past work to generalize to family-involved mental health care more broadly." It is unclear what "more broadly" means: Comorbidity? Special populations? Non-symptom outcomes?	We have clarified this in the Introduction
On page 33, the authors state "For studies of AUD, all trials report better outcomes for BCT or BMT than IBT post-treatment and all follow-up time points, but many of these differences were not statistically significant." The authors should allow that only the statistically significant findings are actually reportable as "better outcomes."	We have removed discussion of non-significant differences between conditions.
On page 34, the authors discussion the controversy over Fals-Stewart's findings very economically and fairly. They need to provide a citation for the public charges of fabrication and of his death, a reputable news source, for example (a Google search will yield one fairly quickly).	We have included a citation of both the NY State Attorney General's press release and a copy of the felony complaint filed by the AG's office.
Page 39, last line "(Reference)" appears in the text when it likely [should list the author/year citation].	Corrected.
On page 58, the authors refer to Table XX, when the next table is 15.	Corrected.
"Baucom (1998)" many times was cited when the correct citation is Baucom et al. (1998).	Corrected.
The evidence base bearing on the questions of interest was, unfortunately, very limited. The studies reviewed covered a wide range of interventions but the number of trials for the same interventions was very few. This means that although there were a number of promising findings from single trials, but evidence in these cases was of low quality, given lack of replication. One finding with moderate strength of evidence, that behavioral couples therapy can slow the rate of relapse for substance abuse disorders, appears to overstate the impact of the intervention, given that findings related to more important outcomes such as abstinence rates were mixed. In the Conclusions section starting on page 60, it is stated that Behavioral Couples Therapy is superior to individual therapy for substance abuse disorders, but this conclusion does not seem warranted given the mixed findings across studies. Behavioral Family Therapy did seem to have a consistently positive effect on family functioning outcomes across all four studies that reported outcomes in this domain; possibly, this finding should be emphasized more in the report. Given the lack of the research base, it may be worth expanding the Future Research section; potentially this report can prompt more methodologically strong research on family interventions within VA research organizations.	Regarding the strength of evidence of BCT, since the initial peer review, we have conducted pooled analyses comparing BCT to individual treatment in improving rates of abstinence and improving family adjustment. These findings are more supportive of BCT then our previous narrative review of the number of studies finding significant versus non-significant differences.

REVIEWER COMMENT	RESPONSE
1. A paragraph (pg. 34) is included regarding work by Fals-Stewart – it may be helpful to provide this background information prior to presenting data regarding studies (Fals-Stewart – 1996, 2002, 2003 etc...)	Thank you for the suggestion. This has been done.
2. Table 15 – may be useful to add borders (gridlines) to facilitate ease of reading.	Done.
3. Cost related outcomes did not appear to be a focus of studies presented. Wonder about this as an outcome for future studies (particularly within VA), and whether it would be useful to include discussion regarding this in the Recommendations for Future Research.	Thank you for your suggestion. We have addressed this in Future Research.
4. Several small typos noted (e.g., page 34 line 2 – Fals-Stewart, 1996, 200, 2002...) – also Higgins 2009 reference appears to be missing from list (this reviewer was interested in this publication so it was looked for all references were not checked).	Thank you for your attention to detail. We have attended closely to these issues in the final report draft.
The exclusive focus on RCT's and patient outcomes is a limitation. Not clear why previous reviews such as meta-analyses were not considered. Numerous sophisticated quantitative reviews have been published.	Our literature search identified systematic reviews and meta-analyses in additions to RCTs. Several recent reviews are mentioned in the report. We also looked at reference lists of recent reviews to identify primary studies our literature search might have missed. We have taken care to be more explicit in integrating these reviews into our results discussion for each set of mental health conditions reviewed.
It is not clear to me what "drug treatment" or "no treatment" means in the comparison condition for KQ1. Does that mean the absence of any alternative active treatment? The reason for asking is that drug treatment would typically come with some kind of support, and that might be mentioned.	We were interested in reviewing the evidence of the efficacy of family involved interventions (compared to no intervention or non-psychosocial interventions), as well as the degree to which family involved interventions are superior to an alternative individually-focused or family involved intervention (i.e., specificity). The 'medication only' conditions involve interventions that were solely pharmacological including medication and monitoring of medication use, but where the medication condition was not intended as a psychosocial treatment or psychotherapy. This has been clarified in the introduction and the wording of the Key Questions. We have also clarified what additional provider contact was included in intervention conditions we considered 'medication only'
I am not sure what this means: "Overall, the studies reviewed appeared to favor comparisons between a family-intervention and an active treatment, limiting our conclusions for this key question. (page 3)." Does that mean that the review didn't consider many of the landmark studies? The review's findings regarding schizophrenia are puzzling given the extensive number of studies and meta-analyses supporting the effectiveness of family psychoeducation.	This is due to the scope of our review. We did not include non-US studies or studies published prior to 1996. However, we highlighted the work prior to our review that established the efficacy of these treatments in Table 1 and discussed our findings within the context of other reviews throughout the document in the executive summary, results, and discussion sections
One issue for consideration is the "lumping" vs "splitting" issue. This review splits studies by diagnosis. However, in practice family interventions are not narrowly offered, and they share techniques. Miklowitz's FFT is similar to FPE for schizophrenia; an alternative way to understand the literature is across diagnoses.	We have addressed this in the limitations section.
The name of the office is Office of Mental Health Services, not just Office of Mental Health	This has been corrected. Thank you.
I appreciated that in the summary of areas for future research in two areas in the paper, the role of nontraditional family constellations was highlighted. In the substance use disorder section, I appreciated that the results were broken into different types of effectiveness re: initiation, attendance, and adherence. On pg 34, although it is a touchy subject, I think it is a good thing that the issues around the work of Drs. Fals-Stewart are addressed.	Thank you for your positive feedback.

REVIEWER COMMENT	RESPONSE
5. Are there any clinical performance measures, programs, quality improvement measures, patient care services, or conferences that will be directly affected by this report? If so, please provide detail.	Thank you – we will share these suggestions with the people responsible for dissemination of the report.
Findings should be of direct relevance to the mission of the VA's Family Services Program	
Every major VA medical center will be affected by this report in that the effectiveness of family involved services, especially in reducing relapse for substance abuse and alcohol disorders	
The report appears to indicate that evidence for most couples and family-based interventions is largely insufficient to warrant widespread implementation within VHA. The intervention that does appear to be supported by consistent evidence, CRAFT, is not very well suited to implementation within VHA because it is delivered by a mental health professional to a family member whose loved on is not seeking treatment. It may have important training implications for community-based providers and possibly staff members of Vet Centers. The other finding with moderate strength of evidence, that behavioral couples therapy can slow the rate of relapse for substance abuse disorders, is not very impressive given the lack of impact of this intervention on arguably more important outcomes such as abstinence rates.	Regarding the strength of evidence of BCT, since the initial peer review, we have conducted pooled analyses comparing BCT to individual treatment in improving rates of abstinence and improving family adjustment. These findings are more supportive of BCT then our previous narrative review of the number of studies finding significant versus non-significant differences.
Would expect that findings would have implications in terms of future VA research funding. May also have implications for current evidence-based treatment rollouts.	
The Office of Mental Health Operations should review to determine if there is any relevance of the information in this report to their Mental Health Information System, which monitors a variety of practices in the field.	
6. Please provide any recommendations on how this report can be revised to more directly address or assist implementation needs.	
I am still struggling with the bottom line – probably effective – won't cause harm? How does the research supporting family interventions compare to the research supporting other interventions currently being used in the VA?	To adequately address how family interventions compare to the population of interventions currently provided by the VA, a systematic review of individually-oriented interventions would be required. This is beyond the scope of the review.

However, we have taken care to better highlight the primary take home points in the executive summary and in our final discussion section. We have included additional pooled analyses of the BCT studies comparing BCT to individual therapy, which provide greater clarity to our conclusions regarding the comparative effectiveness of BCT to individual therapy. |
A potential conclusion from the findings of the report is that the state-of-the-science is that more efficacy and effectiveness research is needed on Veteran-focused family-involved psychosocial treatments to inform dissemination and implementation.	We agree and have highlighted these issues in the discussion section.
The review's scope would have to be expanded significantly to discuss effective implementation strategies, but this would indeed be highly valuable for VA.	We agree that identifying and evaluating effective implementation strategies would be valuable; however, it is outside the scope of this report.
As mentioned above, comorbidity is the rule, rather than the exception, and very few studies address comorbidity. Clinicians have very little guidance as to how to proceed in these circumstances. A brief (and very common) clinical scenario that illustrates the problem: A 34 yo Veteran with PTSD, depression, and TBI violently pushes his wife after weeks of arguments over money, his at-risk alcohol use, and discipline of their children. He recently entered VA care and is open to treatment. Possible interventions include individual alcohol treatment, BCT for alcohol abuse, IBCT, anger management, and cognitive rehabilitation. The couple is asking for couples counseling for their arguing because they realize it upsets their 4 yo son. The Veteran is unconvinced he has a drinking problem.	See above.

REVIEWER COMMENT	RESPONSE
It may be helpful if the authors would recommend research priorities related to the area. Several interventions are promising, but research is very limited and trials with Veterans are lacking. A set of recommendations about which interventions might be prioritized for investigation within VHA research mechanisms might be helpful.	We have included a more expansive future research section and address these issues there.
I think the report could benefit from greater consideration of how family interventions might be used in clinical care and the gap between the research parameters and what is found clinically.	We have included a more direct discussion of the need for studies examining patients with multiple problems (e.g., substance use, TBI, intimate partner violence) in the Future Research section.
See my comments in response to question #3 and #4. I am afraid that the super rigorous limitation of the review to just RCTs may cut off possibilities for identifying promising practices for pilot projects in the field.	See above.

APPENDIX D. EVIDENCE TABLES

Table 1. Study Descriptive Information – Substance Abuse Studies

Study, Year Funding Source	Sample Characteristics	Inclusion/Exclusion Criteria	Treatment Groups	Intervention Characteristics	Outcomes Assessed	Quality
Carroll, 2001[77] Government	N = 127 randomized N = 127 data analysis Gender: 76% male Age: 32.4 years Race/ethnicity: African American 14.4% Hispanic 7% White 77% Marital Status: Single/divorced 65% Education: ≥High school 81% Veterans: NR *Recruitment Method* Completed outpatient detoxification for opioids and seeking tx for opioid dependence *Family Characteristics:* None reported	MH Condition: Substance use Assessed by: DSM clinical interview SO: non-abusing parent, spouse, child, sibling or close friend Inclusion: Seeking tx for opioid dependence Exclusions: Significant medical condition that would contraindicate Naltrexone; did not have significant other; met DSM criteria for schizophrenia or bipolar or was in substance use treatment within past 3 months	1) SO relationship counseling added to standard tx (Naltrexone) with voucher-based contingency management (CM) N=48 2) Standard tx (Naltrexone) with voucher-based contingency management N=35 3) Standard tx (receive Naltrexone) only n=44 *Treatment adherence* 5 did not initiate treatment 10 removed from tx protocol (not clear from which groups they dropped)	Format: Standard tx or contingency management or contingency management plus 6 sessions of reciprocal relationship counseling Manualized: Yes Session: 6 sessions Approach: All participants in all three groups were randomized to receive Naltrexone in addition to cognitive behavioral group therapy. One group was offered reciprocal relationship counseling in addition to group therapy and vouchers redeemable for goods and services contingent on taking Naltrexone and drug-free urine screens (contingency management). A second group received group therapy, Naltrexone and contingency management. The third group received group therapy and Naltrexone only.	Patient Outcomes Symptom Improvement a. Drug free urine b. Opiate free urine c. Cocaine free urine d. % of drug free urine e. PDA opioids f. PDA cocaine g. Maximum PDA Family Outcomes: Psychosocial functioning (including family functioning): a. ASI Intermediate Outcomes: Attendance: a. weeks in treatment Adherence: a. # Naltrexone doses	Allocation concealment: unclear Blinding: treating clinicians and outcome assessors Intention to treat analysis: yes Withdrawals adequately described: yes Treatment integrity: Naltrexone adherence monitored by urine screens. No report of tx integrity for CM or SO sessions. **Study Quality: Good**

Family Involved Psychosocial Treatments for Adult Mental Health Conditions: A Review of the Evidence

Evidence-based Synthesis Program

Study, Year Funding Source	Sample Characteristics	Inclusion/Exclusion Criteria	Treatment Groups	Intervention Characteristics	Outcomes Assessed	Quality
Fals-Stewart, 1996[66] Government	N = 80 randomized N = 80 data analysis Gender: 100% male (husbands) Age: 34.1 years Race/ethnicity: White 67% Black American 10% Hispanic 3% Marital Status: Married 100% Education (mean years/SD): 11.9(2.4) Veterans: NR *Recruitment Method* Men entering outpatient substance use tx in community based clinics were asked to participate *Family Characteristics:* Spouse/partner Gender: 100% female Age (mean): 33.0 Race/ethnicity: White 69% Black 8% Hispanic 3% Education (mean yrs/SD): 11.7 (2.3)	MH Condition: Substance use Assessed by: Diagnostic interview SO: wives Inclusions: Husband: between 20 and 60; married at least 1 year or in stable relationship for 2; met abuse or dependence criteria for at least one psychoactive substance use, primary drug not alcohol; medical clearance for tx; refrain from using; refrain from additional treatment except self help meetings; Exclusions: wife met DSM criteria for substance use; husband or wife had delusional disorder; husband or wife in methadone program and looking for adjunctive outpatient support	1) Behavioral couple therapy (BCT) N=40 2) Individual treatment - behavioral therapy for husbands N=40	1) Format: Couple Manualized: Yes Sessions: 56 BCT Approach: Treatment included IBT through group (once weekly) and individual counseling (once weekly) plus BCT through one conjoint (once weekly) 2) Format: Individual Manualized: Yes Sessions: 56 Approach: Cognitive-Behavioral Treatment included group (once weekly) and individual counseling (twice weekly)	Patient Outcomes Symptom Improvement a. Urine screens b. PDA (alcohol and drugs) c. Blood alcohol Intermediate Outcomes: Attendance: a. Sessions attended Satisfaction with care a. CSQ-8 Family Outcomes: Couple functioning: a. MAT b. ACQ c. % of days separated Conflict: a. Response to conflict	Allocation concealment: no Blinding: no Intention to treat analysis: no Withdrawals adequately described: yes Treatment integrity: PI supervised 1 hr week and reviewed progress notes **Study Quality: Poor**
Fals-Stewart, 2000[84]	Same as Fals-Stewart 1996	Same as Fals-Stewart 1996	Same as Fals-Stewart 1996	Same as Fals-Stewart 1996	Patient Outcomes Symptom Improvement a. PDA Family Outcomes: Couple functioning: a. Locke Wallace Marital adjustment test (MAT)	Same as Fals-Stewart 1996

109

Family Involved Psychosocial Treatments for Adult Mental Health Conditions: A Review of the Evidence

Study, Year Funding Source	Sample Characteristics	Inclusion/Exclusion Criteria	Treatment Groups	Intervention Characteristics	Outcomes Assessed	Quality
Fals-Stewart, 2002[85]	Same as Fals-Stewart 1996	Same as Fals-Stewart 1996	Same as Fals-Stewart 1996	Same as Fals-Stewart 1996	Patient Outcomes Symptom Improvement a. % of days of alcohol or drug use Family Outcomes: Couple functioning: a. MAT Intimate Partner Violence: a. CTS – male to female	Same as Fals-Stewart 1996
Fals-Stewart, 2001[67] Government	N = 43 randomized N = 36 data analysis Gender: 100% male Age: 38.1 (7.5) years Race/ethnicity: White 50 % Black 42% Hispanic 8% Marital Status: Married or cohabitating 100% Education (mean years): 12.0 (2.0) Veterans: NR_ *Recruitment Method* Subjects recruited from patients entering substance abuse treatment at one of two community based methadone maintenance clinics. *Family Characteristics:* 100% female wives or significant others Age: 36.0 (7.3) years Race/ethnicity: White 56 % Black 39% Hispanic 5% Education (mean years): 12.2 (2.3)	MH Condition: Abuse or dependence for a psychoactive substance use disorder (intravenous opiate users) Assessed by: DSM-III-R interview SO: Inclusion: male; age 21-60 years; married ≥1 year or living with significant other ≥2 years; medical clearance to engage in methadone maintenance treatment; refrain from seeking other substance abuse treatment except for self help meetings during duration of treatment (unless recommended by primary therapist) Exclusions: if female partner met DSM-III-R criteria for psycho-active substance use disorder in last six months; either partner met DSM-III-R criteria for organic mental, paranoid, or other psychotic disorder or schizophrenia; either partner had plans for imminent departure from geographic region	1) BCT treatment package N= 21 2) IBMM services (Individual based methadone maintenance), standard treatment N=22 Treatment adherence 1) 19/21 (90%) remained in treatment through analysis 2) 17/22 (77%) remained in treatment through analysis	1) Format: BCT Manualized: Yes Sessions: 2 sessions weekly for 12 weeks Approach: In addition to an individual weekly session (similar to IBMM below), partners met conjointly with a therapist once weekly for 60 minute sessions. Verbal agreement made to have a daily "sobriety trust discussion." Weekly homework reinforcing session content. 2) Format: IBMM Manualized: Yes Sessions: 2 sessions weekly for 12 weeks Approach: Subject met with therapist alone, twice weekly; adapted from cognitive behavioral treatment programs for alcoholism; emphasis on coping skills training. Standard methadone dose of 60 mg/day, increased at patient's request or when opiate positive urine sample.	Patient Outcomes Symptom Improvement a. ASI - alcohol and drug composite b. Urine samples Family Outcomes: Couple functioning: a. DAS b. ASI (family-social composite) Intermediate Outcomes: Satisfaction a. CSQ Attendance a. # sessions attended	Allocation concealment: NR Blinding: NR Intention to treat analysis: no Withdrawals adequately described: yes Treatment integrity: Manualized; counselors supervised weekly for consistent treatment techniques; randomly audiotaped sessions Study Quality: Fair

Study, Year Funding Source	Sample Characteristics	Inclusion/Exclusion Criteria	Treatment Groups	Intervention Characteristics	Outcomes Assessed	Quality
Fals-Stewart, 2003[68] Government Foundation	N = 124 randomized N = 124 data analysis Gender: 100% male Age: 32.35 years Race/ethnicity: White 40.5 % Black 15.5% Hispanic 2.5% Other 3.5% Marital Status: Married 49% Education (mean years/SD): 13.2 Veterans: NR *Recruitment Method* Opioid dependent men seeking outpatient treatment in community based clinics were asked to participate. *Family Characteristics:* Family member Gender: NR Age: NR Race/ethnicity: NR Spouse 49% Parent 36.5% Sibling 15%	MH Condition: substance use Assessed by: Structured clinical interview SO: family member Inclusions: Men with opioid dependence; living with someone not abusing drugs/alcohol and without diagnosis of serious mental illness; able to forgo any other substance use counseling except for self-help groups Exclusion: Physical condition that could interfere with tx; allergic to Naltrexone; dependent on other psychoactive drug other than opioid that requires inpatient hospitalization for detoxification; suicidal or homicidal; in methadone tx within 30 days of tx.	1) Naltrexone + Behavioral Family Therapy (BFT) N=62 2) Naltrexone + individual based therapy (IBT) N=62	1) Format: Behavioral Family Therapy Manualized: Yes Session: 56 sessions for IBT; 16 additional BFT Approach: BFT Approach: Treatment included IBT through group (once weekly) and individual counseling (once weekly) plus BFT through one conjoint session (once weekly) 2) Format: Individual Manualized: Yes Sessions: 56 Approach: Treatment individual cognitive behavior therapy through group (once weekly) and individual counseling (twice weekly)	*Patient Outcomes* Symptom Improvement a. Abstinence – opioid free urine screens b. Abstinence – drug free urine screens c. PDA opioids d. PDA cocaine e. PDA alcohol f. PDA drugs g. Length of continuous abstinence *Family Outcomes:* Family functioning a. ASI sub-scale *Intermediate Outcomes:* Attendance: a. Sessions attended Adherence: a. # days took Naltrexone Satisfaction with care a. CSQ	Allocation concealment: NR Blinding: NR Intention to treat analysis: yes Withdrawals adequately described: yes Treatment integrity: Recorded sessions; counselors assessed for adherence (NS); counselors assessed for competence (NS) Study Quality: Fair

Family Involved Psychosocial Treatments for Adult Mental Health Conditions: A Review of the Evidence

Study, Year Funding Source	Sample Characteristics	Inclusion/Exclusion Criteria	Treatment Groups	Intervention Characteristics	Outcomes Assessed	Quality
Fals-Stewart, 2005[69] Government	N = 100 randomized N = 100 data analysis Gender: 100% male Age: 34.8 years Race/ethnicity: White 58% Black 24% Hispanic 13% Other 7% Marital or cohabitating: 100% Education (mean years/SD): 13.4 Veterans: NR Recruitment Method Alcohol dependent married men entering outpatient treatment were asked to participate. Family Characteristics: Spouse/partner Gender: 100% female Age: NR Race/ethnicity: NR Spouse 49% Parent 36% Sibling 15%	MH Condition: substance use Assessed by: NR SO: wife/intimate partner Inclusions: Men, 20-60 yrs old; married ≥1 yr or cohabitating ≥2 yrs.; meet DSM criterion for alcohol dependence; medical clearance; agreed to abstain from drugs/alcohol; restrain from other tx programs; Exclusions: Any psychoactive drug dependence within last 6 months, any serious mental illness for participant and/or SO.	1) Brief Relationship Therapy N=25 2) Standard Behavioral Couples Therapy N=25 3) Individual based therapy (IBT) N=25 4) Psychoeducational attention control treatment (PACT) N=25	1) Format: Brief Relationship Therapy Manualized: Yes Session: 18 Approach: Group session weekly and an additional session with partner every other week; focus on couple communication, problems solving and reinforcing sobriety 2) Format: Standard Behavioral Couples Therapy Manualized: Yes Session: 24 Approach: One 12-step group and 1 conjoint (with spouse) session weekly. Conjoint session focused on focused on couple communication, problems solving and reinforcing sobriety. 3) Format: IBT Manualized: Yes Session: 18 Approach: One group session/week and 1 individual counseling every other week 4) Format: PACT Manualized: Yes Session: 18 Approach: One group session weekly and 6 additional sessions with partner every other week. Partner was a passive participant, listening to lectures on substance use.	Patient Outcomes Symptom Improvement a. PDHD Family Outcomes: Couple functioning: a. DAS Intermediate Outcomes: Attendance: a. Sessions attended Satisfaction with care a. CSQ	Allocation concealment: NR Blinding: NR Intention to treat analysis: unclear Withdrawals adequately described: yes Treatment integrity: All sessions were audiotaped; 20% of sessions rated for competence and adherence; manualized; no significant differences across groups Study Quality: Fair

112

Family Involved Psychosocial Treatments for Adult Mental Health Conditions: A Review of the Evidence

Study, Year Funding Source	Sample Characteristics	Inclusion/Exclusion Criteria	Treatment Groups	Intervention Characteristics	Outcomes Assessed	Quality
Fals-Stewart, 2006[74] Government	N = 138 randomized N = 138 data analysis *Gender:* 100% female *Age:* 33.4 years *Race/ethnicity:* White 59 % Black 30.3% Hispanic 6.7% Other 2.3% *Marital or cohabitating:* 100% *Education (mean years/SD):* 12.8 Veterans: NR *Recruitment Method* Alcohol dependent married/cohabitating women entering outpatient treatment for alcohol dependence were asked to participate. *Family Characteristics:* Spouse/partner *Gender:* 100% male *Age:* 35.8 years Education (years): 12.9 *Race/ethnicity:* White 56% Black 30.3% Hispanic 8.3% Other 4.3%	*MH Condition:* alcohol use *Assessed by:* Structured clinical interview *SO:* husband/intimate male partner *Inclusions:* Women, 20-60 yrs old; married ≥1 yr or cohabitating ≥2 yrs.; meet DSM criterion for alcohol dependence; have alcohol as primary drug of abuse; agreed to abstain from drugs/alcohol; restrain from other tx programs *Exclusions:* Male partner met DSM criteria for any psychoactive drug dependence, any serious mental illness for participant and/or SO	1) Standard Behavioral Couples Therapy (S-BCT) N=46 2) Individual based therapy (IBT) N=46 3) Psychoeducational attention control tx (PACT) N=46	1) *Format:* S-BCT *Manualized:* Yes *Session:* 32 *Approach:* 20 individual sessions and 12 conjoint (with spouse) sessions. Conjoint session focused on couple communication, problems solving and reinforcing sobriety. 2) *Format:* IBT *Manualized:* Yes *Session:* 32 *Approach:* 32 individual sessions 3) *Format:* PACT *Manualized:* Yes *Session:* 32 *Approach:* 20 individual sessions and 12 conjoint (with spouse) sessions. Conjoint sessions were designed so partner was a passive participant, listening to lectures about alcoholism and sobriety.	*Patient Outcomes* Symptom Improvement a. PDA *Family Outcomes:* Couple functioning: a. DAS Partner violence a. TLFB-Spousal Violence *Intermediate Outcomes:* Attendance: a. Sessions attended Satisfaction with care b. CSQ	<u>Allocation concealment:</u> yes <u>Blinding:</u> NR <u>Intention to treat analysis:</u> unclear <u>Withdrawals adequately described:</u> yes <u>Treatment integrity:</u> Sessions audiotaped, reviewed and rated. **<u>Study Quality:</u> Good**

Family Involved Psychosocial Treatments for Adult Mental Health Conditions: A Review of the Evidence

Evidence-based Synthesis Program

Study, Year Funding Source	Sample Characteristics	Inclusion/Exclusion Criteria	Treatment Groups	Intervention Characteristics	Outcomes Assessed	Quality
Fals-Stewart, 2008[78] Funding source not reported	N =184 randomized N =184 data analysis Gender: 73% male, 27% female Age: 34.4 years Race/ethnicity: White 58 % Black 24% Hispanic 13% Other 7% Marital or cohabitating: 100% Education (mean years/SD): 13.4 Veterans: NR Recruitment Method Drug dependent married/ cohabitating men and women entering outpatient treatment were asked to participate. Family Characteristics: Spouse/partner Gender: 27% male, 73% female Age: 28.8 years Education (years): 14.4 Race/ethnicity: White 51% Black 17.3% Hispanic 3.3% Other 5.5%	MH Condition: substance use Assessed by: NR SO: spouse/intimate partner Inclusions: Men or women, 20-60 yrs old; married ≥1 yr or cohabitating ≥2 yrs.; meet DSM criterion for psychoactive substance use disorder and be dependent on a drug other than alcohol or nicotine; medical clearance; agreed to abstain from drugs/ alcohol; restrain from other tx programs; Exclusions: Partners met DSM criteria for any psychoactive drug dependence within last 6 months, any serious mental illness for participant and/or SO.	1) Brief BCT N=46 2) Standard BCT N=46 3) Individual based therapy (IBT) N=46 4) Psychoeducational attention control treatment (PACT) N=46	1) Format: B-BCT Manualized: Yes Session: 18 Approach: 12 group sessions and 6 conjoint sessions with partner, where partner is an active participant. Conjoint sessions focused on couple communication, problems solving and reinforcing sobriety. 2) Format: BCT Manualized: Yes Session: 24 Approach: 12 group sessions and 12 conjoint sessions with partner, where partner is an active participant. Conjoint sessions focused on couple communication, problems solving and reinforcing sobriety. 3) Format: IBT Manualized: Yes Session: 18 Approach: 12 group sessions and 6 individual counseling sessions 4) Format: PACT Manualized: Yes Session: 18 Approach: 12 group sessions and 6 conjoint sessions with partner, but partner is a passive participant. Conjoint sessions were lecture based sessions about alcoholism	Patient Outcomes Symptom Improvement a. PDA Family Outcomes: Couple functioning: a. DAS Intermediate Outcomes: Attendance: a. Sessions attended Satisfaction with care a. CSQ	Allocation concealment: NR Blinding: NR Intention to treat analysis: unclear Withdrawals adequately described: yes Treatment integrity: Recorded; 20% assessed for adherence and competence Study Quality: Fair

114

Study, Year Funding Source	Sample Characteristics	Inclusion/Exclusion Criteria	Treatment Groups	Intervention Characteristics	Outcomes Assessed	Quality
Fals-Stewart, 2009[79] Government	TWO GROUPS: 1) GAY MALES: N = 52 randomized N = 52 data analysis Gender: 100% male Age: 31.3 years Race/ethnicity: White: 77% Black: 8% Hispanic: 2% Other: 2% Marital Status: NR Education(years): 15.0 Veterans: NR *Family Characteristics:* Partners Gender: 100% male 2) LESBIANS: N =48 randomized N =48 data analysis Gender: 100% female Age: 27.7 years Race/ethnicity: White: 77% Black: 10% Hispanic: 6% Other: 6% Marital Status: NR Education (years): 13.3 Veterans: NR *Family Characteristics:* Partners Gender: 100% female *Recruitment Method* Gays or lesbians entering tx for alcohol use disorder at community health center were approached and asked to participate.	MH Condition: current alcohol abuse or dependence Assessed by: Structured interview with DSM-IV criteria SO: gay or lesbian partner Inclusions: gay or lesbian sexuality, alcohol as primary drug of abuse, living with SO in stable relationship ≥1 year; ≥18 yrs old; agreed to refrain from alcohol/drugs during treatment; not in any other SA treatment. Exclusions: if partner met DSM-IV criteria for any current substance use disorder (except nicotine), or if either pt or partner had schizophrenia or psychotic disorder	1) Behavioral Couples Therapy N = NR 2) Individual based treatment N=NR	1) Format: Behavioral Couples Therapy treatment Manualized: Yes Sessions: 32 x 60 minutes Txt Length: 20 weeks Approach: Same program as IBT for 20 sessions (individual therapy); remaining 12 conducted with partner (substance and relationship focused interventions) 2) Format: Individual treatment Manualized: modified from Individual Drug Counseling Manual Sessions: 32 x 60 minutes Txt Length: 20 weeks Approach: Individual therapy, using 12 step facilitation; participants encouraged total abstinence	Patient Outcomes Symptoms: a. PDHD Family Outcomes Couple functioning: a. DAS Intermediate Outcomes Attendance: a. # sessions attended Treatment Satisfaction a. CSQ	Allocation Concealment: NR Blinding: NR Intention-to-treat analysis: yes Withdrawals adequately described: no Treatment Integrity Limitation; 80% of participants refused to be video-taped. Study Quality: Poor

Study, Year Funding Source	Sample Characteristics	Inclusion/Exclusion Criteria	Treatment Groups	Intervention Characteristics	Outcomes Assessed	Quality
Jones, 2011[70] Government	N = 62 randomized N = 62 data analysis Gender: 100% male Age: 33.3 (6.7) years Race/ethnicity: White 51% Non-white: 49% Marital Status: Married: 17% Unmarried: 86% Education (mean years): 11.7 (1.1) Veterans: NR *Recruitment Method* Subjects recruited from Center for Addiction and Pregnancy clinic. *Family Characteristics:* Gender: 100% female	MH Condition: Opioid use Assessed by: Self report SO: Pregnant partner Inclusion: Eligibility initially based on eligibility of a pregnant partner. Pregnant woman needed to be age ≥18, ≤30 weeks pregnant, meet DSM-IV criteria for current opioid dependence. With referral from pregnant woman, her male partner then became subject. His eligibility requirements: male; age ≥18 years; see the pregnant woman ≥thrice weekly; no evidence of physical violence toward woman, self reported opioid use of ≥4 days/week each week in the past month. Exclusions: either pregnant woman or partner if diagnosed with a medical or psychiatric condition that contraindicated study participation or signing informed consent.	Drug abusers 1) HOPE: Helping Other Partners Excel N=45 2) Usual care N= 17	1) Format: HOPE (couples based) Manualized: Yes Sessions: 22 weeks; 6 individual male partner sessions, then 12 manualized couples education. Approach: Four components – motivational enhancement therapy for male partners, case management and proactive counseling, 12 weeks couple's group therapy and education sessions, contingency management to initiate and sustain drug abstinence. 2) Format: Usual care Manualized: NR Sessions: 22 weeks; 1 60 minute weekly session Approach: Weekly support group for male partner only; drug education and other topics. Couples' counseling available upon request. Free methadone maintenance for 6 months; or inpatient detoxification followed by 6 months of outpatient care provided to male partners in both groups (subject choice)	Patient Outcomes Symptom Improvement a. ASI b. Days use, past 30 days (heroin) c. % with heroin use Global Functioning: a. Depression (BDI) Family Outcomes: Couple functioning: a. Partner Support Questionnaire (based on Norbeck Social Support Questionnaire) b. Relationship Assessment form	Allocation concealment: NR Blinding: NR Intention to treat analysis: yes Withdrawals adequately described: yes Treatment integrity: Weekly supervision, training of counselors, feedback on audiotaped sessions. **Study Quality:** Fair

Study, Year Funding Source	Sample Characteristics	Inclusion/Exclusion Criteria	Treatment Groups	Intervention Characteristics	Outcomes Assessed	Quality
Kelley, 2002[63] Government	N = 135 randomized N = 127 data analysis All subjects (both alcohol and drug abusers): Gender: 100% male Age: 32.35 years Race/ethnicity: White 63 % Black 32% Hispanic 5% Marital Status: Married or cohabitating 100% Education (mean years): 12.2 Veterans: NR Recruitment Method Subjects recruited from clinics specializing in treatment of alcohol or drug abuse. Family Characteristics: 100% female wives or significant others Age: 36.6 Race/ethnicity: White 67 % Black 25% Hispanic 8% Education (mean years): 12.1	MH Condition: Abuse or dependence for a psychoactive substance use disorder Assessed by: DSM-III-R criteria SO: wives or female SO Inclusion: male; age 20-60 years; married ≥1 year or living with significant other ≥2 years; medical clearance to engage in abstinence oriented treatment; agree to refrain from alcohol or illicit drugs during treatment, refrain from seeking other substance abuse treatment except for self help meetings; have at least one child age 6-16 living in household for whom one or both adults were legal guardians. Exclusions: if female partner met DSM-III-R criteria for psycho-active substance use disorder in last six months; either partner in methadone maintenance program; either partner met DSM-III-R criteria for organic mental, paranoid, or other psychotic disorder or schizophrenia.	Alcohol abusers 1) BCT N=25 2) IBT only N= 22 3) Psychoeducational attention control treatment (PACT) N= 24 Drug abusers 1) BCT N=22 2) IBT only N= 22 3) PACT N= 21	1) Format: BCT Manualized: Yes Sessions: 32 Approach: Both partners attend 12 treatment sessions, used to help male partners remain abstinent, teach effective communication, increase positive exchanges, eliminate aggression. In remaining 20 sessions, subjects participated in individual CBT. 2) Format: IBT Manualized: Yes Sessions: 32 Approach: After a baseline assessment, the partner no longer participated in treatment. Subject alone attended 20 IBT sessions (same as BCT group), followed by 12 coping skills based sessions. 3) Format: PACT Manualized: Yes Sessions: 32 Approach: Subject alone attended 20 IBT sessions (same as BCT and groups), followed by 12 educational lectures that both partners attended (not couples therapy).	Patient Outcomes Symptom Improvement a. PDA Family Outcomes: Couple functioning: a. DAS Intermediate Outcomes: a. Session attendance	Allocation concealment: NR Blinding: NR Intention to treat analysis: yes; missing data imputation described Withdrawals adequately described: yes Treatment integrity: Manualized Study Quality: Fair

117

Family Involved Psychosocial Treatments for Adult Mental Health Conditions: A Review of the Evidence

Study, Year Funding Source	Sample Characteristics	Inclusion/Exclusion Criteria	Treatment Groups	Intervention Characteristics	Outcomes Assessed	Quality
Kirby, 1999[80] Government	N = 36 randomized N = 30 for data analysis (due to drop outs following randomization) _Gender:_ 6% male _Age:_ 39.6 years _Race/ethnicity:_ White 75% Black 21.9% Hispanic NR Other 3.1% _Marital Status:_ NR _Education:_ NR Veterans:_ NR _Family Characteristics:_ Spouse/partner: 56.3% Parent 37.5% Sibling 6.3% _Recruitment Method_ Recruited from newspaper ads.	_Participants:_ Family or significant other of drug abuser (FSO) _MH Condition:_ FSO report of family member drug abuse _Assessed by:_ Condition was assessed by FSO self-report _SO:_ drug user not involved in intervention _Inclusions:_ FSOs were over 18, had contact with drug user >3 times/week, concern about illicit drug user, drug user not in tx, FSO not in tx.	1) Individual counseling and psychoeducation (community reinforcement training intervention or CRT) 2) Self help (Narcotics Anonymous)	1) _Format:_ CRT _Manualized:_ No _Session:_ 14X60 minutes _Txt Length:_ 10 weeks _Approach:_ Individual counseling sessions, that includes motivation to change, communication, coping strategies, and developing social support 2) _Format:_ Self-help group _Manualized:_ Yes _Session:_ 10X75 minutes _Txt Length:_ 10 weeks _Approach:_ Group counseling sessions that included discussion of 12 steps, self-esteem, views about addiction, responsibility and detachment.	_Patient Outcomes_ Symptoms: a. FSO ratings of patient drug use during after treatment Health Care Utilization: a. % of patient entry into treatment during FSO treatment _Family Outcomes:_ Family functioning: a. SAS family unit subscale Couple functioning: a. SAS marital subscale _Intermediate Outcomes_ Attendance: a. FSO attendance, b. Treatment completion	<u>Allocation concealment:</u> Unclear <u>Blinding:</u> Unclear <u>Intention to treat analysis:</u> No <u>Withdrawals adequately described:</u> Drop outs after randomization discussed; no explanation of what was done with missing data <u>Treatment Integrity</u> Supervised counseling **Study Quality:** **Poor**

118

Family Involved Psychosocial Treatments for Adult Mental Health Conditions: A Review of the Evidence

Evidence-based Synthesis Program

Study, Year Funding Source	Sample Characteristics	Inclusion/Exclusion Criteria	Treatment Groups	Intervention Characteristics	Outcomes Assessed	Quality
Lam, 2009[71] Government	N = 30 randomized N = 30 data analysis Gender: 100% male Age: 34.1 years Marital Status: Married or cohabitating: 100% Race/ethnicity: White 63% Black 23% Hispanic 7% Other 7% Education (years): 12.9 Veterans: NR *Family Characteristics:* Wives/partners (children not actively involved in treatment) Gender: 100% Age: 33.0 years Education (years): 13.6 Race/ethnicity: White 66.6 Black 13.3 Hispanic 6.6 Other 13.3 *Recruitment Method* Heterosexual married men entering tx for alcohol dependence with a child were asked to participate within 1 week of admission to tx.	MH Condition: alcohol use disorder per DSM-IV criteria Assessed by: structured clinical interview (for both pt and SO) SO: female partners (wife or SO) Inclusions: Male, ≥18, married ≥1 year or cohabitating ≥2 years; female partner did NOT mean DSM-IV criteria for substance abuse or dependence, had legal guardianship of at least one child between ages 8-12 living in the home. Exclusions: N/A	1) PSBCT (Parent Skills with Behavioral Couples Therapy) N = 10 2) Behavioral Couples Therapy (BCT) N= 10 3) Individual based treatment (IBT) N=10	1) Format: PSBCT. Manualized: Yes Sessions: 24 Txt Length: 12 weeks (2/wk x 60 minutes) Approach: 12 individual sessions plus 6 core BCT plus 6 parent skills training sessions. Partner attended the BCT and parent sessions with participant. 2) Format: BCT Manualized: Yes Sessions: 24 Txt Length:12 weeks (2/wk x 60 minutes) Approach: 12 individual sessions plus 12 manualized BCT sessions. Partner attended the BCT with participant; BCT included communication and problem solving skill building. 3) Format: IBT Manualized: yes Sessions: 24 Txt Length:12 weeks (2/wk x 60 minutes) Approach: 12 individual plus 12 individual based coping sessions using Cognitive Behavioral Therapy (CBT) All three treatment groups received 12 weekly standard CBT sessions; the second weekly session content differed by treatment group.	Patient Outcomes Symptoms: a. PDA Family Outcomes Couple functioning a. DAS Inter-personal Violence: a. TLFB –Spousal Violence Intermediate Outcomes Attendance: a. % of sessions attended	Allocation Concealment: NR Blinding: NR Intention-to-treat analysis: Yes Withdrawals adequately described: No; not defined by treatment group Treatment integrity: Videotaped training sessions for each therapist reviewed for guideline adherence and competency. Study Quality: Fair

Family Involved Psychosocial Treatments for Adult Mental Health Conditions: A Review of the Evidence

Study, Year Funding Source	Sample Characteristics	Inclusion/Exclusion Criteria	Treatment Groups	Intervention Characteristics	Outcomes Assessed	Quality
McCrady, 1996[72] Government	N = 90 randomized N = 88 data analysis Gender: 100% male Age: 39.4 (10.3) years Race/ethnicity: NR Marital Status: NR Education (years): 13.4 (2.3) Veterans: NR *Family Characteristics:* Spouse/partners Gender: 100% female Age: 37.4 (10.3) years Education (years): 13.7 (2.0) *Recruitment Method* Male alcoholics and female partners recruited through outpatient treatment program, community referrals and advertisements for low-fee couple therapy for alcoholism.	MH Condition: alcohol dependence Assessed by: Structured clinical screening interview SO: female partners Inclusions: Men who were married or in cohabitating relationship >6 months, met criteria for alcohol dependence or abuse; not dependent on other drug; not psychotics; without signs of severe organic brain syndrome; partners did not have alcohol problems, drug dependence or psychosis.	1) Alcohol focused spouse involvement plus behavioral marital therapy (ABMT) N=30 2) Alcohol focused spouse involvement plus behavioral marital therapy (ABMT) PLUS AA/Al Anon N=31 3) Alcohol focused spouse involvement plus behavioral marital therapy plus relapse prevention N=29	1) Format: ABMT Manualized: Yes Sessions: 15 Txt Length: 15 weeks (1/wk x 90 minutes) Approach: BMT that included behavioral self-recording, stimulus and consequence control procedures; communication and problem solving skill Partner attended the BCT with participant. 2) Format: ABMT/AA Manualized: Yes Sessions: 15 Txt Length: 15 weeks (1/wk x 90 minutes) Approach: BMT that included communication and problem solving skill, encouragement to go to AA/Al-Anon, homework and used common language to AA. 3) Format: ABMT/AA/RP Manualized: Yes Sessions: 19 minimum Txt Length: 15 weeks (1/wk x 90 minutes) Approach: BMT that included communication and problem solving skill, encouragement to go to AA/Al Anon, homework and used common language to AA plus 4 maintenance sessions over 12 months to reduce relapse.	Patient Outcomes Symptoms: a. Mean % drinking days b. Mean # drinks per drinking day Intermediate Outcomes Attendance a. Session attendance b. Homework completed	Allocation concealment: NR Blinding: NR Intention to treat analysis: No Withdrawals adequately described: Yes Treatment integrity: Manualized; audiotaped treatment adherence assessed rigorously Study Quality: Fair

Study, Year Funding Source	Sample Characteristics	Inclusion/Exclusion Criteria	Treatment Groups	Intervention Characteristics	Outcomes Assessed	Quality
McCrady, 1999[86] Government	Same as McCrady 1996[72]	Same as McCrady 1996[72]	Same as McCrady 1996[72]	Same as McCrady 1996[72]	<u>Patient Outcomes</u> Symptoms: a. PDA b. PDHD c. Mean length of drinking episodes d. % continuous abstinent e. % non-problem drinking f. % drinking, but improved g. % unimproved <u>Intermediate Outcomes</u> Attendance a. Mean # sessions attended b. Mean #days in treatment	Same as McCrady 1996[72]
McCrady, 2004[87] Government	Same as McCrady 1996[72]	Same as McCrady 1996[72]	Same as McCrady 1996[72]	Same as McCrady 1996[72]	<u>Patient Outcomes</u> Symptoms: a. PDA <u>Family Outcomes</u> Couple functioning a. MHS	Same as McCrady 1996[72]

Family Involved Psychosocial Treatments for Adult Mental Health Conditions: A Review of the Evidence

Study, Year Funding Source	Sample Characteristics	Inclusion/Exclusion Criteria	Treatment Groups	Intervention Characteristics	Outcomes Assessed	Quality
McCrady, 2009[75] Government	N = 109 randomized N = 102 analyzed Gender: 100% female Age: 45.1 years Race/ethnicity: White: 95% Not white: 5% Hispanic: NR Marital Status: Married: 89% Not married: 11% Education (years): 14.91 Veterans: NR Family Characteristics: Husbands: 89% Male Significant Others(SO): 11% Children: 0 Recruitment Method Women recruited through advertisements in the community and referrals from local alcohol tx programs.	MH condition: current alcohol abuse or dependence Assessed by: Structured clinical Interview for DSM-IV SO: male partner _ Inclusions: Female, married, cohabitating for >6 months, or committed relationship for >1 year (with intent to continue). Exclusions: Neither party <25 on MMSE , signs of psychotic disorder, current drug or physiological dependence, no evidence of domestic abuse in past 12 months OR if aggression reported on Modified CTS, a) victim does not fear retribution & b) violence occurred only when intoxicated or resulted in no injuries.	1) Alcohol Behavior Couples Therapy (N =50) 2) Alcohol Behavior Individual Therapy (N=52)	1) Format: Couples Manualized: Yes Sessions: 20 x 90 minutes Txt Length: Maximum 6 months Approach: CBT, same as individual plus intervention for partner to support abstinence and improve couple relationship. 2) Format: Individual Manualized: Yes Sessions: 20 x 60 minutes Txt Length: Maximum 6 months Approach: CBT including self monitoring, functional analysis of drinking, coping skills.	Patient Outcomes Symptoms: a. PDA b. PDHD c. % complete abstinence after treatment d. % no heavy drinking days Health Care Utilization: a. % pts receiving additional formal treatment. b. # day's treatment. Family Outcomes Couple functioning: a. % separated during treatment. b. Days length of separation Intermediate Outcomes Attendance: a. % Attended all sessions. b. # sessions Treatment adherence a. % Homework completed (patient)	Allocation Concealment: Yes Blinding: none Intention-to-treat analysis: No Withdrawals adequately described: Yes Treatment integrity: Therapists met weekly to review cases, audiotapes reviewed randomly; MATCH Treatment rating scale used (no significant differences). Study Quality: Good

122

Study, Year Funding Source	Sample Characteristics	Inclusion/Exclusion Criteria	Treatment Groups	Intervention Characteristics	Outcomes Assessed	Quality
Meyers, 2002[83] Funding NR	N = 90 randomized N = 90 in data analysis Gender: NR Age: NR Marital Status: NR Relationship length: over 20 years Race/ethnicity: NR Education: NR Veterans: NR Family Characteristics: Female intimate partner: 30% Parents: 53% Close friend/other family member: 17% Had children: NR Recruitment Method SOs were recruited through newspaper ads offering help with tx-refusing, drug abusing loved one.	MH Condition: psychoactive substance use disorder other than alcohol Assessed by SCI for DSM-IV SO: a first-degree relative, spouse, intimate partner, or someone who lives with the IP; who has contact with the patient on at least 40% of the last 90 days. Inclusions: ≥ age 18; live within 60 miles of the project; describe the loved one in a manner consistent with the DSM-IV diagnoses for a psychoactive substance use disorder other than alcohol; consent to participate. Exclusions: SOs of an individual with a substance use disorder who would be interested in entering treatment.	1) Community Reinforcement and Family Training (CRAFT) N = 29 2) CRAFT + aftercare N = 30 3) Al-Anon or Narcotics Anonymous facilitation therapy N = 31 *Skills taught in CRAFT: domestic violence precautions, motivational strategies, assessment of the context of the patient's use, communication training, positive-reinforcement training, discouragement of drug use, training CSOs to reward themselves, and suggesting treatment to the patient	1) Format: CRAFT in individual sessions with the SO Manualized: Yes Sessions: 1 2-14 Txt Length: NR Approach: SO taught skills* for impacting drinker's alcohol use and decision to enter treatment and improving their own quality of life 2) Format: CRAFT conducted in individual sessions with the SO Manualized: Yes Sessions: 12-14 + aftercare group therapy for up to 6 months Txt Length: NR Approach: See above + open-ended groups for after care for up to 6 months; aftercare used same CRAFT principles 3) Format: Al-Anon or Narcotics Anonymous facilitation therapy Manualized: Yes Sessions: 1 2 Txt Length: NR Approach: parallels 12-step program and adds emphasis on getting patient to enter formal treatment	Patient Outcomes Health Care Utilization a. % of patients who came to treatment after their significant others were recruited for the study	Allocation Concealment: NR Blinding: NR Intention-to-treat analysis: NR Withdrawals adequately described: No Treatment integrity: Weekly supervision; sample of sessions were videotaped and reviewed. Study Quality: Fair

Family Involved Psychosocial Treatments for Adult Mental Health Conditions: A Review of the Evidence

Study, Year Funding Source	Sample Characteristics	Inclusion/Exclusion Criteria	Treatment Groups	Intervention Characteristics	Outcomes Assessed	Quality
Miller, 1999[81] Government	N = 130 SOs randomized N = 130 data analysis Gender: 91% female Age: 47 years Marital Status: NR Relationship length: 22 years (range 1 to 57 years) Race/ethnicity: White/non-Hispanic: 53% Hispanic: 39% Native American: 6% Other: 1% Education (years): 14 Veterans: NR Family Characteristics: Spouse: 59% Parent: 30% Boy/Girlfriend: 8% Adult Child: 1.5% Grandparent: 1.5% Had children: NR Recruitment Method SOs seeking advice or help with the drinking behaviors of someone with whom they lived. Referrals primarily came from announcements in local news media.	MH Condition: alcohol use disorder Assessed by: SO report using the Structured Clinical Interview for the DSM-III-R SO: close relative (parent, child, grandchild, sibling) or a spouse or unmarried intimate partner Inclusions: Concerned SO must be 1) living with a problem drinker who is a close relative or intimate partner, 2) within 60 miles of research site, 3) in contact with drinker on at least 40% of the past 90 days, with no planned change (e.g., separation) in the next 90 days, 4) age ≥18 (both SO and drinker), 5) willing to participate in research, 6) describes the drinker in a manner consistent with DSM-III diagnostic criteria for alcohol abuse or dependence, and 7) evidence that the drinker refused to seek treatment and had not received and treatment (other than detoxification) for alcohol or drug problems in the past 3 months	1) CRAFT N = 45 (44 completed) 2) Johnson Institute intervention N = 40 (36 completed) 3) Alcoholics-Anonymous N = 45 (42 completed) *Skills taught in CRAFT: awareness training (incorporating the style of motivational interviewing), contingency management, communication skills training, planned activities that compete with drinking, outside activities for SO self-care, handling dangerous situations, suggesting counseling, and functional analysis of triggers and reinforcers for nondrinking	1) Format: CRAFT in individual sessions with the SO Manualized: Yes Sessions: 12 1-hr sessions Approach: SO taught skills* for impacting drinker's alcohol use and decision to enter treatment and improving their own quality of life 2) Format: Johnson Institute intervention Manualized: Yes Sessions: 6 2-hr sessions Approach: Special form of family intervention; family members are prepared to confront problem drinking with their own experiences and observations about drinking and related problems, encourage treatment entry in a supportive manner, and apply sanctions if the drinker fails to enter tx 3) Format: Alcoholics-Anonymous Manualized: Yes Sessions: 812-hr sessions Approach: parallels 12-step program – philosophy that SO is powerless to control drinker, must detach, and instead accept Al-Anon and strengthen own mental health	Primary outcomes Utilization a. Patient engagement in at least an initial assessment and one treatment session of substance use treatment Family Outcomes Family functioning a. FES (Family cohesion) b. RHS Conflict a. FES (Family conflict) Intermediate Outcomes Attendance: a. session attendance	Allocation Concealment: NR Blinding: NR Intention-to-treat analysis: Yes Withdrawals adequately described: Yes Treatment integrity: Therapists thoroughly trained, certified in tx, and then supervised. All sessions videotaped and randomly selected tapes were monitored. Study Quality: Good

Study, Year Funding Source	Sample Characteristics	Inclusion/Exclusion Criteria	Treatment Groups	Intervention Characteristics	Outcomes Assessed	Quality
O'Farrell, 1998a[4] Government	N = 59 randomized N = 59 data analysis Gender: 100% male Age 44.4 years Marital Status: Married 100% Race/ethnicity: White: NR Education (years): 12.73 Veterans: 100% Family Characteristics: Spouses Gender: 100% female Age: 41.6 years Race/ethnicity: NR Education (years): 13.0 Recruitment Method Participants recruited from VA inpatient detoxification units (for alcohol) and outpatients in alcohol rehabilitation program, and from newspaper and media announcements.	MH Condition: Alcohol Abuse or Dependence Assessed by: MAST SO: Wife/female cohabitating partner Inclusions: Legally married male alcoholics with non-alcoholic spouses or in stable common law marriage for at least 3 yrs; living together; ages 25-60 yrs.; husband met DSM criteria for alcohol dependence; had consumed alcohol sometime 120 prior to initial assessment; score >7 on MAST; accepted abstinence as goal; refrained from other tx or counseling during trial. Exclusions: Wife abused alcohol or had been abstinent< 6 months; wife or husband had psychoactive substance use disorder (other than alcohol); serious mental illness; separated and not willing to reconcile for trial.	1) Behavioral Marital Therapy (BMT) + Relapse Prevention (RP) N = 30 2) Behavioral Marital Therapy N = 29	1) Format: BMT + RP Manualized: Yes Sessions: BMT NR + 15 Relapse Prevention sessions Txt Length: 5-6 months for BMT + 1 year Approach: Couple therapy delivered first with only the couple and provider then in groups of couples later in the treatment + couples therapy for relapse prevention with only the couple and the provider Behavioral marital therapy with Antabuse contracts to promote abstinence, behavioral assignments, and communication /negotiation training + relapse prevention to maintain behaviors and gains, deal with unresolved problems, to develop and rehearse a relapse prevention plan 2) Format: BMT only Manualized: Yes Sessions: NR Txt Length: 5-6 months Approach: Couple therapy delivered first in with only the couple and provider then in groups of couples later in the treatment. Behavioral marital therapy with Antabuse contracts to promote abstinence, behavioral assignments, and communication/ negotiation training	Patient Outcomes Symptoms a. PDA Family Outcomes Couple functioning a. Marital Adjustment Test b. CBQ (marital behaviors scale) Intermediate Outcomes Adherence: a. CBQ (participation in Antabuse contract scale)	Allocation Concealment: No Blinding: no Intention-to-treat analysis: No Withdrawals adequately described: Yes Treatment integrity: Extensive training, weekly supervision, co-author leading or observing 80% of sessions Study Quality: Fair

Family Involved Psychosocial Treatments for Adult Mental Health Conditions: A Review of the Evidence

Study, Year Funding Source	Sample Characteristics	Inclusion/Exclusion Criteria	Treatment Groups	Intervention Characteristics	Outcomes Assessed	Quality
O'Farrell, 1998b[65] Government	N = 36 randomized N = 34 data analysis Gender: 100% male Age: 42.4 years Marital Status: 100% Yrs married (mean): 15.79 Race/ethnicity: White: NR Education (years): 12.47 Veterans: 100% (n=34) Family Characteristics: Wife/partner Gender: 100% female Age: 40.4 years Education (years): 12.4 Recruitment Method Married male alcoholics in the first month of tx in the VA Alcoholism Outpatient Clinic were contacted to participate.	MH Condition Alcohol Use Disorder Assessed by: MAST SO: wife/female partner Inclusions: Legally married male alcoholics with non-alcoholic spouses; living together; no older than 60yrs.; score >7 on MAST. Exclusions: Patient refused to accept sobriety as goal; had psychotic or had organic memory deficits; wife had drinking problem, nervous disorder, or was psychotic.	1) Behavioral Marital Therapy N = 10 2) Interactional Couples Therapy N = 12 3) Individual treatment only N = 12	1) Format: Individual treatment for alcoholism + BMT Manualized: Yes Sessions: 10 Txt Length: 10 weeks/2hrs. Approach: Used behavioral rehearsal and homework to decrease drinking and alcohol related interactions; develop communication skills 2) Individual treatment for alcoholism + Interactional Couples therapy Manualized: No Sessions: 10 Txt Length: 10 weeks/2 hrs. Approach: less structured group; not manualized or pre-planned; emphasized mutual support, sharing of feelings, problem solving through discussion and providing verbal insight on the relationship 3) Format: Individual treatment for alcoholism only Manualized: NA Sessions/Txt Length: NA Approach: NA	Family Outcomes Couple functioning a. Sexual Adjustment Questionnaire – multiple subscales	Allocation Concealment NR Blinding: Yes Intention-to-treat analysis: No Withdrawals adequately described: No Treatment integrity: Audiotaped, supervised sessions. Ratings of tx integrity used. Study Quality: Fair

Study, Year Funding Source	Sample Characteristics	Inclusion/Exclusion Criteria	Treatment Groups	Intervention Characteristics	Outcomes Assessed	Quality
O'Farrell, 2008[64] Government	N = 46 randomized N = 45 data analysis (one died after randomization) Gender: 96 % male Age: 47.8 years Race/ethnicity: White: 93% Black: 7% Hispanic: 0% Marital Status: NR Education: <HS or GED: 9% HS: 51% >HS: 40% Veterans: NR Family Characteristics: NR Recruitment Method Patients admitted to a hospital-based inpatient substance abuse detoxification unit were recruited.	MH Condition: Alcohol dependence (with or without comorbid drug diagnosis) Assessed by: inpatient unit/ medical records SO: wives, parents, or SO partner Inclusions: admitted to a inpatient detoxification unit, ages 21-65; living with wife, parent(s) or female partner prior to admit, live within 45 minutes driving distance of treatment center, no evidence of schizophrenia, organic mental disorder, paranoid disorder, other psychotic disorder Exclusions: None	1) Brief Family Treatment Intervention N=24 2) Treatment as usual (TAU) N=21 3) Brief Family Treatment subset N=9	1) Format: Brief Family Treatment Manualized: Yes Sessions: 2 session Txt Length: NR Approach: First session was in person or in depth telephone conference with patient and family member to develop a strategy for continuing care and to review options; help make practical plans for continuing care. Second call was phone call 2 weeks after detoxification discharge to find out success and troubleshoot continuing care 2) Format: TAU Manualized: No Sessions: NA Txt Length: 3–4 days inpatient detoxification Approach: Participants admitted for substance use detoxification; to assist with withdrawal symptoms; monitor risks for developing serious problems during withdrawal. Family not involved during detoxification unit stay (confirmed by medical record review). 3) Subset of Brief Family treatment group that compared in-person session to phone delivered session	Patient Outcomes Symptoms: a. % days substance use Utilization: a. % entered continuing care post inpatient detoxification b. Days attended continuing care	Allocation Concealment: Yes - um Blinding: NR Intention-to-treat analysis: Yes Withdrawals adequately described: Yes Treatment integrity: Counselors provided detailed steps for tx; cases reviewed weekly Study Quality: Poor

Family Involved Psychosocial Treatments for Adult Mental Health Conditions: A Review of the Evidence

Study, Year Funding Source	Sample Characteristics	Inclusion/Exclusion Criteria	Treatment Groups	Intervention Characteristics	Outcomes Assessed	Quality
O'Farrell, 2010[82] Government	N = 29 randomized N = 28 data analysis Gender: 55% male Age: 29.1 years Marital Status: Married/cohabitating: NR Race/ethnicity: White: 89.8% Education(years): 12.9 Veterans: NR Family Characteristics: Parent: 93% Sibling: 75 Age: 55.3 years Race/ethnicity: White: 89.5% Education(years): 14.1 Recruitment Method Patients who were living with a family member other than a spouse and who entered an outpatient clinic for tx for substance use were recruited.	MH Condition: Substance use Assessed by: unclear SO: non-spouse with whom patient lives. Inclusions: (a) age 18-65; living with adult family member other than a spouse or partner for at least 6 months in prior year, participant meets DSM criteria for alcohol or drug dependence or both; family member without current drug or alcohol dependence; patient and family member without serious mental illness, suicidal ideation or homicide risk; agreement to refrain from other substance use counseling except for self-help; agree to abstinence during study period. Exclusions: History in past 3 years of domestic violence when not using drugs/alcohol or if family voiced fear of violence due to tx; opioid use or maintenance in past 12 months; dependence on alcohol, heroin or other opioids that required detox; history of drug overdose or attempted suicide.	1) BFT+IBT (n=15) 2) IBT only (n=14)	1) Format: BFT+IBT Manualized: Yes Sessions: 24 (2/week, 60 min): 12 BFT, 12 IBT Txt Length: 12 weeks Approach: Patient and family members attended one session/ week which included "daily trust discussion." Tx emphasized daily support of abstinence, less on relationships enhancement to fit non-spousal relationship. IBT used Project MATCH manual 2) Format: IBT Manualized: Yes Sessions: 24 (2/week, 60 min) Txt Length: 12 weeks (2/week) Approach: Participants attended therapy by themselves. Project MATCH manual used (repeating each session twice).	Patient Outcomes Symptoms: a. PDA b. % days primary substance use Family Outcomes a. RHS-dyad score Intermediate Outcomes Attendance a. mean # sessions attended -	Allocation Concealment: NR Blinding: NR Intention-to-treat analysis: Yes Withdrawals adequately described: Yes Treatment integrity: Weekly supervision; review of audiotaped sessions Study Quality: Poor

Family Involved Psychosocial Treatments for Adult Mental Health Conditions: A Review of the Evidence

Study, Year Funding Source	Sample Characteristics	Inclusion/Exclusion Criteria	Treatment Groups	Intervention Characteristics	Outcomes Assessed	Quality
Walitzer, 2004[73] Government	N = 64 randomized N = 64 data analysis _Gender:_ 100% male _Age:_ 42.0 (11.3) years _Race/ethnicity:_ Non-Hispanic White: 98% _Marital Status:_ Married: 81% Unmarried, but cohabitating: 19% _Education (years):_ NR Veterans: NR _Recruitment Method_ Newspaper advertisements for "Couples Drinking Reduction Program" _Family Characteristics:_ _Gender:_ 100% female _Age:_ 39.3 (9.6) years _Race/ethnicity:_ Non-Hispanic White: 95%	_MH Condition:_ Alcohol abuse _Assessed by:_ Medical evaluation _SO:_ wife or cohabitating partner _Inclusion:_ Male subject drank ≥10 drinks/week; both subject and spouse willing to accept subject's goal of reduced drinking. _Exclusions:_ Subject psychiatric hospitalization in past 5 years, or multiple lifetime psych hospitalizations. For both subject and partner: 1) no alcohol related arrests in past year or no more than 2 lifetime alcohol related arrests; 2) concurrent alcohol treatment (other than self help group; 3) history of alcohol related hospitalization or detox; 4) serious domestic violence; 5) current separation; and 6) for unmarried couples, living together <6 months.	1) C/AF – couples with alcohol focus N=21 2) C/AF + BCT – couples with alcohol focus + Behavior Couples Therapy N=21 3) PDO – problem drinker only N=22 _Treatment adherence_ NR by group	1) _Format:_ C/AF _Manualized:_ Yes _Sessions:_ 10 weeks x 2 hours weekly _Approach:_ During first hour strategies to reduce alcohol consumption, strategies to increase spouse behaviors supportive of drinking reduction; last hour, alcohol and health lectures, with encouraged discussion between partners. 2) _Format:_ C/AF +BCT _Manualized:_ Yes _Sessions:_ 10 weeks x 2 hours weekly _Approach:_ During first hour strategies to reduce alcohol consumption, strategies to increase spouse behaviors supportive of drinking reduction; last hour, BCT series of treatment components to equip couples with skills to increase cohesion and positive relationship aspects, enhance communication and conflict resolution. 3) _Format:_ PDO _Manualized:_ Yes _Sessions:_ 10 weeks x 2 hours weekly _Approach:_ During first hour-strategies to reduce alcohol consumption, last hour-alcohol and health lectures	_Patient Outcomes_ Symptom Improvement a. TLFB – heavy days drinking/month b. TLFB – abstinent/light days drinking/month c. TLFB – time to heavy drinking episode Global Functioning a. Drinker Inventory of Consequences _Family Outcomes:_ Couple functioning: a. Partner Interaction Questionnaire b. Significant Other Behavior Questionnaire c. DAS	<u>Allocation concealment:</u> NR <u>Blinding:</u> NR <u>Intention to treat analysis:</u> Yes <u>Withdrawals adequately described:</u> Yes <u>Treatment integrity:</u> Weekly supervision, training of counselors, sessions audiotaped and checked against a session checklist. <u>**Study Quality:**</u> Fair

Family Involved Psychosocial Treatments for Adult Mental Health Conditions: A Review of the Evidence

Evidence-based Synthesis Program

Study, Year Funding Source	Sample Characteristics	Inclusion/Exclusion Criteria	Treatment Groups	Intervention Characteristics	Outcomes Assessed	Quality
Winters, 2002[76] Government	N = 75 randomized N = 75 data analysis Gender: 100% female Age: 32.9 years Marital Status: Married/cohabitating:100% Race/ethnicity: White: 70% Black: 24% Hispanic: 1% Education (years): 12.3 Veterans: NR Family Characteristics: Male Intimate Partner: 100% Age: 35.2 years Marital Status: Married/cohabitating:100% Race/ethnicity: White 61% Black 31% Hispanic 8% Recruitment Method Married and cohabitating women entering tx for substance use were asked to participate.	MH Condition: Drug Abuse Assessed by: Diagnostic clinical interview SO: Male intimate partner Inclusions: age 20-60; married ≥ 1 yr or living with SO in a stable common law relationship ≥ 2 yrs; meet abuse or dependence criteria for ≥ 1 psychoactive substance use disorder (not nicotine), primary drug of abuse not alcohol; agree to refrain from psychoactive substances during treatment; no additional substance-abuse treatment except self-help meetings during treatment unless recommended by primary individual therapists Exclusions: male partner met criteria for psychoactive substance use disorder in past 6 months; male or female partners met criteria for organic mental disorder, schizophrenia, delusional (paranoid) disorder, or other psychotic disorders; or female partners were in a methadone maintenance program and seeking treatment for adjunctive outpatient support.	1) Behavior Couples Therapy and Individual Behavioral Therapy N = 37 2) Individual Behavioral Therapy N = 38	1) Format: Individual and group counseling + couple therapy Manualized: Yes Sessions: 56; Weeks 1-12: 1 group; 1 individual; 1 couple therapy session per week; Weeks 13-20: 1 individual session per week; emergency sessions as needed Txt Length: 20 weeks Approach: Individual cognitive-behavioral therapy for skills building + Behavioral Couples Therapy including a sobriety contract daily between couples, communication skills, and positive behavioral exchange 2) Format: Group, individual, and behavioral couples therapy Manualized: Yes Sessions: 56; Weeks 1-12: 1 group; 2 individual per week; Weeks 13-20: 1 individual session per week; emergency sessions as needed Txt Length: 20 weeks Approach: Individual cognitive-behavioral therapy for skills building	Patient Outcomes Symptoms a. PDA Family Outcomes Couple functioning a. DAS b. MHS Intermediate Outcomes Attendance a. session attendance Treatment Satisfaction a. CSQ	Allocation Concealment: NR Blinding: NR Intention-to-treat analysis: Yes Withdrawals adequately described: Yes Treatment integrity: Trained and supervised Study Quality: Good

NR = not reported; HS = high school; SO = significant other or family member included; DSM = Diagnostic and Statistical Manual of Mental Disorders; CM = Contingency Management; tx = treatment; BCT=Behavioral couple therapy; PDA = percent days abstinent; ASI = Addiction Severity Index; CSQ =Client Satisfaction Questionnaire; MHS = Marital Happiness Scale; ACQ=Areas of Change Questionnaire; PI = Principal Investigator; MAT=Locke Wallace Marital adjustment test; CTS =Conflict Tactics Scale; IBMM = Individual Based Methadone Maintenance; ns = not significant; BFT = Behavioral Family Therapy; IBT = Individual Based Therapy; PACT = Psychoeducational Attention Control Treatment; PDHD=percent days heavy drinking; DAS=Dyadic Adjustment Scale; S-BCT=Standard Behavioral Couples Therapy; TLFB=Time Line Follow Back interview; HOPE = Helping Other Partners Excel; BDI = Beck Depression Inventory; CRT= Community reinforcement training intervention; PSBCT = Parent Skills with Behavioral Couples Therapy; BMT = Behavioral Marital Therapy; ABMT = Alcohol focused spouse involvement plus behavioral marital therapy; AA = Alcoholics Anonymous; RP = Relapse prevention; MMSE = Mini mental Status Exam; CRAFT= Community Reinforcement and Family Training; CSO = concerned significant other; FES = Family Environment Scale; RHS = Relationship Happiness Scale; CBQ = Couples Behaviors Questionnaire; TAU = Treatment as usual; C/AF = couples with alcohol focus; PDO= problem drinker only; MAST = Michigan Alcoholism Screening Test

Table 2. Patient Outcomes – Substance Abuse Studies

Study, Year Interventions Sample	Baseline	Post-Treatment	Short-term Follow-up	Long-term Follow-up
SYMPTOM IMPROVEMENT				
Carroll, 2001[77] 1) SO+CM+Naltrexone 2) CM+Naltrexone 3) Naltrexone only	Drug Free Urine Screens 1) 16.7 (15.1) N=48 2) 13.6 (13.6) N=35 3) 8.9 (12.0) N=44 1) vs. 2) (p=0.35) **1) & 2) vs. 3) (p=0.02)**	Opiate Free Urine Screens 1) 20.2 (15.5) N=48 2) 18.9 (13.7) N=35 3) 13.5 (12.0) N=44 1) vs. 2) (p=0.48) **1) & 2) vs. 3) (p=0.04)**		
		Cocaine Free Urine Screens 1) 18.5 (15.0) N=48 2) 16 (13.5) N=35 3) 12.2 (12.6) N=44 1) vs. 2) (p=0.44) 1) & 2) vs. 3) (p=0.06)		
		% Drug-Free Urine 1) 59.7% (39.7) 2) 57.4% (39.1) 3) 45.2% (39.3) 1) vs. 2) (p=.77) 1) & 2) vs. 3) (p=0.08)		
		PDA, Opioids 1) 89% (20.3) 2) 87.5% (20.9) 3) 79.8% (25.5) 1) vs. 2) (p=.37) 1) & 2) vs. 3) (p=0.06)		
		PDA, Cocaine 1) 88.6% (14.9) 2) 84.3% (24.5) 3) 82.6% (23.0) 1) vs. 2) (p=.77) 1) & 2) vs. 3) (p=0.06)		
		Maximum PDA, Opioids 1) 53.4% (36.5) 2) 49.1% (32.7) 3) 37.7% (32.8) 1) vs. 2) (p=0.60) **1) & 2) vs. 3) (p=0.05)**		

Family Involved Psychosocial Treatments for Adult Mental Health Conditions: A Review of the Evidence

Study, Year Interventions *Sample*	Baseline	Post-Treatment	Short-term Follow-up	Long-term Follow-up
Fals-Stewart, 1996,[66] 2002,[85] 1) BCT 2) IBT *Per protocol analysis*		Maximum PDA, Cocaine 1) 51.7% (35.4) 2) 49.1% (32.7) 3) 37.7% (32.8) 1) vs. 2) (p=0.39) 1) & 2) vs. 3) (p=0.09)		
	PDA, drugs 1) 37.9% (30.1) 2) 38.4% (30.4) p=ns	PDA, drugs 1) 97.1% (9.2) 2) 94.1% (8.6) p=ns	PDA, drugs 1) 84.4% (25.3) 2) 73.2% (23.3) (authors reported significant difference, but p-value NR)	PDA, drugs 1) 76.6% (27.7) 2) 69.4% (22.1) (authors reported significant difference, but p-value NR)
	PDA, alcohol 1) 78.3% (46.5) 2) 79.4% (40.7) p=ns	PDA, alcohol 1) 97.4% (21.1) 2) 96.3% (20.4) p=ns	PDA, alcohol 1) 84.3% (28.7) 2) 78.6% (29.9) p=ns	PDA, alcohol 1) 77.4% (34.9) 2) 71.6% (33.6) p=ns
	PDA, alcohol and drugs 1) 31.3% (38.6) 2) 28.2% (34.4) p=ns	PDA, alcohol and drugs 1) 95.4% (15.4) 2) 91.1% (14.1) p=ns	PDA, alcohol and drugs 1) 81.5% (28.6) 2) 70.4% (24.5) (authors reported significant difference, but p-value NR)	PDA, alcohol and drugs 1) 73.2% (29.8) 2) 65.1% (26.9) (authors reported significant difference, but p-value NR)
				% change in days abstinent % improved 1) 83% 2) 60% p=.03 % Unchanged 1) 17% 2) 40% p=NR
	% days alcohol/drug use 1) 68.7% (38.6) 2) 71.8% (34.4), p=ns			% days alcohol/drug use 1) 19.0% (26.9) 2) 29.7% (26.1) (authors reported significant difference, but p-value NR)
	% days drug use 1) 62.1% (30.1) 2) 61.7% (30.4) p=ns			% days drug use 1) 16.5% (25.1) 2) 26.1% (24.0) (authors reported significant difference, but p-value NR)
	% days alcohol use 1) 21.7% (46.5) 2) 20.6% (40.7) p=ns			% days alcohol use 1) 16.4% (30.3) 2) 22.3% (29.9) (authors reported significant difference, but p-value NR)
	% days heavy alcohol use 1) 17.9% (31.2) 2) 18.3% (33.6) p=ns			% days heavy alcohol use 1) 8.4% (19.2) 2) 16.9% (20.4) (authors reported significant difference, but p-value NR)

Family Involved Psychosocial Treatments for Adult Mental Health Conditions: A Review of the Evidence

Study, Year Interventions *Sample*	Baseline	Post-Treatment	Short-term Follow-up	Long-term Follow-up
Fals-Stewart, 2001[67] 1) BCT 2) IBMM *Completers*	Alcohol composite score of ASI 1) 0.32 (.06) N=19 2) 0.33 (.07) N=17 p=ns	Alcohol composite score of ASI 1) 0.27 (.06) N=19 2) 0.34 (.08) N=17 Paired t-test, p=ns for both BCT and IBMM		
	Drug composite score of ASI 1) 0.44 (.08) N=19 2) 0.41 (.09) N=17 p=ns	Drug composite score of ASI 1) **0.16 (.09) N=19** 2) **0.28 (.08) N=17** **p<0.01**		
Fals-Stewart, 2003[68] 1) Naltrexone + BFT 2) Naltrexone + IBT *ITT*				PDA from opioids 1) **69.3% (21.4)** 2) **56.3% (20.2)** **p<.01**
				PDA from cocaine 1) **74.4% (22.9)** 2) **61.8% (24.2)** **p<0.05**
				PDA from alcohol 1) **69.4% (23.2)** 2) **60.1% (24.2)** **p<0.05**
				PDA from drugs 1) **59.6% (26.4)** 2) **49.3% (28.4)** **p<0.05**
Fals-Stewart, 2005[69] 1) BBCT 2) S-SBT 3) IBT 4) PACT *ITT*	PDHD 1) 56.32% (22.41) 2) 58.91% (24.34) 3) 59.47% (25.23) 4) 57.46% (26.12) p=NR	PDHD 1) 5.0% (12.2) 2) 5.2% (14.3) 3) 4.9% (15.1) 4) 5.0% (17.0) p=NR	PDHD 1) 15.0% (18.0) 2) 14.1% (19.3) 3) 23.6% (15.0) 4) 24.3% (15.0) p=NR	PDHD 1) 19.5% (20.2) 2) 19.2% (38.2) 3) 38.2% (25.6) 4) 37.3% (27.0) p=NR
		Piecewise growth model for effect of tx condition on PDHD: **Equivalence test between:** **1) vs. 2): z=0.16, p<0.05** Group differences between: 1) vs. 3): z=-0.06, p=ns 1) vs. 4): z=-0.01, p=ns		*Piecewise growth model for effect of tx condition on PDHD after tx:* **Equivalence test between:** **1) vs. 2): z=0.13, p<0.05** **Group differences between:** **1) vs. 3): z=-2.02, p<0.05** **1) vs. 4): z=2.34, p<0.05**

Family Involved Psychosocial Treatments for Adult Mental Health Conditions: A Review of the Evidence

Study, Year Interventions Sample	Baseline	Post-Treatment	Short-term Follow-up	Long-term Follow-up
Fals-Stewart, 2006[74] 1) BCT 2) IBT 3) PACT ITT	PDA 1) 44.21% (35.10) 2) 40.82% (34.26) 3) 43.70% (30.64) p=ns	PDA 1) 96.3% (16.3) 2) 93.6% (17.7) 3) 94.5% (14.8) p=ns *Piecewise growth model for effect of tx condition on PDA:* **Group differences between:** **1) vs. 2): z=1.02, p=ns** **1) vs. 3): z=0.99, p=ns**	PDA 1) 85.9% (18.1) 2) 75.0% (20.3) 3) 74.4% (22.5) p=ns	PDA 1) 79.3% (29.7) 2) 60.2% (20.9) 3) 62.1% (21.6) p<0.01 *Piecewise growth model for effect of tx condition on linear rate of change in PDA after tx:* **Group differences between:** **1) vs. 2): z=-3.3, p<0.05** **1) vs. 3): z=2.4, p<0.05**
Fals-Stewart, 2008[78] 1) BBCT 2) BCT 3) IBT 4) PACT ITT	PDA 1) 36.2% (29.4) 2) 38.3% (32.1) 3) 37.0% (30.5) 4) 34.0% (32.2) p=NR	PDA 1) 93.7% (12.6) 2) 94.1% (13.4) 3) 88.3% (13.0) 4) 89.6% (14.1) p=NR *Piecewise growth model for effect of tx condition on PDA:* **Equivalence test between:** **1) vs. 2): z=0.02, p<0.05** Group difference between: 1) vs. 3): z=0.2, p=ns 1) vs. 4): z=0.1, p=ns	PDA 1) 83.4% (27.2) 2) 84.1% (26.5) 3) 70.3% (27.1) 4) 69.5% (25.1) p=NR	PDA 1) 75.6% (26.7) 2) 74.1% (25.8) 3) 60.2% (27.3) 4) 58.9% (31.2) p=NR *Piecewise growth model for effect of tx condition on PDHD after tx:* **Equivalence test between:** **1) vs. 2): z=0.2, p<0.05** Group differences between: 1) vs. 3): z=2.1, p<0.05 1) vs. 4): z=2.3, p<0.05
Fals-Stewart, 2009[79] 1) BCT 2) IBT	TLFB – PDHD (men) 1) 41.9 (18.7) N=NR 2) 43.8 (21.6) N=NR p=NR TLFB – PDHD (women) 1) 38.6 (16.4) N=NR 2) 39.8 (19.7) N=NR p=NR	TLFB – PDHD (men) 1) 6.0 (13.6) N=NR 2) 5.3 (14.9) N=NR p=NR TLFB – PDHD (women) 1) 5.1 (14.1) N=NR 2) 5.3 (14.1) N=NR p=NR *Multi-level growth model for effect of tx condition on PDHD (men):* **Group difference between:** 1) vs. 2): z=-1.1, p=ns *Multi-level growth model for effect of tx condition on PDHD (women):* **Group difference between:** 1) vs. 2): z= 0.4, p=ns	TLFB – PDHD (men) 1) 13.6 (18.9) N=NR 2) 25.4 (21.1) N=NR p<0.05 TLFB – PDHD (women) 1) 11.9 (15.8) N=NR 2) 20.6 (18.2) N=NR p<0.05	TLFB – PDHD (men) 1) 18.0 (20.5) N=NR 2) 32.2 (23.5) N=NR p<0.05 TLFB – PDHD (women) 1) 15.7 (20.4) N=NR 2) 27.9 (20.6) N=NR p<0.05 *Multi-level growth model for effect of tx condition on PDHD after tx (men):* **Group difference between:** **1) vs. 2): z= -2.1, p<0.05** *Multi-level growth model for effect of tx condition on PDHD after tx (women):* **Group difference between:** **1) vs. 2): z= 2.4, p<0.05**

Family Involved Psychosocial Treatments for Adult Mental Health Conditions: A Review of the Evidence

Study, Year Interventions *Sample*	Baseline	Post-Treatment	Short-term Follow-up	Long-term Follow-up
Jones, 2011[70] 1) HOPE 2) Usual Care *ITT*	Days of heroin use 1) 27.3 (1.4) N=45 2) 26.6 (2.4) N=17 p>0.8	Days of heroin use (mid-tx 4 weeks) 1) **4.9 (1.7)** 2) **16.2 (2.6)** **p<0.001**	Days of heroin use 1) **9.8 (1.9)** 2) **3.4 (6.2)** **p<0.001**	
	Heroin use past 30 days 1) 100% N=45 2) 100% N=17 p=n/a	Heroin use past 30 days (mid tx – 4 weeks) 1) 63% (0.40) 2) 91% (1.05) p=NR	Heroin use past 30 days 1) 53% (0.40) 2) 61% (1.16) p=0.25	
	ASI Composite, Drugs 1) 0.36 (0.02) N=45 2) 0.34 (0.03) N=17 p=NR	ASI Composite, Drugs (mid tx – 4 weeks) 1) 0.19 (0.02) 2) 0.23 (0.04) p=NR	ASI Composite, Drugs 1) 0.20 (0.03) 2) 0.12 (0.08) p=0.32	
Kelley, 2002[63] 1) BCT 2) IBT 3) PACT *ITT*	PDA (alcohol abusing pts) 1) 40.0 (35.5) N=25 2) 36.9 (33.3) N=22 3) 27.4 (29.2) N=24 p=ns	PDA (alcohol abusing pts) 1) 90.2 (21.9) 2) 86.6 (17.4) 3) 87.4 (18.2) p=ns	PDA (alcohol abusing pts) 1) **80.6 (27.2) vs. 2) 71.4 (26.2)** 1) **80.6 (27.2) vs. 3) 70.4 (25.3)** **p<0.05**	PDA (alcohol abusing pts) 1) **70.9 (25.6) vs. 2) 60.4 (22.4)** 1) **70.9 (25.6) vs. 3) 57.9 (32.1)** **p<0.05**
	PDA (drug abusing pts) 1) 30.4 (33.7) N=22 2) 32.7 (33.6) N=22 3) 34.9 (36.9) N=21 p=ns	PDA (drug abusing pts) 1) 85.9 (22.7) 2) 81.8 (26.2) 3) 83.4 (24.4) p=ns	PDA (drug abusing pts) 1) **77.6 (25.8) vs. 2) 63.6 (24.3)** 1) **77.6 (25.8) vs. 3) 61.5 (26.8)** **p<0.05**	PDA (drug abusing pts) 1) **66.9 (35.6) vs. 2) 53.4 (24.8)** 1) **66.9 (35.6) vs 3) 51.2 (32.2)** **p<0.05**
Kirby, 2009[80] 1) CRT 2) Self Help		**SO knowledge of current drug use (5=sure he is using; 1=sure he is not using)** 1) 2.20 2) 2.43 p=ns		
Lam, 2009[71] 1) PSBCT 2) BCT 3) IBT *ITT*	PDA 1) 38.3 (28.1) N=10 2) 39.2 (25.4) N=10 3) 37.6 (29.7) N=10 p=NR r≥0.5 large 1) vs. 3): z=0.24, ns; r=0.03 1) vs. 2): z=0.11; ns; r-0.02	PDA 1) 90.1 (18.6) N=10 2) 92.3 (15.2) N=10 3) 88.3 (16.7) N=10 p=NR r≥0.5 large 1) vs. 3): z=-0.28, ns; r=0.03 1) vs. 2): z=0.39; ns; r-0.23	PDA 1) 84.3 (22.4) N=10 2) 85.1 (20.7) N=10 3) 78.2 (22.6) N=10 p=NR r≥0.5 large 1) vs. 3): z=-1.08, ns; r=0.23 1) vs. 2): z=0.13; ns; r-0.02	PDA 1) 78.6 (19.4) N=10 2) 77.8 (20.2) N=10 3) 70.2 (18.6) N=10 p=NR r≥0.5 large 1) vs. 3): z=-1.4, ns; r=0.33 1) vs. 2): z=0.10; ns; r-0.02

Family Involved Psychosocial Treatments for Adult Mental Health Conditions: A Review of the Evidence

Study, Year Interventions Sample	Baseline	Post-Treatment	Short-term Follow-up	Long-term Follow-up
McCrady, 1996,[72] 1999[86] 1) ABMT 2) AA/ABMT 3) RP/ABMT	Mean % drinking days 1) 15.1 (24.6) N=22 2) 19.4 (21.1) N=23 3) 9.8 (11.1) N=22 p=ns			
	Mean # drinks per drinking days 1) 7.3 (9.7) N=14 2) 5.9 (5.0) N=19 3) 4.6 (2.7) N=17 p=ns			
	PDA 1) 36.7 (32.0) N=21 2) 33.4 (24.3) N=26 3) 46.3 (30.0) N=24 p=ns	PDA 1) 80.0 (27.2) 2) 83.2 (22.7) 3) 87.6 (20.6) p=ns	PDA 1) 82.4 (25.3) N=21 2) 72.8 (33.6) N=26 3) 82.6 (24.5) N=24 p=ns	
		PDHD 1) 10.0 (19.1) 2) 9.4 (15.7) 3) 6.6 (16.9) p=ns	PDHD 1) 6.1 (11.3) N=14 2) 17.1 (25.2) N=15 3) 9.0 (17.0) N=16 p=ns	
	Mean Length of Drinking Episodes 1) 5.4 (7.6) vs. 2) 8.4 (14.6) 3) 1.9 (1.7) vs. 2) 8.4 (14.6) p<0.05			
		% participants continuously abstinent 1) 31.8 N=22 2) 41.7 N=24 3) 41.7 N=24 p=NR		
		% non-problem drinking, mostly controlled 1) 18.2 N=22 2) 4.2 N=24 3) 8.3 N=24 p=NR		
		% drinking but improved 1) 18.2 N=22 2) 8.3 N=24 3) 25.0 N=24 p=NR		
		% unimproved (pre to post-6 months) 1) 31.8 N=22 2) 45.8 N=24 3) 25.0 N=24 p=NR		

Family Involved Psychosocial Treatments for Adult Mental Health Conditions: A Review of the Evidence

Study, Year Interventions Sample	Baseline	Post-Treatment	Short-term Follow-up	Long-term Follow-up
McCrady, 2004[87] 1) ABMT 2) AA/ABMT 3) RP/ABMT *Not ITT*			PDA 1) 79.51 (29.6) N=20 2) 70.41 (37.32) N=24 3) 80.63 (30.28) N=22 p=NR	PDA 1) 82.7 (30.7) N=20 2) 78.7 (33.4) N=24 3) 83.1 (29.4) N=22 p=NR
McCrady, 2009[75] 1) ABCT 2) ABIT *Completers*	PDA 1) 35.0 (29.2) N=50 2) 32.0 (28.0) N=52 p=NR	PDA 1) 80.5 (27.7) N=50 2) 74.2 (35.0) N=52 p=NR	PDA 1) 75.7 (34.3) N=50 2) 61.4 (39.5) N=52 p=NR	PDA 1) 75.4 (34.7) N=50 2) 63.1 (37.6) N=52 p=NR
				Latent growth curve models for PDA: Differences between groups: d =0.31 (small effect), p=ns
	PDHD 1) 56.8 (28.9) N=50 2) 57.3 (32.3) N=52 p=NR	PDHD 1) 10.5 (22.2) N=50 2) 18.7 (34.6) N=52 p=NR	PDHD 1) 12.3 (27.4) N=50 2) 23.8 (37.6) N=52 p=NR_	PDHD 1) 12.8 (26.2) N=50 2) 22.7 (34.2) N=52 p=NR
				Latent growth curve models for PDHD: Differences between groups: d =0.19 (small effect), p=ns
		% complete abstinence after treatment 1) 36.0 N=50 2) 34.6 N=52 p=NR		% complete abstinence after treatment 1) 16 N=50 2) 15.4 N=52 p=NR (ns)
			% no heavy drinking days 1) 60.0 N=50 2) 55.8 N=52 p=NR	% no heavy drinking days 1) 26.0 N=50 2) 28.8 N=52 p=NR
O'Farrell, 1998a[4] 1) BMT/RP 2) BMT *Sample Unclear*	PDA 1) 33.7 (27.6) 2) 29.2 (25.4) p=ns	PDA 1) 98.9 (4.4) 2) 98.0 (6.6) p=ns	PDA **1) 96.9 (6.9)** **2) 87.6 (21.2)** **p=0.03**	PDA 1) 84.9 (25.3) 2) 82.7 (26.1) p=ns
O'Farrell, 2008[64] 1) Brief Family Treatment 2) Brief Family Treatment-in person 3) TAU *Completers*	TLFB - % days alcohol/ drug use 1) NR N=24 3) NR N=19 p=NR	TLFB - % days alcohol/drug use 1) NR N=24 3) NR N=19 p=NR r=NR	TLFB - % days alcohol/drug use 1) 22.6 (36.3) N=24 3) 36.1 (40.3) N=19 p=0.25 r=0.17 small	
	TLFB - % days alcohol or drug use (in person subset) 2) NR N=9 3) NR N=19 p=NR	TLFB - % days alcohol or drug use (in person subset) 2) NR N=9 3) NR N=19 p=NR r: NR	TLFB - % days alcohol or drug use (in person subset) 2) 10.6 (28.3) N=9 3) 36.1 (40.3) N=19 p= 0.07 r=0.33 medium	

Family Involved Psychosocial Treatments for Adult Mental Health Conditions: A Review of the Evidence

Study, Year Interventions *Sample*	Baseline	Post-Treatment	Short-term Follow-up	Long-term Follow-up
O'Farrell, 2010[82] 1) BFT+IBT 2) IBT *ITT*	PDA 1) 32.5 (33.42) 2) 35.2 (27.3) p=ns PDPSU 1) 51.9 (29.5) 2) 55.8 (27.7) p=ns	PDA 1) 71.1(37.0) 2) 43.6 (41.9) p=ns PDPSU 1) 19.9 (27.5) 2) 41.1 (37.3) p=ns	PDA 1) 57.7 (40.4) 2) 46.4 (32.0) p=ns PDPSU 1) 29.2 (41.4) 2) 38.7 (30.6) p=ns	
Walitzer, 2004[73] 1) C/AF+BCT (family tx) 2) C/AF 3) PDO (individual tx) *Completers*	Abstinent/light days drinking/month 1) 17.8 (7.7) N=21 2) 17.7 (7.1) N=21 3) 15.7 (9.1) N=22 p=NR Heavy days drinking/month 1) 4.9 (4.2) N=21 2) 3.6 (3.9) N=21 3) 6.7 (8.8) N=22 p=NR	Abstinent/light days drinking/month 1) 22.2 (4.9) N=20 2) 21.4 (7.0) N=21 3) 16.2 (8.9) N=22 p=NR Heavy days drinking/month 1) 1.5 (1.8) N=20 2) 1.8 (2.3) N=21 3) 4.7 (4.5) N=22 p=NR	Abstinent/light days drinking/month 1) 21.2 (7.8) N=20 2) 20.8 (6.7) N=21 3) 16.7 (9.6) N=21 p=NR Heavy days drinking/month 1) 3.1 (4.9) N=20 2) 2.1 (3.2) N=21 3) 5.5 (6.1) N=21 p=NR	Abstinent/light days drinking/month 1) 22.9 (5.4) N=20 2) 20.1 (8.0) N=21 3) 17.1 (10.4) N=20 p=NR Heavy days drinking/month 1) 2.6 (4.7) N=20 2) 1.9 (2.5) N=21 3) 5.8 (7.7) N=20 p=NR
Winters, 2002[76] 1) BCT+ICBT 2) ICBT *ITT*	PDA 1) 42.3 (29.2) 2) 45.2 (28.3) p=ns	PDA 1) 94.2 (6.4) 2) 90.2 (8.0) p=ns	PDA 1) **81.9 (16.3)** 2) **71.9 (17.9)** **p<0.05**	PDA 1) 74.2 (22.2) 2) 65.4 (26.1) p=ns

HEALTH CARE UTILIZATION

Study, Year Interventions *Sample*	Baseline	Post-Treatment	Short-term Follow-up	Long-term Follow-up
Kirby, 1999[80] 1) CRT 2) Self Help	% of pt entry into treatment during FSO treatment 1) **64%** 2) **17%** **p<0.01**			
McCrady, 2009[75] 1) ABCT 2) ABIT *Completers*				% pts receiving add'l tx 1) 18.0 2) 11.5 p=NR (ns) Days add'l tx 1) 37.6 (26.6) 2) 24.7 (24.7) p= NR
Meyers, 2002[83] 1) CRAFT 2) CRAFT+Aftercare 3) AA/AL-NAR Facilitation Therapy		Pt completes a baseline assessment and schedules a substance use tx session 1) **58.6%** 2) **76.7%** 3) **29.0%**, **p<0.01** Both CRAFT conditions (1 & 2) better than condition 3, but no significant differences between conditions 1 and 2		

Study, Year Interventions *Sample*	Baseline	Post-Treatment	Short-term Follow-up	Long-term Follow-up
Miller, 1999[81] 1) CRAFT 2) Johnson Institute 3) AA *ITT*			% completing at least an initial assessment and 1 substance use treatment session **1) 64.4% vs. 2) 30.0% 1) 64.4% vs. 3) 13.3% p<0.001**	% completing at least an initial assessment and 1 substance use treatment session **1) 66.7% vs. 2) 35.0% 1) 66.7% vs. 3) 20.0% p<0.001**
O'Farrell, 2008[64] 1) Brief Family Treatment 2) Brief Family Treatment+in person subgroup 3) TAU			% continued care in 30 day period post detoxification (1 month post-treatment) **1) 92% N=24 2) 62% N=21 p=0.02; r=0.36 medium** Days attended continuing care in 3 months post tx (3 months post-treatment) 1) 12.4 (11.4) N=24 2) 7.2 (11.3) N=19 p=0.13; r=0.22 small	
GLOBAL FUNCTIONING				
Jones, 2011[70] 1) HOPE 2) UC *ITT*	Beck Depression Inventory 1) 13.7 (1.5) N=45 2) 18.7 (2.4) N=17 p=0.10	Beck Depression Inventory Mid-treatment (4 weeks): 1) 6.6 (1.7) 2) 14.3 (2.6) p=NR	Beck Depression Inventory 1) 9.7 (5.6) 2) 7.5 (1.9) p=0.56	
Walitzer, 2004[73] 1) C/AF+BCT (family tx) 2) C/AF 3) PDO (individual tx) *Completers*	Drinker Inventory of Consequences 1) 19.7 (9.9) N=19 2) 20.4 (1.7) N=21 3) 21.9 (18.4) N=21 p=NR		Drinker Inventory of Consequences 1) 12.2 (13.2) N=16 2) 13.5 (11.9) N=18 3) 15.5 (12.1) N=17 p=NR	Drinker Inventory of Consequences 1) 12.8 (14.4) N=17 2) 15.6 (16.1) N=18 3) 11.6 (8.4) N=15 p=NR

Outcomes reported as mean (standard deviation) unless otherwise noted.

Short-term follow up = 6 months post-treatment, unless otherwise noted; Long term=12 months post-treatment, unless otherwise noted. If an outcome had a final measure reported beyond 12 months, it is reported in long term follow up column and noted.

Measures listed in the study descriptive tables but not reported here if either 1) the authors did not report findings from these measures or 2) they did not test for differences between conditions on these measures.

ns = not significant (at 5% level); NR = not reported; N/A = not applicable; tx = treatment; Completers = findings for analyses conducted only with treatment completers; ITT = findings for analyses using an intent-to-treat approach.

BCT = Behavioral Couple/Marital Therapy; BFT = Behavioral Family Therapy ; CBT = Individual Cognitive-Behavioral Therapy; BBCT = Brief Behavioral Couples Therapy; IBT = Individual Based Treatment; ACT = Assertive Community Treatment; MFG = Multiple Family Group; SAS-FV = Social Adjustment Scale III, Family Version; AFM = Applied Family Management; SFM = Supportive Family Management; SC = Standard care; MSANS = Modified Scale for Assessment of Negative Symptoms; PDA = Percent Days Abstinent; PDHD = Percent Days Heavy Drinking; FSO = family member or significant other; CRT = Community Reinforcement Training; PSBCT = Parent Skills with Behavioral Couples Therapy; ABMT = Alcohol focused behavioral marital therapy; AA = Alcoholics Anonymous/Al-Anon; RP = relapse prevention; TAU = Treatment as usual.

Table 3. Family Outcomes – Substance Abuse Studies

Study, Year Interventions Sample	Baseline	Post-Treatment	Short-term Follow-up	Long-term Follow-up
FAMILY FUNCTIONING				
Carroll, 2001[77] 1) SO + CM + Naltrexone 2) CM + Naltrexone 3) Naltrexone only		Addiction Severity Index (z-score) **1) vs. 2) 2.30 p=0.02 1) vs. 2) & 3) = -2.4, p=0.02**		
Fals-Stewart, 2003[68] 1) BFT 2) IBT	Family functioning subscale of Addiction Severity Index **1) 0.4 (.08) 2) 0.5 (.09) authors reported significant difference, but p-value NR**	Family functioning subscale of Addiction Severity Index **1) 0.2 (.1) 2) 0.3 (.1) authors reported significant difference, but p-value NR**		
Kirby, 1999[80] 1) CRT 2) 12-step		Social Adjustment Scale (family unit subscale, pre-post change) 1) -.64 2) -.54 p=ns		
Miller, 1999[81] 1) CRAFT 2) Johnson Institute 3) Al-Anon *ITT*	SO's report of Family Environment Scale – Family Cohesion 1) 5.6 (2.6) 2) 4.4 (2.2) 3) 5.3 (2.9) p=ns	SO's report of Family Environment Scale – Family Cohesion 1) 6.2 (2.8) 2) 5.2 (3.0) 3) 5.8 (2.7) p=ns	SO's report of Family Environment Scale – Family Cohesion 1) 6.8 (2.3) 2) 5.9 (2.6) 3) 5.7 (2.9) p=ns	
	SO's report of Relationship Happiness Scale 1) 4.9 (2.8) 2) 4.8 (2.0) 3) 5.6 (2.3) p=ns	SO's report of Relationship Happiness Scale 1) 5.9 (2.8) 2) 4.8 (2.6) 3) 5.6 (2.7) p=ns	SO's report of Relationship Happiness Scale 1) 6.4 (2.7) 2) 5.9 (2.6) 3) 6.3 (2.8) p=ns	

Family Involved Psychosocial Treatments for Adult Mental Health Conditions: A Review of the Evidence

Study, Year Interventions Sample	Baseline	Post-Treatment	Short-term Follow-up	Long-term Follow-up
COUPLE FUNCTIONING				
Fals-Stewart, 1996, [66, 84, 85] 1) BCT 2) IBT	Marital Adjustment Test **1) 67.5 (20.1)** **2) 66.9 (20.8)** **authors reported significant difference, but p-value NR**	Marital Adjustment Test **1) 97.3 (17.2)** **2) 70.8 (17.5)** **authors reported significant difference, but p-value NR**	Marital Adjustment Test 1) 71.7 (19.3) 2) 70.2 (18.4) p=ns	Marital Adjustment Test 1) 71.6 (21.2) 2) 70.2 (18.8) p=ns
	Areas of Change Questionnaire **1) 34.4 (10.9)** **2) 36.2 (13.0)** **authors reported significant difference, but p-value NR**	Areas of Change Questionnaire **1) 20.0 (11.9)** **2) 32.7 (13.8)** **authors reported significant difference, but p-value NR**	Areas of Change Questionnaire 1) 35.0 (11.7) 2) 38.7 (12.1) p=ns	Areas of Change Questionnaire 1) 34.1 (11.8) 2) 37.0 (12.0) p=ns
	% days separated 1) 19.8 (17.7) 2) 17.6 (18.4) p=NR	% days separated 1) 3.5 (4.3) 2) 15.1 (16.3) p=NR	% days separated 1) 7.4 (18.6) 2) 22.4 (24.6) p=NR	% days separated 1) 20.7 (21.4) 2) 22.4 (29.1) p=ns
		% change on Marital Adjustment Test **% Improved** **1) 60%** **2) 35% (p=0.03)** % unchanged 1) 38% 2) 50% (p=0.26) **deteriorated** **1) 2%** **2) 15% (p=0.05)**		
	Aggregated MAT scores **1) 67.5 (20.1)** **2) 66.9 (20.8)** **authors reported significant difference, but p-value NR**			Aggregated MAT scores **1) 76.0 (20.4)** **2) 69.9 (19.0)** **authors reported significant difference, but p-value NR**
	Aggregated ACQ scores 1) 34.4 (10.9) 2) 36.2 (13.0) p=ns			Aggregated ACQ scores 1) 32.4 (11.9) 2) 37.3 (13.4) p=ns
Fals-Stewart, 2001[67] 1) BCT 2) IBMM *Completers*	Dyadic Adjustment Scale 1) 72.8 (18.1) N=19 2) 75.1 (19.4) N=17 p=ns	Dyadic Adjustment Scale* **1) 97.9 (16.4) N=19** **2) 79.2 (18.1) N=17** **p<0.01** *using baseline DAS as a covariate		

Family Involved Psychosocial Treatments for Adult Mental Health Conditions: A Review of the Evidence

Study, Year Interventions Sample	Baseline	Post-Treatment	Short-term Follow-up	Long-term Follow-up
	ASI – Family-Social Composite Score 1) 0.47 (0.08) N=19 2) 0.54 (0.09) N=17 p=NR	ASI – Family-Social Composite Score* 1) 0.23 (0.06) N=19 2) 0.46 (0.08) N=17 p<0.05		
Fals-Stewart, 2005[69] 1) BRT 2) S-BFT 3) IBT 4) PACT *Male partner only*	Dyadic Adjustment Scale 1) 88.26 (21.64) 2) 89.94 (22.61) 3) 90.61 (24.27) 4) 89.21 (22.61) p=NR	Dyadic Adjustment Scale 1) 114.3 (14.0) 2) 119.3 (11.9) 3) 104.6 (11.6) 4) 106.3 (13.0) p=NR	Dyadic Adjustment Scale 1) 109.4 (15.3) 2) 112.6 (16.2) 3) 98.4 (11.6) 4) 97.9 (13.2) p=NR	Dyadic Adjustment Scale 1) 107.3 (16.3) 2) 109.3 (17.2) 3) 96.0 (19.3) 4) 93.0 (20.2) p=NR
		Piecewise growth model for effect of tx condition on DAS: Equivalence test between: 1) vs 2): z=1.7, p=ns **Group differences between:** **1) vs 3): z=-2.6, p<.01** **1) vs 4): z=-2.5, p<.01**		*Piecewise growth model for effect of tx condition on DAS after tx:* Equivalence test between: 1) vs 2): z=1.0, p=ns **Group differences between:** **1) vs 3): z=-2.2, p<0.05** **1) vs 4): z=2.0, p<0.05**
Fals-Stewart, 2006[74] 1) BCT 2) IBT 3) PACT *Female patients only*	Dyadic Adjustment Scale 1) 94.64 (19.36) 2) 96.11 (18.44) 3) 95.34 (18.40) p=NR	Dyadic Adjustment Scale 1) 123.0 (12.1) 2) 111.2 (18.6) 3) 109.8 (13.3) p=NR	Dyadic Adjustment Scale 1) 117.2 (13.7) 2) 102.2 (14.4) 3) 100.1 (15.2) p=NR	Dyadic Adjustment Scale 1) 112.4 (14.0) 2) 98.0 (18.8) 3) 98.0 (16.2) p=NR
		Piecewise growth model for effect of tx condition on DAS: **Group differences between:** **1) vs. 2): z=2.6, p<.01** **1) vs. 3): z=2.7, p<.01**		*Piecewise growth model for effect of tx condition on linear rate of change in DAS after tx:* **Group differences between:** **1) vs. 2): z=2.2, p<0.05** **1) vs. 3): z=2.0, p<0.05**

Study, Year Interventions *Sample*	Baseline	Post-Treatment	Short-term Follow-up	Long-term Follow-up
Fals-Stewart, 2008[78] 1) BBCT 2) BCT 3) IBT 4) PACT *Participants*	Dyadic Adjustment Scale 1) 85.0 (16.7) 2) 83.8 (17.1) 3) 86.8 (20.8) 4) 85.9 (21.0) p=NR	Dyadic Adjustment Scale 1) 112.3 (15.2) 2) 114.2 (15.1) 3) 101.9 (13.6) 4) 100.1 (11.8) p=NR	Dyadic Adjustment Scale 1) 107.2 (15.3) 2) 109.8 (16.0) 3) 94.1 (14.8) 4) 93.0 (15.9) p=NR	Dyadic Adjustment Scale 1) 104.4 (16.9) 2) 106.9 (16.5) 3) 87.3 (17.2) 4) 88.7 (18.6) p=NR
		Piecewise growth model for effect of tx condition on DAS: Test of equivalence between: 1) vs. 2): z=1.6, p=ns **Group differences between:** **1) vs. 3): z=-2.9, p<.01** **1) vs. 4): z=2.8, p<.01**		*Piecewise growth model for effect of tx condition on DAS after tx:* Test of equivalence between: 1) vs 2): z=-0.8, p=ns **Group differences between:** **1) vs. 3): z=-2.8, p<0.01** **1) vs. 4): z=2.0, p<0.05**
Fals-Stewart, 2009[79] 1) BCT 2) IBT	DAS (men) 1) 88.2 (22.9) N=NR 2) 86.8 (23.1) N=NR p=NR DAS (women) 1) 92.7 (20.4) N=NR 2) 93.2 (23.1) N=NR p=NR	DAS (men) 1) 119.4 (13.6) N=NR 2) 110.4 (14.2) N=NR p<0.05 DAS (women) 1) 111.4 (12.7) N=NR 2) 103.2 (15.2) N=NR p<0.05	DAS (men) 1) 109.5 (16.2) N=NR 2) 95.4 (18.2) N=NR p <0.05 DAS (women) 1) 104.9 (17.5) N=NR 2) 95.4 (19.5) N=NR p <0.05	DAS (men) 1) 106.0 (22.8) N=NR 2) 92.0 (20.3) N=NR p<0.05 DAS (women) 1) 101.4 (22.8) N=NR 2) 92.0 (22.7) N=NR p <0.05
		Multi-level growth model for effect of tx condition on DAS (men): **Group differences between:** **1) vs. 2): z=-2.8, p<.01**		*Piecewise growth model for effect of tx condition on linear rate of change in DAS after tx (men):* **Group differences between:** **1) vs. 2): z=2.0, p<0.05**
		Multi-level growth model for effect of tx condition on DAS (women): **Group differences between:** **1) vs. 2): z=2.1, p<.05**		*Piecewise growth model for effect of tx condition on linear rate of change in DAS after tx (men):* Group differences between: 1) vs. 2): z=1.4, p=ns
Jones, 2001[70] 1) HOPE 2) Usual Care *ITT*	Partner Support Quest. (mean, SE) 1) 3.3 (0.2) N=45 2) 3.5 (0.3) N=17 p>0.4	Partner Support Quest.(mid-tx -4 weeks) 1) 3.6 (0.2) 2) 2.6 (0.3) p=NR	Partner Support Quest. 1) 2.6 (0.2) 2) 3.4 (0.8) p=NR	

Study, Year Interventions *Sample*	Baseline	Post-Treatment	Short-term Follow-up	Long-term Follow-up
	Relationship Assessment score (mean, SE) 1) 61.8 (1.7) 2) 59.0 (2.9) p>0.4	Relationship Assessment score (mid-tx 4 weeks) 1) 62.5 (2.0) 2) 62.1 (3.1) p=NR	Relationship Assessment score 1) 68.5 (2.2) 2) 65.6 (6.9) p=0.83	
Kelley, 2002[63] 1) BCT 2) IBT (Individual) 3) PACT (couples, no BCT) *ITT*	DAS (alcohol abusing pts) 1) 85.3 (21.4) N=25 2) 84.6 (22.2) N=22 3) 83.3 (22.4) N=24 p=ns	DAS (alcohol abusing pts) 1) 115.4 (18.2)* 2) 102.2 (19.1) 3) 104.6 (21.6) p<0.05 (significantly higher than baseline) *significantly higher than the other treatment groups	DAS (alcohol abusing pts) 1) 103.9 (16.2)* 2) 86.7 (19.2) 3) 85.8 (23.0) p<0.05 (significantly higher than baseline) *significantly higher than the other treatment groups	DAS (alcohol abusing pts) 1) 91.4 (19.9)* 2) 82.1 (20.7) 3) 80.0 (19.6) p<0.05 (significantly higher than baseline) *significantly higher than the other treatment groups
	DAS (drug abusing pts) 1) 75.2 (22.7) N=22 2) 77.3 (19.8) N=21 3) 74.4 (20.2) N=21 p=ns	DAS (drug abusing pts) 1) 103.6 (22.1)* 2) 88.7 (16.4) 3) 86.4 (21.7) p<0.05 (significantly higher than baseline)	DAS (drug abusing pts) 1) 93.6 (17.2)* 2) 77.8 (18.7) 3) 80.0 (19.2) p<0.05 (significantly higher than baseline) *significantly higher than the other treatment groups	DAS (drug abusing pts) 1) 907 (22.3)* 2) 75.8 (20.4) 3) 77.2 (21.6) p<0.05 (significantly higher than baseline) *significantly higher than the other treatment groups
Kirby, 1999[80] 1) CRT 2) 12-step *ITT*		SAS (marital subscale, pre-post change) 1) -.18 2) -.05 (p=ns)		
Lam, 2009[71] 1) PSBCT 2) BCT 3) IBT *ITT*	Dyadic Adjustment scale 1) 86.7 (19.1) N=10 2) 84.2 (20.6) N=10 3) 83.6 (22.4) N=10 p=NR	Dyadic Adjustment Scale 1) 112.3 (18.6) N=10 2) 114.4 (16.8) N=10 3) 98.1 (17.9) N=10 p=NR Within group over time: 1) r≥0.5 large 2) r≥0.5 large 3) r≥0.3 medium Paired contrasts: 1) vs. 3) medium 2) vs. 3) medium 1) vs. 2) negligible	Dyadic Adjustment Scale 1) 104.0 (19.2) N=10 2) 105.9 (19.6) N=10 3) 93.9 (20.2) N=10 p=NR Within group over time: 1) r≥0.5 large 2) r≥0.5 large 3) r≥0.2 clinically meaningful Paired contrasts: 1) vs. 3) medium 2) vs. 3) medium 1) vs. 2) negligible	Dyadic Adjustment Scale 1) 98.3 (20.2) N=10 2) 99.8 (20.3) N=10 3) 88.9 (22.0) N=10 p=NR Within group over time: 1) r≥0.3 medium 2) r≥0.3 medium 3) r=negligible Paired contrasts: 1) vs. 3) medium 2) vs. 3) medium 1) vs. 2) negligible

144

Family Involved Psychosocial Treatments for Adult Mental Health Conditions: A Review of the Evidence

Study, Year Interventions *Sample*	Baseline	Post-Treatment	Short-term Follow-up	Long-term Follow-up
McCrady, 2004[87] 1) ABMT 2) AA/ABMT 3) RP/ABMT				Marital Happiness Scale (18 months) 1) 5.2 (1.0) 2) 5.0 (1.0) 3) 5.1 (1.1) p=ns
McCrady, 2009[75] 1) ABCT 2) ABIT *Completers*				% separated during follow up 1) 20.0% 2) 11.5% p=NR
				Length separation (days) 1) 251.0 (186.4) 2) 128.2 (125.0) p=NR
O'Farrell, 1998a[4] 1) BMT+RP 2) BMT *Sample Unclear*	Marital Adjustment Test (husband report, patient) 1) 96.1 (20.4) 2) 86.6 (31.7) p=ns	Marital Adjustment Test (husband report, patient) 1) 108.3 (21.9) 2) 104.1 (30.0) p=ns	Marital Adjustment Test (husband report, patient) 1) 112.7 (22.4) 2) 102.4 (30.6) p=ns	Marital Adjustment Test (husband report, patient) 1) 112.4 (19.3) 2) 96.7 (36.1) p=ns Final (30 months): 1) 102.5 (29.9) 2) 89.8 (39.6) p=ns
	CBQ (marital behaviors) – Average couple response 1) 3.5 (0.7) 2) 3.3 (0.8) p=ns	CBQ (marital behaviors) – Average couple response 1) 2.5 (0.9) 2) 2.2 (0.9) p=ns		CBQ (marital behaviors) – Average couple response 1) 2.5 (0.9) 2) 2.2 (1.0) p=ns Final (30 months): 1) 2.1 (1.1) 2) 1.9 (1.1) p=ns

145

Study, Year Interventions Sample	Baseline	Post-Treatment	Short-term Follow-up	Long-term Follow-up
O'Farrell, 1998b[65] 1) BMT 2) ICT 3) Individual Tx Only Sample Unclear	Sexual Adjustment Questionnaire - satisfaction with privacy and context 1) 2.9 (0.9) 2) 3.3 (1.2) 3) 3.7 (3.9) p=ns	Sexual Adjustment Questionnaire - satisfaction with privacy and context 1) **3.8 (1.3)*** 2) 3.5 (1.2) 3) 3.9 (1.2) p=0.003 *changes for group 1 were significant, but not other groups		
	Sexual Adjustment Questionnaire - frequency of intercourse 1) 4.2 (1.9) 2) 5.0(1.5) 3) 5.0 (2.1) p=ns	Sexual Adjustment Questionnaire - frequency of intercourse 1) 4.7 (2.0) 2) 5.1 (1.7) 3) 4.0 (1.9) p=ns		
O'Farrell, 2010[82] 1) BFT+IBT 2) IBT	RHS dyad score 1) 42.4 (19.5) 2) 42.5 (11.9) p=NR	RHS dyad score 1) 58.8 (13.9) 2) 54.8 (11.7) p=NR; r=0.07	RHS dyad score 1) 52.8 (17.6) 2) 51.2 (15.2) p=NR; r=0.07	
Walitzer, 2004[73] 1) C/AF 2) C/AF+BCT (family) 3) PDO (individual) ITT	Dyadic Adjustment Scale 1) 104.1 (12.3) N=20 2) 107.6 (13.3) N=19 3) 108.5 (22.0) N=21 p=ns	Dyadic Adjustment Scale 1) 103.7 (15.7) N=19 2) 108.4 (14.4) N=19 3) 105.4 (26.2) N=21 p=ns	Dyadic Adjustment Scale 1) 106.0 (12.4) N=18 2) 107.8 (12.7) N=16 3) 108.3 (25.6) N=15 p=ns	Dyadic Adjustment Scale 1) 109.0 (10.1) N=17 2) 101.2 (15.9) N=17 3) 113.6 (23.0) N=14 p=ns
Winters, 2002[76] 1) BCT+IBCT 2) IBCT ITT/Female patients	Dyadic Adjustment Scale 1) 81.4 (32.7) 2) 83.6 (31.8) p=ns	Dyadic Adjustment Scale 1) **105.3 (13.2)** 2) **97.2 (16.1)** **p=0.05**	Dyadic Adjustment Scale 1) 93.4 (22.7) 2) 84.3 (23.6) p=ns	Dyadic Adjustment Scale 1) 86.2 (25.2) 2) 82.8 (25.9) p=ns

Study, Year Interventions Sample	Baseline	Post-Treatment	Short-term Follow-up	Long-term Follow-up
INTIMATE PARTNER VIOLENCE				

Fals-Stewart, 1996,[74] 2000,[84] 2002[85]
1) BCT
2) IBT
	<u>Male to female partner violence</u>
	(p = NR for all)
	a. Twisted partner' arm:
	  1) 8% vs. 2) 10%
	b. Pushed, grabbed partner:
	  1) 25% vs. 2) 30%
	c. Slapped partner:
	  1) 10% vs. 2) 13%
	d. Forced sex on partner:
	  1) 13% vs. 2) 15%
	e. Shaken partner:
	  1) 20% vs. 2) 23%
	f. Thrown partner:
	  1) 3% vs. 2) 3%
	g. Thrown object at partner:
	  1) 10% vs. 2) 13%
	h. Choked / strangled partner:
	  1) 0% vs. 2) 0%
	i. Kicked, bitten, hit partner:
	  1) 18% vs. 2) 18%
	j. Hit or tried to hit partner:
	  1) 20% vs. 2) 23%
	k. Beaten up partner:
	  1) 0% vs. 2) 3%
	l. Threatened partner with knife
	  or gun:
	  1) 0% vs. 2) 0%
	m. Used knife or gun on partner:
	  1) 0% vs. 2) 0%
	
	p=NR
				<u>Male to female partner violence</u>
				(p = NR for all)
				Male to female partner violence
				(p = NR for all)
				a. Twisted partner' arm:
				  1) 3% vs. 2) 8%
				b. Pushed, grabbed partner:
				  1)10% vs. 2) 23%
				c. Slapped partner:
				  1) 8% vs. 2) 8%
				d. Forced sex on partner:
				  1) 5% vs. 2) 13%
				e. Shaken partner:
				  1) 5% vs. 2) 23%
				f. Thrown partner:
				  1) 0% vs. 2) 3%
				g. Thrown object at partner:
				  1) 5% vs. 2) 10%
				h. Choked / strangled partner:
				  1) 0% vs. 2) 0%
				i. Kicked, bitten, hit partner:
				  1) 5% vs. 2) 15%
				j. Hit or tried to hit partner:
				  1) 8% vs. 2) 15%
				k. Beaten up partner:
				  1) 0% vs. 2) 0%
				l. Threatened partner with
				  knife or gun:
				  1) 0% vs. 2) 0%
				m. Used knife or gun on partner:
				  1) 0% vs. 2) 0%

Fals-Stewart, 2006[74] 1) BCT 2) IBT 3) PACT *Female patients only*				p=NR TLFB-SV, Male-to-Female **1) 1.7 (4.9)** **2) 3.4 (4.2)** **3) 3.9 (9.7)** **p<0.05** TLFB-SV, Female to Male_ **1) 1.7 (3.8) vs. 2) 4.0 (4.2)** **1) 1.7 (3.8) vs 3) 4.1 (4.4)** **p<0.05**

147

Family Involved Psychosocial Treatments for Adult Mental Health Conditions: A Review of the Evidence

Study, Year Interventions Sample	Baseline	Post-Treatment	Short-term Follow-up	Long-term Follow-up
Lam, 2009[71] 1) PSBCT 2) BCT 3) IBT *ITT*	TLFB –SV M-to-F, % days 1) 2.4 (3.0) N=10 2) 2.4 (2.5) N=10 3) 2.4 (2.5) N=10 p=NR	TLFB –SV M-to-F, % days 1) 1.3 (1.9) N=10 2) 1.2 (2.2) N=10 3) 1.4 (2.2) N=10 p=NR Within group over time: 1) r≥0.2 clinically meaningful 2) r≥0.2 clinically meaningful 3) r=negligible Paired contrasts: 1) vs. 3) negligible 2) vs. 3) negligible 1) vs. 2) negligible	TLFB –SV M-to-F, % days 1) 1.5 (1.9) N=10 2) 1.5 (2.0) N=10 3) 1.7 (2.8) N=10 p=NR Within group over time: 1) r≥0.2 clinically meaningful 2) r≥0.2 clinically meaningful 3) r=negligible Paired contrasts: 1) vs. 3) negligible 2) vs. 3) negligible 1) vs. 2) negligible	TLFB –SV M-to-F, % days 1) 1.4 (1.7) N=10 2) 1.4 (2.2) N=10 3) 1.8 (2.5) N=10 p=NR Within group over time: 1) r≥0.2 clinically meaningful 2) r≥0.2 clinically meaningful 3) r=negligible Paired contrasts: 1) vs. 3) negligible 2) vs. 3) negligible 1) vs. 2) negligible
CONFLICT				
Fals-Stewart, 1996,[74] 2000,[84] 2002[85] 1) BCT 2) IBT	Response to conflict scale 1) 112.4 (30.8) 2) 107.6 (27.3) p=NR	Response to conflict scale 1) 79.8 (26.1) 2) 102.3 (26.9) p=ns	Response to conflict scale 1) 106.4 (30.0) 2) 103.4 (27.2) p=ns	Response to conflict scale 1) 106.9 (27.7) 2) 103.9 (21.9) p=ns
Miller, 1999[81] 1) CRAFT 2) Johnson Institute 3) Al-Anon *ITT*	SO's report of Family Environment Scale – Family Conflict 1) 3.4 (2.5) 2) 3.6 (2.0) 3) 3.5 (2.5) p=ns	SO's report of Family Environment Scale – Family Conflict 1) 2.7 (2.4) 2) 2.8 (1.9) 3) 3.2 (2.3) p=ns	SO's report of Family Environment Scale – Family Conflict 1) 2.5 (2.1) 2) 2.9 (2.3) 3) 2.8 (2.4) p=ns	

Outcomes reported as mean (standard deviation) unless otherwise noted.

Short-term follow up = 6 months post-treatment, unless otherwise noted; Long term=12 months post-treatment, unless otherwise noted. If an outcome had a final measure reported beyond 12 months, it is reported in long term follow up column and noted.

Measures listed in the study descriptive tables but not reported here if either 1) the authors did not report findings from these measures or 2) they did not test for differences between conditions on these measures.

ns = not significant (at 5% level); NR = not reported; N/A = not applicable; tx = treatment; Completers = findings for analyses conducted only with treatment completers; ITT = findings for analyses using an intent-to-treat approach.

BCT = Behavioral Couples Therapy; BFT = Behavioral Family Therapy; ICBT = Individual Couple Behavioral Therapy; IBT = Individual Based Treatment; ICT = Individual Couple Therapy;; BFT=Behavioral Family Counseling; BBCT = Brief Behavioral Couples Therapy; S-BFT=Standard Behavioral Couples Therapy; BMT = Behavioral Marital Therapy; BRT = Brief Relationship Therapy; PACT= Psychoeducational Attention Control Treatment; FSO = family member/significant other ; PSBCT = Parent Skills with Behavioral Couples Therapy; ABMT = Alcohol Focused Behavioral Marital Therapy; AA= Alcoholics Anonymous; AA/Al-Anon; RP = Relapse prevention; ABCT= Alcohol Behavior Couples Therapy; ABIT= Alcohol Behavior Individual Therapy; CRAFT = Community Reinforcement and Family Training; ACQ = Area of Change Questionnaire; ASI = Addiction Severity Index; DAS= dyadic adjustment scale; TLFB-SV = Time Line Follow Back Interview , Spousal Violence; M-to-F= male to female; FES = Family Environment Scale; CBQ = Couples Behaviors Questionnaire, RHS = Relationship Happiness Scale; SO = Significant Other

Table 4. Intermediate Outcomes – Substance Abuse Studies

Study, Year Interventions *Sample*	Outcome Post-Treatment[1]
ATTENDANCE	
Carroll, 2001[77] 1) Significant Other+Contingency Management+Naltrexone 2) Contingency Management+Naltrexone 3) Naltrexone	# weeks in therapy 1) 7.4 (5.1); 2) 7.4 (4.4); 3) 5.6 (4.5) 1) vs. 2) ns **1) & 2) vs. 3) p=0.05**
Fals-Stewart, 1996[66] 1) Behavioral Couples Therapy 2) Individual Based Treatment	# sessions attended 1) 42.9 (13.2); 2) 42.5 (12.2) p=ns
Fals-Stewart, 2001[67] 1) Behavioral Couples Therapy 2) Individual based methadone maintenance *ITT*	Session attendance 1) 20.3 (4.2) N=21; 2) 19.6 (5.4) N=22 p=ns
Fals-Stewart, 2003[68] 1) Naltrexone+Brief Family Treatment 2) Naltrexone+Individual Based Treatment	# sessions attended **1) 34.2 (14.9); 2) 26.5 (15.2)** **p<0.05**
Fals-Stewart, 2005[69] 1) Brief Relationship Therapy 2) Standard Behavioral Couples Therapy 3) Individual Based Treatment 4) Psychoeducational Attention Control Treatment	# sessions attended 1) 0.8 (0.2); 2) 0.8 (0.2); 3) 0.9 (0.2); 4) 0.8 (0.2) p=ns
Fals-Stewart, 2006[74] 1) Standard Behavioral Couples Therapy 2) Individual Based Treatment 3) Psychoeducational Attention Control Treatment	# sessions attended 1) 23.9 (4.0); 2) 25.6 (4.1); 3) 23.6 (4.8) p=ns
	#emergency sessions attended 1) 1.1 (2.0); 2) 1.0 (0.8); 3) 1.2 (1.3) p=ns
Fals-Stewart, 2008[78] 1) Brief Behavioral Couples Therapy 2) Behavioral Couples Therapy 3) Individual Based Treatment 4) Psychoeducational Attention Control Treatment	#sessions attended 1) 0.8 (0.2); 2) 0.8 (0.2); 3) 0.8 (0.2); 4) 0.8 (0.2) p=ns
Fals-Stewart, 2009[79] 1) Behavioral Couples Therapy 2) Individual Based Treatment	# sessions attended (men) 1) 24.3 (3.6); 2) 23.0 (3.0) p=ns
	# sessions attended (women) 1) 22.7 (4.9); 2) 24.9 (5.1) p=ns
Kelley, 2002[63] 1) Behavioral Couples Therapy 2) Individual Based Treatment 3) Psychoeducational Attention Control Treatment *ITT*	# of sessions (alcohol-abusing pts) 1) 23.7 (4.2) N=25; 2) 22.8 (4.0) N=22; 3) 23.0 (4.2) N=24 p=ns
	# of sessions (drug-abusing pts) 1) 22.4 (5.7) N=22; 2) 22.9 (5.1) N=22 3) 22.6 (4.0) N=21 p=ns
Kirby, 1999[80] 1) Community Reinforcement Training Intervention 2) Self Help	# weeks for FSO **1) 8.6; 2) 5.2** **p<0.001**
	% FSOs completing therapy **1) 85.7%; 2) 38.8%** **p<0.01**

Study, Year Interventions *Sample*	Outcome Post-Treatment[1]
Lam, 2009[71] 1) Parent Skills Behavioral Couples Therapy 2) Behavioral Couples Therapy 3) Individual Based Treatment	Attendance rates 1) 84%; 2) 86%; 3) 83% p=ns
McCrady, 1996,[72] 1999[86] 1) Alcohol Focused Spouse Involvement+ Behavioral Marital Therapy 2) Alcohol Focused Spouse Involvement+ Behavioral Marital Therapy+AA/Al-Anon 3) Alcohol Focused Spouse Involvement+ Behavioral Marital Therapy+Relapse Prevention	# therapy sessions attended (patients) 1) 10.5 (6.0) N=30; 2) 10.6 (5.8) N=31 3) 11.1 (5.7) N=29 p=ns
	# patients who dropped therapy (≤5 session) 1) 26.7 N=8; 2) 22.6 N=7; 3) 24.1 N=7 p=ns
	# therapy sessions attended (couples) 1) 10.4 (5.9) N=15; 2) 10.6 (5.8) N=14; 3) 11.1 (5.7) N=16 p=ns
	# days in therapy attended (couples) 1) 155.9 (42.5) N=15; 2) 145.9 (42.7) N=14; 3) 172.8 (44.3) N=16 p=ns
McCrady, 2009[75] 1) Alcohol Behavioral Couples Therapy 2) Alcohol Behavior Individual Therapy *Completers*	% attended all sessions **1) 24%; 2) 44%** **p<0.05**
	# sessions attended 1) 12.4 (6.4); 2) 14.9 (6.5) p=0.05
Miller, 1999[81] 1) Community Reinforcement and Family Training 2) Johnson Institute 3) Al-Anon	Session attendance by SOs (mean #/#sessions, %) 1) 10.7/12 (89%); 2) 3.2/6 (53%); 3) 11.4/12 (95%) p=NR
O'Farrell, 2010[82] 1) Behavioral Family Counseling +Individual Based Treatment 2) Individual Based Treatment *ITT*	Session attendance **1) 17.1 (6.7); 2) 12.0 (6.3)** **p=0.05**
Winters, 2002[76] 1) Behavioral Couples Therapy+Individual Behavioral Therapy 2) Individual Couple Behavioral Therapy *ITT*	Session attendance 1) 39.5 (10.6); 2) 38.4 (12.2) p=ns
ADHERENCE	
Carroll, 2001[77] 1) Significant other +contingency management+Naltrexone 2) Contingency management+Naltrexone 3) Naltrexone	# doses in therapy 1) 19.4(15.4); 2) 17.8 (13.4); 3) 14.2 (12.4) 1) vs. 2) = ns 1) & 2) vs. 3) = ns
Fals-Stewart, 2003[68] 1) Naltrexone+Brief Family Treatment 2) Naltrexone+Individual Based Treatment	# days on Naltrexone **1) 102.6 (41.3); 2) 79.4 (46.3)** **p<0.01**
McCrady, 1996,[72] 1999[86] 1) Alcohol Focused Spouse Involvement+ Behavioral Marital Therapy 2) Alcohol Focused Spouse Involvement+ Behavioral Marital Therapy+AA/Al-Anon 3) Alcohol Focused Spouse Involvement+ Behavioral Marital Therapy+Relapse Prevention	% homework completed 1) 76.9%; 2) 66.4%; 3) 66.7% p=ns
McCrady, 2009[75] 1) Alcohol Behavioral Couples Therapy 2) Alcohol Behavior Individual Therapy *Completers*	% homework completed (among treatment completers) 1) 72.8% (16.6); 2) 73.7% (24.2) p=NR

Study, Year Interventions *Sample*	Outcome Post-Treatment[1]
O'Farrell, 1998a[4] 1) Behavioral Marital Therapy + Relapse Prevention 2) Behavioral Marital Therapy	Couples Behaviors Questionnaire (participation in Antabuse contract learned in BMT), averaged across the dyad Post-treatment 1) 4.2 (1.2); 2) 4.5 (0.8) p = NR Short-term Follow-up (6 months) **1) 2.9 (1.8); 2) 1.6 (1.9)** **p=0.008** Long-term Follow-up (12 months) **1) 2.0 (2.0); 2) 0.8 (1.2)** **p=0.004** Final Follow-up (30 months) 1) 0.9 (1.6); 2) 0.4 (0.8) p=ns
SATISFACTION WITH CARE	
Fals-Stewart, 1996[66] 1) Behavioral Couples Therapy 2) Individual Based Treatment	Client Satisfaction Questionnaire 1) 25.3 (5.2); 2) 26.4 (6.0) p=ns
Fals-Stewart, 2001[67] 1) Behavioral Couples Therapy 2) Individual based methadone maintenance *ITT*	Client Satisfaction Questionnaire 1) 27.9 (6.4) N=21; 2) 25.5 (6.7) N=22 p=ns
Fals-Stewart, 2003[68] 1) Naltrexone+Brief Family Treatment 2) Naltrexone+Individual Based Treatment	Client Satisfaction Questionnaire-8 1) 23.2 (3.8); 2) 24.4 (4.0) p=ns
Fals-Stewart, 2005[69] 1) Brief Relationship Therapy 2) Standard Behavioral Couples Therapy 3) Individual Based Treatment 4) Psychoeducational Attention Control Treatment	Client Satisfaction Questionnaire-8 1) 24.7 (2.9); 2) 26.2 (3.9); 3) 24.1 (4.1); 4) 24.0 (4.0) p=ns
Fals-Stewart, 2006[74] 1) Behavioral Couples Therapy 2) Individual Based Treatment 3) Psychoeducational Attention Control Treatment	Client Satisfaction Questionnaire 1) 24.3 (4.5); 2) 25.0 (5.2); 3) 23.0 (6.4) p=ns
Fals-Stewart, 2008[78] 1) Brief Behavioral Couples Therapy 2) Behavioral Couples Therapy 3) Individual Based Treatment 4) Psychoeducational Attention Control Treatment	Client Satisfaction Questionnaire-8 1) 23.8 (4.0); 2) 24.3 (4.1); 3) 25.0 (4.4); 4) 23.1 (4.6) p=ns
Fals-Stewart, 2009[79] 1) Behavioral Couples Therapy 2) Individual Based Treatment	Client Satisfaction Questionnaire-8 (Men) 1) 23.74 (3.91); 2) 24.00 (4.12) p=ns
	Client Satisfaction Questionnaire-8 (Women) 1) 22.9 (4.5); 2) 24.0 (4.9) p=ns
Winters, 2002[76] 1) Behavioral Couples Therapy+ Individual Behavioral Therapy 2) Individual Couple Behavioral Therapy *ITT*	Client Satisfaction Questionnaire 1) 24.1 (3.7); 2) 22.9 (4.4) p=ns

Outcomes reported as mean (standard deviation) unless otherwise noted.
ns = not significant (at 5% level); NR = not reported; N/A = not applicable; Completers = findings for analyses conducted only with treatment completers;
ITT = findings for analyses using an intent-to-treat approach.
[1]Outcomes are reported post-treatment, unless otherwise noted.

Table 5. Study Descriptive Information – Bipolar Disorder Studies

Study, Year Funding Source	Sample Characteristics	Inclusion and Exclusion Criteria	Treatment Groups	Intervention	Outcomes Assessed	Quality
Clarkin, 1998[94] Government, Foundation	N = 46 randomized N = 33 analyzed Gender: 54% male Age: 47.7 years Race/ethnicity: NR Marital status: NR Education: NR Veterans: NR Family Characteristics: significant other of opposite sex Recruitment Method: patients consecutively admitted to inpatient and outpatient services were considered for inclusion	MH Condition: major affective disorder or bipolar disorder, manic, depressed, or mixed Assessed by: Interview using Schedule for Affective Disorders and Schizophrenia SO: spouse or partner of opposite sex, married or living together ≥ 6 months Inclusions: 21 to 65 years old; admission diagnosis of major affective disorder or bipolar disorder, manic, depressed, or mixed; married or living with significant other of opposite sex ≥6 months Exclusions: organic brain syndrome, current primary diagnosis of alcohol or drug abuse, pregnancy, contraindications to use of lithium or carbamazepine	1) Medical management + marital intervention (N=18) 2) Medical management only (N=15) Randomized: N=46 Analysis: Baseline: N = 33 Post-treatment (Final 11 months): N=33	Format: marital therapy Manualized: Yes Session: 25 (one weekly for first 10; then bimonthly) Txt Length: 11 months Approach: psychoeducational NOTE: all patients received standardized medications in each of 3 classes: mood stabilizers, antidepressants, and antipsychotics	Patient Outcomes: Symptoms a. SADS-C Functioning a. Global Assessment Scale Intermediate Outcomes: a. Medication Adherence using study developed scale (1-6 rating, poor to excellent) Family Outcomes: None Outcome timeframe: Baseline Post-treatment (Final): 11months	Allocation concealment: Unclear Blinding: Unclear Intention to treat analysis: No Withdrawals adequately described: No Treatment Integrity: audio tapes of marital intervention sessions were sampled for adherence to procedures outlined in manual Study Quality: Poor

Study, Year Funding Source	Sample Characteristics	Inclusion and Exclusion Criteria	Treatment Groups	Intervention	Outcomes Assessed	Quality
Miklowitz, 2000[90] Government, Foundation	N = 101 randomized N = 79 analyzed Gender: 37% male Age: 35.6 yrs Race/ethnicity: White 84% Marital Status: 55% married or cohabiting Education: NR Veterans: NR *Family Characteristics:* 37% parents, 55% spouses, 7% siblings, 1% adult offspring *Recruitment Method:* Recruited from 4 psychiatric inpatient units or referred to study as outpatients.	MH Condition: Bipolar I disorder, manic, mixed, or depression Assessed by: Structured Clinical Interview for DSM-III-R SO: "close relatives" including parents, spouses, siblings Inclusions: DSM-II-R diagnosis of bipolar I disorder, manic, mixed, or depressed episode in previous 3 months; age 18-60 yrs; no neurologic disorder or developmental disability; no DSM-III-R drug or alcohol disorders in previous 6 months; living with or in regular contact (4+ hrs/ wk) with close relative; willing to commit to pharmacotherapy with mood stabilizers or antipsychotic medications; English speaking; patient and relative willing to consent Exclusions: no additional criteria reported	1) Family-focused treatment with pharmacotherapy (N=31) 2) Crisis management with pharmacotherapy (N=70) ("treatment as usual" condition with 2 home-based family education sessions, emergency counseling as needed, minimum of monthly telephone call to monitor status) Randomized: N=101 Analysis: Baseline: N=101 Long term (Final): 12 months: N=79	Format: Family-focused (family or marital) Manualized: Yes Session: up to 21 sessions, 1 hour, in the family's home Txt Length: 9 months Approach: psychoeducation, communication skills, problem definition and solution	Patient Outcomes: Symptoms a. SADS-C b. Relapse c. Survival Intermediate Outcomes: a. Medication Compliance Family Outcomes: None Outcome timeframe: Baseline Long Term (Final): 12 months	Allocation concealment: Unclear Blinding: Yes (medication intensity and compliance ratings) Intention to treat analysis: No Withdrawals adequately described: Yes Treatment Integrity: audio tapes reviewed for adherence **Study quality:** **Good**
Miklowitz, 2003[5] Government, Foundation	Same as Miklowitz 2000[90]	Same as Miklowitz 2000[90] MH Condition: Assessed by: SO: Inclusions: Exclusions: Same as Miklowitz 2000[90]	Same as Miklowitz 2000[90] 1) Family-focused treatment with pharmacotherapy (N = 22 completed 2 years) 2) Crisis management with pharmacotherapy (N = 43 completed 2 years)	Same as Miklowitz 2000[90]	Same as Miklowitz 2000[90] 2 year outcomes	Same as Miklowitz 2000[90]

153

Family Involved Psychosocial Treatments for Adult Mental Health Conditions: A Review of the Evidence

Study, Year Funding Source	Sample Characteristics	Inclusion and Exclusion Criteria	Treatment Groups	Intervention	Outcomes Assessed	Quality
Miklowitz, 2007[92] Government All patients were enrolled in Systematic Treatment Enhancement Program for Bipolar Disorder (STEP-BD) study NOTE: included patients in 26-wk trial of mood stabilizer + placebo or mood stabilizer + antidepressant (RAD) and willing to be randomized to psychosocial treatment; initiated study (PAD) with patients ineligible for pharmacotherapy trial due to previous poor response to agents	N = 293 randomized N = 293 analyzed Gender: 41% male Age: 40.1 yrs Race/ethnicity: Caucasian 94% African American 4% Native American <1% Asian/Pacific Islander 1% Other 1% Marital Status: Married 33% Unmarried 37% Separated 31% Veterans: NR *Family Characteristics:* Not specified – "typically spouses, parents, or siblings" *Recruitment Method:* Referrals from Systematic Treatment Enhancement Program for Bipolar Disorder (STEP-BD)	MH Condition: Bipolar I or II disorder and current major depressive episode Assessed by: Structural Clinical Interview for DSM-IV and Mini-International Neuropsychiatric Interview SO: Family members Inclusions: 18+ years; DSM-IV criteria for current bipolar I or II disorder and a current major depressive episode; current treatment with mood stabilizer or willing to start treatment; no current psychotherapy (or willing to discontinue or taper); English speaking, able to consent Exclusions: require immediate treatment for DSM-IV substance or alcohol abuse or dependence disorder (except nicotine); pregnant or planned pregnancy in next yr; history of intolerance, nonresponse, or medical contraindication to paroxetine or buproprion; required initiation or dose changes of antipsychotic medications	1) Family-focused treatment (FFT)* (N=26) 2) Interpersonal and social rhythm therapy (IPSRT) (N=62) 3) Cognitive behavior therapy (CBT) (N=75) 4) Collaborative care (CC) – control group (N=130) NOTE: All patients received pharmaco-therapy *Assignment to FFT possible only if willing family members Randomized: N=293 Analysis: Baseline: N=293 Long term (Final): 12 months: N=293	1) Format: FFT Manualized: Yes Session: up to 30 50-min sessions Txt Length: 9 months Approach: psychoeduca-tion, communication en-hancement, problem solv-ing 2) Format: IPSRT Manualized: Yes Session: up to 30 50-min sessions Txt Length: 9 months Approach: Social Rhythm Metric for stable social rhythms, problem resolu-tion, rehearsed strategies 3) Format: CBT Manualized: Yes Session: up to 30 50-min individual sessions Txt Length: 9 months Approach: psychoeduca-tion, life events scheduling, cognitive restructuring, problem-solving, detection and intervention for mood episodes, interventions for comorbidities 4) Format: CC Manualized: Yes Session: 3 50-min individual sessions Txt Length: 6 weeks Approach: psychoeduca-tion	Patient Outcomes: 1) Recovery 2) Time to recovery Clinical Monitoring Form - depression and mania items used to define recovery (≤2 moderate symptoms for ≥8 of the previous weeks) and compute time to recovery and total time in recovery over 1 year of observation Intermediate Outcomes: Attendance Family Outcomes: None Outcome timeframe: Baseline Long Term (Final): 12 months	Allocation concealment: Unclear Blinding: unclear Intention to treat analysis: Yes Withdrawals adequately described: Yes Treatment Integrity: audio tapes rated for adherence to treatment **Study quality: Good**

Study, Year Funding Source	Sample Characteristics	Inclusion and Exclusion Criteria	Treatment Groups	Intervention	Outcomes Assessed	Quality
Miklowitz, 2007[95] NOTE: Data from subset of patients from Miklowitz 2007 with baseline assessment with LIFE-RIFT) tool	N = 152 Gender: 41 % male Age: 41.1 yrs Race/ethnicity: White 95% Marital Status: Married 31% Unmarried 37% Separated 32% Veterans: NR Family Characteristics: Husbands Children:	Same as Miklowitz 2007[92] MH Condition: Assessed by: SO: Inclusions: Exclusions:	1) Psychosocial Treatment (combined FFT, IPSRT, and CBT groups) (N=84) 2) Collaborative Care (CC) (N=68)	Same as Miklowitz 2007[92]	Patient Outcomes: a. Functioning (LIFE-RIFT total score) Intermediate Outcomes: None Family Outcomes: a. Relationship functioning & satisfaction domains (LIFE-RIFT) Outcome timeframe: Baseline Long term (Final): 9 months	Same as Miklowitz 2007[92]
Miller, 2004[89] Government	N = 92 randomized N = 92 analyzed Gender: 43% male Age: 39 years Race/ethnicity: NR Marital Status: Married 67% Never married 15% Separated/divorced/ Widowed 18% Education (years): 13 Veterans: NR Family Characteristics: Spouses 62% Parents 17% Other adults 21% Recruitment Method: In-patients, partial hospital patients, and outpatients from a university-affiliat-ed psychiatry clinic	MH Condition: Bipolar I disorder mood episode (mania, major depression, or mixed) Assessed by: Structured Clinical Instrument for DSM-III-R-Patient Version SO: patient and family members Inclusions: current bipolar I disorder mood episode; no DSM-III-R alcohol or drug dependence within 12 months of enrollment; age 18-65 yrs; living with or in regular contact with relative or significant other; English speaking Exclusions: no additional criteria reported	1) Pharmacotherapy + family therapy (N=33) 2) Pharmacotherapy + multifamily psychoedu-cational group (MFG) therapy (N=30) 3) Pharmacotherapy alone (N=29) Randomized: N=92 Analysis: Baseline: N=92 Long term (Final): 28 months: N=92	1) Format: Family therapy Manualized: Yes Session: 6 to 10 50-min sessions Txt Length: NR* Approach: Problem Centered Systems Therapy of the Family 2) Format: MFG therapy (4-6 patients and family members > 12 yrs) Manualized: Yes Session: 6 90-min ses-sions Txt Length: 6 weeks* Approach: Psychoeduca-tional 3) Format: Pharmaco-therapy Manualized: Yes Session: weekly for 1 mo then every 3 months Txt Length: NR* Approach: medication ad-justment, support, encour-agement	Patient Outcomes: Symptoms a. Recovery (defined as 2 consecutive months scores of <7 on HAM-D and <6 on BRMS) Intermediate Outcomes: a. Pharmaco-therapy sessions attended Family Outcomes: None Outcome timeframe: Baseline Long Term (Final): 28 months	Allocation concealment: Unclear Blinding: Yes (rating of pharmacotherapy) Intention to treat analysis: Yes Withdrawals adequately described: No Treatment Integrity: Treatments monitored and evaluated at weekly meetings of study clinicians and investigators Study Quality: Fair

Family Involved Psychosocial Treatments for Adult Mental Health Conditions: A Review of the Evidence

Study, Year Funding Source	Sample Characteristics	Inclusion and Exclusion Criteria	Treatment Groups	Intervention	Outcomes Assessed	Quality
Miller, 2008[98] Funding source not reported	N = 91* Gender: 57% male Age: 39.5 years Race/ethnicity: NR Marital Status: NR Education: NR Veterans: NR Family Characteristics: NR for this analysis *One family did not complete MCRS at baseline Recruitment Method: Inpatients, partial hospital patients, and outpatients from a university-affiliated psychiatry clinic (96% while hospitalized)	Same as Miller 2004[89] Analysis using proportional measures of long-term course of illness and based on level of family impairment according to McMaster Clinical Rating Scale (MCRS) Additional Exclusions reported: DSM-IIIR for alcohol/drug dependence in the last year; mood disorder secondary to a general medical condition; illness that contraindicates mood stabilizer use; pregnant, or not using contraception.	Same as Miller 2004[89] Baseline N = 91 High impairment: N = 60 (66%) Low impairment N = 31 (34%) Final (28 months) N= 82 High impairment: N = 55 (67%) Low impairment N = 27 (33%)	Same as Miller 2004[89] except indicates target was 10-15 family-therapy sessions (vs. 6-10)	Patient Outcomes: a. Recovery/ relapse (% who recovered and relapsed based on HAM-D and BRMS for high and low family impairment subgroups) Intermediate Outcomes: None Family Outcomes: None Outcome timeframe: Baseline Long Term (Final): 28 months	Same as Miller 2004[89]

Family Involved Psychosocial Treatments for Adult Mental Health Conditions: A Review of the Evidence

Evidence-based Synthesis Program

Study, Year Funding Source	Sample Characteristics	Inclusion and Exclusion Criteria	Treatment Groups	Intervention	Outcomes Assessed	Quality
Perlick, 2010[93] Government	Patients: N = 46 Gender: 37% male Age: 34.7 Race/ethnicity: Caucasian 75% African American 7.5% Hispanic 17.5% Marital Status: Married/cohabiting 15% Widowed/divorced/ separated 30% Never married 55% Veterans: 2 caregivers from VA Medical Center Caregivers: N = 46 Gender: 16% male Age: 52.8 yrs Race/ethnicity: Caucasian 77% African American 5% Hispanic 16% Other 2% Marital Status: Married/cohabiting 44% Widowed/divorced/ separated 33% Never married 23% Family Characteristics: Parents 70%; Spouse or SO 14%; Adult child 14%; Friend or neighbor 2% Recruitment Method: Referred by mental health clinicians	MH Condition: Bipolar I or II disorder Assessed by: Structured Clinical Interview for DSM-IV Axis I Disorders SO: Caregiver Inclusions: age 18+; primary caregiver of relative with bipolar I or II; meet at least 3 (2 for non-relatives) criteria: a) spouse or parent, b) more frequent contact than any other caregiver, c) helps support patient financially, d) is contacted by treatment staff for emergencies, e) involved in patient's treatment; current physical and mental health problems Exclusions: no additional criteria reported	1) Family-Focused Treatment-Health Promoting Interven-tion (FFT-HPI) (N=25 caregivers) 2) Health education (HE) (N=21 caregivers) NOTE: recruited caregivers who were primary caregiver of relative with condition Randomized: N = 46 caregivers of 46 patients Analysis: Baseline: N=43 care-givers of 40 patients Post-treatment (Final): 5 months: N = 43 caregivers of 40 patients	1) Format: Family focused (but only the caregiver was involved) Manualized: Yes Session: 12-15 sessions Txt Length: approx 5 months Approach: Psychoedu-cation and goal setting, behavioral analysis of self-care barriers 2) Format: Individual (via DVD) Manualized: Session: 8-12 sessions via DVD Txt Length: approx 5 months Approach: health educa-tion	Patient Outcomes: Symptom Improvement a. HAM-D b. YMRS Intermediate Outcomes: None Family Outcomes: None Outcome timeframe: Baseline Post-treatment (Final): 5 months	Allocation concealment: Yes Blinding: Yes (assessor and participants during administration of the initial assessment; post-test assessment) Intention to treat analysis: No Withdrawals adequately described: No Treatment Integrity: Randomly selected treatment tapes rated for competence and adherence Study quality: Fair

157

Family Involved Psychosocial Treatments for Adult Mental Health Conditions: A Review of the Evidence

Study, Year Funding Source	Sample Characteristics	Inclusion and Exclusion Criteria	Treatment Groups	Intervention	Outcomes Assessed	Quality
Rea, 2003[91] Government	N = 53 randomized N = 53 analyzed Gender: 43% male Age: 25.6 yrs Race/ethnicity: Caucasian 60% African American 23% Asian American 9% Other 9% Marital Status: Single 76% Married 15% Divorced 9% Veterans: NR Family Characteristics: 74 family members (29 mothers, 22 fathers, 1 stepfather, 9 spouses, 7 siblings, 1 grandmother, 1 uncle, 4 aunts Recruitment Method: inpatients in 3 large hospitals	MH Condition: Bipolar disorder, manic type Assessed by: DSM-III-R with confirmation by Present State Examination (PSE) with supplementary mania items SO: "close family member"; 66% had one relative to participated, 34% had multiple relatives Inclusions: diagnosis of bipolar disorder, manic type; age 18-45, able to give consent, currently taking mood-regulating medications; at least one close family member available to participate Exclusions: evidence of organic central nervous system disorder or chronic alcohol or substance abuse/dependence	1) Family-focused treatment with pharma-cotherapy (N=28) 2) Individually focused patient treatment with pharmacotherapy (N=25) Randomized: N=53 Analysis: Baseline: N=53 Post-treatment: N=53 Long term (Final): 24 months: N=29	1) Format: Family-focused or individual Manualized: Yes Session: 21 one-hour sessions over 9 months (medication management continued to 12 months)[a] Txt Length:12 months[a] Approach: psychoeduca-tion, communication enhancement training, problem-solving training 2) Format: Individually focused patient treatment Manualized: Not stated Session: 21 30-min sessions over 9 months (medication management continued to 12 months)[a] Txt Length:12 months[a] Approach: supportive, problem-focused, educa-tional [a]At 12 months, patients were referred to and assisted in transitioning to community providers	Patient Outcomes: a. Relapse (based on BPRS and supplementary items from SADS-C) b. Rehospitalization (Patient and relative reports verified by inpatient records where possible) Intermediate Outcomes: a. Medication Compliance (Psychiatrist-completed form) Family Outcomes: None Outcome timeframe: Baseline Post-treatment Long term (Final): 24 months	Allocation concealment: Unclear Blinding: Yes (outcomes) Intention to treat analysis: No Withdrawals adequately described: Yes Treatment Integrity: Videotapes rated for therapist adherence and competence Study quality: Good

Family Involved Psychosocial Treatments for Adult Mental Health Conditions: A Review of the Evidence

Study, Year Funding Source	Sample Characteristics	Inclusion and Exclusion Criteria	Treatment Groups	Intervention	Outcomes Assessed	Quality
Solomon, 2008[97] Government	N = 53 Gender: 43% male Age: 41 yrs Race/ethnicity: NR Marital Status: 66% Married or living with partner 66% Never married 19%, Separated/divorced/ widowed 15% Education (years): 13 Veterans: NR Family Characteristics: NR for subgroup Recruitment Method: Inpatients, partial hospital patients, and outpatients from a university-affiliated psychiatry clinic	Same as Miller 2004[89] Analysis of recurrence of mood episodes and hospitalizations for 53 subjects who recovered from intake mood episode	Same as Miller 2004[89]	Same as Miller 2004[89]	Patient Outcomes: Symptoms: a. Frequency of mood episode recurrence (based on HAM-D>15 or BRMS>5) Utilization: a. Hospitalization Intermediate Outcomes: None Family Outcomes: None Outcome timeframe: Baseline Long Term (Final): 28 months	Same as Miller 2004[89]

NR = not reported; SO = significant other or family member included; SADS-C = Schedule for Affective Disorders and Schizophrenia-Change Version; DSM = Diagnostic and Statistical Manual of Mental Disorders; tx = treatment; BRMS = Bech-Rafaelsen Mania Scale; HAM-D = Hamilton Depression Rating Scale; LIFE-RIFT = Longitudinal Interval Follow-Up Evaluation – Range of Impaired Functioning Tool; YMRS = Young Mania Rating Scale; DVD = digital video disk; BPRS = Brief Psychiatric Rating Scale
*Study patients were treated on outpatient basis for up to 28 months

Family Involved Psychosocial Treatments for Adult Mental Health Conditions: A Review of the Evidence

Table 6. Patient Outcomes - Bipolar Disorder Studies

Study, Year Interventions Sample	Outcome Baseline	Post-Treatment	Short-term Follow-up	Long-term Follow-up
SYMPTOM IMPROVEMENT				
Clarkin, 1998[94] 1) Medication management + marital intervention 2) Medication management only *Completers only*	SADS-C 1) 55.9 N=18 2) 62.0 N=15	SADS-C 1) 49.8 N=18 2) 54.8 N=15 p=ns for test of differences between treatment groups over time		
Miklowitz, 2000,[90] 2003[5] *(2 year results)* 1) Family-focused with medication 2) Crisis mgmt with medication *Completers or ITT (as noted)*	SADS-C (Total affective symptoms) 1) 2.2 (0.6) N=28 2) 2.2 (0.6) N=51 *Completers only* p = NR	SADS-C 1) 1.9 (0.6) N=28 2) 2.2 (0.8) N=51 p = NR	SADS-C 1) 2.0 (0.7) N=28 2) 2.2 (0.8) N=51 p = NR p=ns for treatment **p=0.05 for test of differences between treatment groups over time at 12 months**	**p=0.007 for test of differences between treatment groups over time at 24 months (15 months post-treatment)**
			Relapse 1) 8/31 (26%) 2) 27/70 (39%) p=NR *ITT analysis*	
			Survival (no relapse) **1) 71% 2) 47% p=0.04** *Drop-outs excluded*	
				Relapse (24 months or 15 months post-treatment) **1) 11/31 (35%) (3 patients terminated early) 2) 38/70 (54%) (16 patients terminated early) p<0.005** *ITT analysis*
Miklowitz, 2000,[90] 2003[5] *(2 year results)* 1) Family-focused with medication 2) Crisis mgmt with medication *Completers or ITT (as noted)*				Mean survival without relapse (24 months or 15 months post-treatment) **1) 73.5 wks 2) 53.2 wks Hazard Ratio=0.37 (95%CI 0.19-0.72)** *ITT analysis*

Family Involved Psychosocial Treatments for Adult Mental Health Conditions: A Review of the Evidence

Study, Year Interventions *Sample*	Outcome Baseline	Post-Treatment	Short-term Follow-up	Long-term Follow-up
Miklowitz, 2007[92] 2007[95] 1) Family-focused 2) Inter-personal and social rhythm therapy 3) CBT 4) Collaborative care *ITT analysis*			Recovery (based on SADS-C) 1) **20/26 (77%) (HR relative to 4 = 1.87)** 2) 40/62 (65%) (HR=1.48) 3) 45/75 (60%) (HR=1.34) 4) **67/130 (52%)** No differences 1, 2, 3 (1, 2, & 3 combined vs. 4, p=0.01) **1 vs 4, p=0.02** Confidence intervals not reported for HRs	
			Time to recovery (median among those who recovered, N=172) 1) 103 days 2) 128 days 3) 112 days 4) 146 days No differences 1, 2, 3	
			Recovery (in subsample with family availability, N=159) 1) 20/26 (77%) (HR=1.40) 2) 17/30 (57%) (HR=1.16) 3) 23/39 (59%) (HR=0.98) 4) 37/64 (58%) No differences 1, 2, 3 1 vs. 4, p=0.10	
Miller, 2004[89] 1) Medication + Family Therapy (FT) 2) Medication + multiple-family group therapy (MFG) 3) Medication only *ITT analysis*				Recovery (2 consecutive months with BRMS < 6 and MHRSD < 7) 1) 16/33 (48%) 2) 21/30 (70%) 3) 16/29 (55%) p=0.21 *(at 28 months – final)*
Miller, 2008[98] 1) Medication + FT 2) Medication + MFG 3) Medication only *Stratify Miller 2004 results by degree of family impairment (N=82 with family impairment data; N=51 with impairment who recovered)*				Recovery Low family impairment (N=27) 1) 2/5 (40%) 2) 7/9 (78%) 3) 11/13 (85%) High family impairment (N=55) 1) 12/24 (50%) 2) 14/18 (78%) 3) 5/13 (39%) p=ns for main effects (family impairment or treatment condition) Interaction p=ns *(at 28 months – final)*

Family Involved Psychosocial Treatments for Adult Mental Health
Conditions: A Review of the Evidence

Evidence-based Synthesis Program

Study, Year Interventions *Sample*	Outcome Baseline	Post-Treatment	Short-term Follow-up	Long-term Follow-up
				Relapse after recovery Low family impairment (N=20) 1) 1/2 (50%) 2) 4/7 (57%) 3) 7/11 (64%) High family impairment (N=31) 1) 8/12 (67%) 2) 9/14 (64%) 3) 3/5 (60%) p=ns for main effects (family impairment or treatment condition) Interaction p=ns **Significant (all p<0.05) family impairment by tx interaction for:** a) # depressive episodes/yr b) % time in any mood episode c) % time in depressive episode **High impairment families:** 1) significant differences - MFG vs. medication only for a), b), and c) 2) significant difference between FT vs. medication only for a) **Low impairment families:** No difference between tx groups *(at 28 months – final)*
Perlick, 2010[93] 1) Family-focused, health promoting 2) Health education *Completers only*	HAM-D 1) 15.6 (10.3) N=22 2) 14.9 (5.7) N=18 p=0.26 YMRS 1) 8.8 (9.7) N=22 2) 9.2 (9.2) N=18 p=0.15	**HAM-D** **1) 5.6 (6.1) N=22** **2) 11.2 (9.1) N=18** **p=0.025, d=0.67** **YMRS** **1) 1.6 (2.4) N=22** **2) 5.8 (9.0) N=18** **p=0.037, d=0.34**		

Study, Year Interventions *Sample*	Outcome Baseline	Post-Treatment	Short-term Follow-up	Long-term Follow-up
Rea, 2003[91] 1) Family-focused with medication 2) Individual therapy with medication *ITT for active tx year, n=39 for post-treatment year.*		Relapse (% with at least 1 relapse based on BPRS and supplementary items from SADS-C) 1) 46% 2) 52% p>0.10 **Interaction with premorbid adjustment – family treatment reduced risk of relapse in patients with poorer premorbid adjustment, p=0.06**		Relapse (% with at least 1 relapse) **1) 28%** **2) 60%** **p<0.05** Interaction with premorbid adjustment, p=ns
		Rehospitalization (% with at least 1 rehospitalization): 1) 29% 2) 40% p>0.10 Interaction with premorbid adjustment, p=ns		Rehospitalization **1) 12%** **2) 60%** **p<0.01** **Interaction with premorbid adjustment, p<0.03**
Solomon, 2008[97] 1) Medication + FT 2) Medication + MFG 3) Medication only *Recurrence and hospitalization data for N=53 from Miller 2004 study who recovered*				Frequency of mood episode recurrence (*MHRSD > 15 or BRMS > 5*) 1) 11/16 (69%) 2) 13/21 (62%) 3) 10/16 (63%) p=0.90 (*at 28 months – final*)
GLOBAL FUNCTIONING				
Clarkin, 1998[94] 1) Medication management + marital intervention 2) Medication management only *Completers only*	GAS 1) 64.4 N=18 2) 64.7 N=15	GAS **1) 73.0 N=18** **2) 65.7 N=15** **p<0.03 (test of treatment group differences over time)**		
Miklowitz, 2007,[92] 2007[95] 1) Family-focused 2) Inter-personal and social rhythm therapy 3) Cognitive Behavioral Therapy 4) Collaborative care *Completers only*		LIFE-RIFT Total Score Difference (9 month and baseline) 1) -3.2 (3.1) 2) -1.6 (4.4) 3) -1.1 (4.7) 4) -0.9 (3.5) 1, 2, & 3 combined vs. 4, p=0.04 (*more negative score = greater improvement*)		

Family Involved Psychosocial Treatments for Adult Mental Health Conditions: A Review of the Evidence

Study, Year Interventions Sample	Outcome Baseline	Post-Treatment	Short-term Follow-up	Long-term Follow-up
HEALTH CARE UTILIZATION				
Solomon, 2008[97] 1) Medication + FT 2) Medication + MFG 3) Medication only *Recurrence and hospitalization data for N=53 from Miller 2004 study who recovered*				Hospitalization frequency **1) 5/16 (31%)** **2) 1/21 (5%)** **3) 6/16 (38%)** **p=0.04 (MFG significantly lower)** *(at 28 months – final)*

Outcomes reported as mean (standard deviation) unless otherwise noted.
Short-term follow up = 6 months post-treatment, unless otherwise noted; Long term=12 months post-treatment, unless otherwise noted. If an outcome had a final measure reported beyond 12 months, it is reported in long term follow up column and noted.
ns = not significant (at 5% level); NR = not reported; N/A = not applicable; Completers = findings for analyses conducted only with treatment completers; ITT = findings for analyses using an intent-to-treat approach; BRMS = Bech-Rafaelsen Mania Scale; GAS = Global Assessment Scale; HAM-D = Hamilton Depression Rating Scale; HR = hazard ratio; LIFE-RIFT = Longitudinal Interval Follow-Up Evaluation – Range of Impaired Functioning Tool; MFG = multiple family group; MHRSD = Modified Hamilton Rating Scale for Depression;
SADS-C = Schedule for Affective Disorders and Schizophrenia–Change Version

Table 7. Family Outcomes - Bipolar Disorder Studies

Study, Year Interventions Sample	Outcome Baseline	Post-Treatment	Short-term Follow-up	Long-term Follow-up
GLOBAL FUNCTIONING /SATISFACTION				
Miklowitz 2007, [92] 2007[95] 1) Family-focused 2) Inter-personal and social rhythm therapy 3) Cognitive Behavioral Therapy 4) Collaborative care *Completers only*		LIFE-RIFT Relationship Functioning Domain *Difference (9 month and baseline)* 1) -0.5 (1.6) 2) -0.3 (2.1) 3) -0.2 (1.3) 4) 0.1 (1.5) **1, 2, and 3 combined vs. 4, p=0.02** *(more negative score = greater improvement)*		
		LIFE-RIFT Satisfaction Domain *Difference (9 month and baseline)* 1) -0.9 (0.9) 2) -0.3 (1.4) 3) -0.1 (1.2) 4) 0.0 (1.3) **1, 2, and 3 combined vs. 4,p=0.048**		

Outcomes reported as mean (standard deviation) unless otherwise noted.
Short-term follow up = 6 months post-treatment, unless otherwise noted; Long term=12 months post-treatment, unless otherwise noted. If an outcome had a final measure reported beyond 12 months, it is reported in long term follow up column and noted.
ns = not significant (at 5% level); NR = not reported; N/A = not applicable; Completers = findings for analyses conducted only with treatment completers; ITT = findings for analyses using an intent-to-treat approach; LIFE-RIFT = Longitudinal Interval Follow-Up Evaluation – Range of Impaired Functioning Tool

Table 8. Intermediate Outcomes – Bipolar Disorder Studies

Study, Year Interventions Sample	Outcome Baseline	Post-Treatment	Short-term Follow-up	Long-term Follow-up
ATTENDANCE				
Miklowitz, 2007,[92] 2007[95] (Am J Psychiatry) 1) Family-focused 2) Inter-personal and social rhythm therapy 3) Cognitive Behavioral Therapy 4) Collaborative care *ITT analysis*			Attendance *mean sessions/# of sessions* 1) 11.5/30 (38%) 2) 16.7/30 (56%) 3) 13.3/30 (44%) 4) 2.2/3 (73%) p=ns (1 vs. 2 vs. 3)	
Miller, 2004[89] *ITT analysis* Solomon, 2008[97] *N=53 who recovered* 1) Medication + Family Therapy (FT) 2) Medication + Multiple-Family Group Therapy 3) Medication only *ITT analysis*				Pharmacotherapy sessions attended *(ITT analysis)* 1) 15 (10) 2) 12 (8) 3) 12 (8) p=ns *(at 28 months – final)*
				Pharmacotherapy sessions attended *(N=53 who recovered)* **1) 20 (9)** **2) 14 (7)** **3) 16 (6)** **p<0.05 (group 1 vs. group 2)** *(at 28 months – final)*
ADHERENCE				
Clarkin, 1998[94] 1) Medication management + marital intervention 2) Medication management only *Completers only*	Study designed med adherence scale 1) NR N=18 2) NR N=17 *scale of 1=poor, 6=excellent*	Study designed med adherence scale **1) 5.7 N=18** **2) 5.2 N=17** **p=0.008**		
Miklowitz, 2003[5] 1) Family-focused with medication 2) Crisis mgmt with medication *Sample not reported*				**1) 2.8 (0.4)** **2) 2.6 (0.5)** **p=0.04** *scale of 1=fully non-adherent, 3=fully adherent*

Family Involved Psychosocial Treatments for Adult Mental Health Conditions: A Review of the Evidence

Study, Year Interventions *Sample*	Outcome Baseline	Post-Treatment	Short-term Follow-up	Long-term Follow-up
Rea, 2003[91] 1) Family-focused with medication 2) Individual therapy with medication *ITT analysis*		Physicians' rating of medication compliance *(7-point Likert-type scale)* 1) 6.2 (1.6) 2) 5.6 (1.9) p=ns		

Outcomes reported as mean (standard deviation) unless otherwise noted.

Short-term follow up = 6 months post-treatment, unless otherwise noted; Long term=12 months post-treatment, unless otherwise noted. If an outcome had a final measure reported beyond 12 months, it is reported in long term follow up column and noted.

ns= not significant (at 5% level); NR = not reported; N/A = not applicable; Completers = findings for analyses conducted only with treatment completers; ITT = findings for analyses using an intent-to-treat approach

Table 9. Study Descriptive Information – Schizophrenia Spectrum Disorder Studies

Study, Year Funding Source	Sample Characteristics	Inclusion/Exclusion Criteria	Treatment Groups	Intervention Characteristics	Outcomes Assessed	Quality
Dyck, 2002[102] Government	N = 106 Gender: 77% male Age: 32.7 years Race/ethnicity: NR Marital Status: Married: 13% Not reported 87% Education: NR Veterans: NR *Recruitment Method:* Enrolled from outpatients enrolled in community mental health services, but living in community. *Family Characteristics:* NR	MH Condition: Schizophrenia or schizoaffective disorder Assessed by: structured clinical interview for DSM-IV criteria diagnosis Inclusions: In addition to diagnosis; age 18-45; enrolled in outpatient community mental health services in Spokane, WA, reside with family of origin, or have regular contact with family; family member and patient agree to consent; minimum attendance by one family member for at least five face to face contacts. [Subjects then stratified by medication status – atypical vs conventional antipsychotic use.] Family member or SO: Any family member	1) Multiple Family Group (MFG) N=55 2) Standard Care (SC) N = 51 No statistical differences at baseline – frequency of substance abuse, use of atypical antipsychotics, or severity of positive or negative symptoms *Analysis:* Baseline (pre and post): N=106	1) Format: Usual care + 1) three weekly sessions with clinicians and families (individually) without patient; 2) then a multiple family educational workshop (again without patient); then 3) bi-weekly multiple family group sessions with patient present. Manualized: Yes Sessions: NR 2 years Approach: multi-disciplinary; psychoeducational, develop a supportive network, formal problem solving techniques. 2) Format: Mental Health multidisciplinary treatment team delivered medication management, case management, some patients therapeutic and rehabilitation services. Manualized: N/A Sessions: N/A Txt Length: N/A Approach: Multidisciplinary	Patient Outcomes: Utilization: a. Hospitalization rate b. Crisis care used c. Outpatient service utilization Outcome timeframe: Pre-treatment (year before baseline) During -treatment (1 year after baseline)	Allocation concealment: NR Blinding: NR Intention to treat analysis: Yes Withdrawals adequately described: Yes Treatment integrity: Study supervisors do systematic review of videotapes for engagement sessions and multiple family group settings; weekly phone consultations, and annual on-site visits. Study Quality: Good

Family Involved Psychosocial Treatments for Adult Mental Health Conditions: A Review of the Evidence

Study, Year Funding Source	Sample Characteristics	Inclusion/Exclusion Criteria	Treatment Groups	Intervention Characteristics	Outcomes Assessed	Quality
Dyck, 2000[101] Government Note: this is the a subset of the study cohort of Dyck 2002[102]	N = 63 Gender: 73% male Age: 33 years Race/ethnicity: White 95% Not white 5% Marital Status: NR Veterans: NR	Same as Dyck, 2002[102]	1) MFG N=32 2) SC N=31 Analysis: 1) MFG N=21 2) SC N=21 (42 participants that received treatment for full 12 months)	Same as Dyck, 2002[102]	Patient Outcomes: Symptoms: a. MSANS Outcome timeframe: Baseline During -treatment (1 year after baseline)	Same as Dyck, 2002[102]
McDonnell, 2006[103] Government Note: Same study as Dyck 2000 and 2002, but different N. These 97 also provided 1 year pre-randomization data.	N = 97 Gender: 76% male Age: 32.8 years Race/ethnicity: European American 90% Not European American 10% Marital Status: NR Veterans: NR	Same as Dyck, 2002,[102] 2000[101]	1) MFG N=53 2) SC N = 44 Analysis: Baseline: N=97 Final: N = 97	Same as Dyck, 2002,[102] 2000[101]	Patient Outcomes: Utilization: a. Hospitalization rate (overall psychiatric, community, state, overall) b. Outpatient service utilization Outcome timeframe: Pre-treatment (year before baseline) Post-treatment (2 years) Final (3 years post baseline, 1 year after post-treatment)	Same as Dyck, 2002,[102] 2000[101]

Family Involved Psychosocial Treatments for Adult Mental Health Conditions: A Review of the Evidence

Study, Year Funding Source	Sample Characteristics	Inclusion/Exclusion Criteria	Treatment Groups	Intervention Characteristics	Outcomes Assessed	Quality
McFarlane, 1996[29] Government	N = 68 Gender: 65% male Age: 29.8 years Race/ethnicity: White 78% Black 15% Hispanic 6% Not reported 1% Marital Status: Married 6% Never Married 84% Separated/divorced/ widowed 9% Not reported 1% Education: NR Veterans: NR Recruitment Method: Subjects selected during admission to inpatient service or acute partial hospital when receiving crisis services for acute psychotic episode. Family Characteristics: NR	MH Condition: Schizophrenia or schizoaffective/ schizophreniform disorders Assessed by: Structured clinical interview DSM-III-R criteria Inclusions: In addition to diagnosis, subjects also needed to have one or more complicating factors: lack of consistent treatment participation; history of violence or suicidality, frequent hospitalization, homelessness, arrests/ convictions, moderate to severe substance use; at least one family member required to participate and give informed consent. Family member or SO: Any family member Exclusions: Acutely violent or suicidal; major medical illness or physical addiction requiring immediate hospitalization (excluded only until subject was stabilized)	1) Multi-family group N=37* 2) Crisis only N = 31* *Both groups are in Assertive community treatment (ACT); ACT consists of manualized program covering eight areas (includes family education and engagement); and one home visit. Analysis: Baseline: N=68 Post-treatment (2 years): N = 68 Family outcomes only: Baseline: N=46 Post-treatment (2 years): N = 46	1) Format: ACT + initial workshop for family only; then multi-family group meetings (6 families and patient is present) Manualized: Yes Session: every 2 wks Txt Length: 2 years Approach: Psychoeducational; Treatment decisions guided by group. Group provides social support, learn formal problem solving technique. 2) Format: ACT + interaction between treatment team and family members only in crisis. No multi-family groups. Manualized: Yes Session: N/A Approach: Psychoeducational	Patient Outcomes Global functioning: a. Employment rates Symptoms: a. PANSS (positive, negative, general) Health Care Utilization a. Re-Hospitalization Family Outcomes: Global Functioning: a. SAS-FV III Dissatisfaction with patient Friction between pt and others Well being of family Outcome timeframe: Baseline Post-treatment	Allocation concealment: No Blinding: NR Intention to treat analysis: No, on family measures. Withdrawals adequately described: No Study Quality: Fair

Family Involved Psychosocial Treatments for Adult Mental Health Conditions: A Review of the Evidence

Study, Year Funding Source	Sample Characteristics	Inclusion/Exclusion Criteria	Treatment Groups	Intervention Characteristics	Outcomes Assessed	Quality
Mueser, 2009[99] Government	N = 108 Gender: 70% male Age: 33.6 years Marital Status: Never married 63% Ever married 37% Race/ethnicity: White 71% Black 7% Other 22% Hispanic NR Education: Completed HS 62% Did not complete HS 38% Veterans: NR *Recruitment Method:* Among patients receiving services at participating mental health agencies, potentially eligible subjects were approached for willingness to participate. *Family Characteristics:* NR	MH condition: Dual disorder; either schizophrenia, schizoaffective or bipolar disorder AND active substance use or dependence within past 6 months Assessed by: Structured clinical interview DSM IV (for both) Family member or SO: a relative, close friend, or other person with a 'caring but non-professional relationship' to subject (e.g. clergy) Inclusions: In addition to diagnosis: ≥18 yrs old; ≥4 hours per week contact with the family member; diagnosis of active substance abuse or dependence within the past six months (based on SCID); subject currently receiving services at one of three mental health agencies participating in study Exclusions: None	1) FIDD - Family Intervention for Dual Disorders N=52 2) FPE – Family Psychoeducation N = 56 Analysis: ITT N=108 up to 36 months.	1) Format: Family member(s) and patient present Manualized: NR Sessions: 20–30 sessions, 1-1.5 hours Txt Length: 9-18 mos Approach: Psycho educational/ behavioral family therapy; education, communication and problem solving, tailored strategies, encouraged attendance at multiple family support groups between end of treatment & 36 months. 2) Format: Family member and patient present Manualized: NR Sessions: 6-8, 1 hour Txt Length: 6-8 weeks Approach: Psychoeducational; basic information about disorders and treatment; encouraged attendance at multiple family support groups between end of treatment & 36 months.	Intermediate Outcomes Adherence: a. Engagement (participation rate in ≥2 sessions) b. Exposure (attended at least 3 problem solving sessions for FIDD or 6 educational sessions for FPE) Outcome timeframe: Post-treatment only	Allocation Concealment: NR Blinding: Yes (assessors) Intention-to-treat analysis: Yes Withdrawals adequately described: Yes Treatment integrity: Interviews were randomly selected and rated by a third interviewer to check on reliability **Study Quality:** **Good**

Study, Year Funding Source	Sample Characteristics	Inclusion/Exclusion Criteria	Treatment Groups	Intervention Characteristics	Outcomes Assessed	Quality
Mueser, *in press*[100] Government	Same as Mueser, 2009[99]	Same as Mueser, 2009[99]	Same as Mueser, 2009[99]	Same as Mueser, 2009[99]	Patient Outcomes Symptom improvement: a. BPRS – total b. BPRS psychosis scale c. TLFB Days Drinking d. TLFB Days using drugs Global functioning: a. GAS b. % stable days in community Intermediate Outcomes Adherence b. Days medication non-adherence Outcome timeframe: Baseline Post-treatment Final (36 months post baseline – 18 months post-treatment for FIDD group; 33 months post-treatment for FPE group)	Same as Mueser, 2009[99]

Family Involved Psychosocial Treatments for Adult Mental Health Conditions: A Review of the Evidence

Study, Year Funding Source	Sample Characteristics	Inclusion/Exclusion Criteria	Treatment Groups	Intervention Characteristics	Outcomes Assessed	Quality
Schooler, 1997[24] Government but medications industry funded	N = 528 randomized, then patients started a stabilization phase (16-24 weeks); N = 313 (maintenance phase) – demographics provided for N=313 Gender: 66% male Age: 29.6 years Race/ethnicity: NR Marital Status: NR Education: NR Veterans: NR *Recruitment Method:* Recruited during hospitalization (93%) or as outpatients during an acute exacerbation *Family Characteristics:* NR	MH Condition: Schizophrenia, schizoaffective/ schizophreniform disorders Assessed by: Structured clinical interview for DSM-III-R diagnosis Family member or SO: Any family member. Inclusions: In addition to diagnosis; age 18-55; willingness to take fluphenazine decanoate injections and not receive other neuroleptic, antidepressant, or mood stabilizing medications; in contact with family of origin or legal guardian > 4 hours per week; subject and family member consent; psychiatric hospitalization or symptom relapse in the past three months. Exclusions: Current physical dependence on alcohol, stimulants, barbiturates, or narcotics, current hospitalization precipitated by substance abuse; current pregnancy; Liver damage, epilepsy or acute brain syndrome, unequivocal liver damage.	Two stage: Assigned to family treatment N = 528 1) Applied family management (AFM) N = 272 2) Supportive Family management (SFM) N = 256 Note: Assigned to a treatment group, then stabilized (stabilization phase for 16-24 weeks); then 2 year maintenance phase. After stabilization, further divided between 3 dose regimens of Fluphenazine. Stabilized, and on to maintenance phase N = 313: 1) AFM N = 157 2) SFM N = 156 Analysis: Baseline: N=313 Post-treatment (2 years) N = 313	1) Format:* Individual family meeting in home, then sessions in home (individual) with patient present; monthly family group meetings and case management that paralleled SFM. Manualized: Yes Sessions: weekly then biweekly then monthly; max of 32 sessions Txt Length: > 2 years Approach: behavioral family therapy, in addition to SFM model - psychoeducational (communication, problem solving, social support) 2) Format:* Monthly group meetings (with patient present), with case management / consultation with treatment team for problem solving (if initiated by family). Manualized: NR Sessions: Monthly Txt Length: > 2 years Approach: psychoeducational (communication, problem solving, social support). Families relied on to initiate contacts with treatment team as needed.	Patient Outcomes Utilization: a. Time to rehospitaliza-tion b. % rehospitalized c. Time to first rescue medication d. Time to psychotic relapse Outcome timeframe: Final (24 months post) Intermediate Outcomes Treatment attendance a. % attended initial workshop b. % attended monthly support meetings Outcome timeframe: Baseline Post-treatment	Allocation concealment: NR Blinding: Medication blinded Intention to treat analysis: No; only those who stabilized shown Withdrawals adequately described: Yes Treatment Integrity: Certification in AFM required for study clinicians based on video sessions; ongoing competency monitored through audio taped sessions & supervisory telephone calls. Study Quality: Fair

172

Family Involved Psychosocial Treatments for Adult Mental Health Conditions: A Review of the Evidence

Study, Year Funding Source	Sample Characteristics	Inclusion/Exclusion Criteria	Treatment Groups	Intervention Characteristics	Outcomes Assessed	Quality
Mueser, 2001[104] Government	Same Study as Schooler, 1997[24]	Same Study as Schooler 1997[24]	Same Study as Schooler 1997[24] Analysis of those who stabilized and went to maintenance phase N = 313 1) AFM, N = 157 2) SFM, N = 156 Analysis: Baseline: N=313 Post-treatment (2 years) N = 313	Same Study as Schooler 1997[24]	Family Outcomes Family Functioning a. SAS-PT Social functioning Family relationship Patient Rejection Scale b. SAS-Interim Patient: Family friction scale Couple functioning: a. SAS-PT Romance-sexual Outcome timeframe: Baseline Post-treatment	Same Study as Schooler 1997[24] Treatment Integrity: Additional information provided: all sessions audio taped, and select sessions evaluated by independent rater.

NR=not reported; HS = high school; DSM=Diagnostic and Statistical Manual of Mental Disorders; SO=significant other or family member included; MFG=Multiple Family Group; SC=Standard Care; NR=not reported; N/A=not applicable; SO=significant other; MANS=Modified Scale for Assessment of Negative Symptoms; ACT=Assertive community treatment; PANSS=Positive and Negative Syndrome Scale; SAS-FV=Social Adjustment Scale – Family Version; FIDD=Family Intervention for Dual Disorders; FPE=Family Psychoeducation; Applied Family management=AFM; Supportive Family Management=SFM; SAS-PT=Social Adjustment Scale Patient; TLFB = Time Line Follow Back; BPRS = Brief Psychiatric Rating Scale; GAS = Global Assessment Scale

*Both groups started with psychoeducational workshop.

Table 10. Patient Outcomes - Schizophrenia Spectrum Disorder Studies

Study, Year Interventions Sample	Pre-treatment (baseline)	During-treatment	Post-Treatment	Long-term follow up
SYMPTOM IMPROVEMENT				
Dyck, 2000[101] 1) Multiple Family Groups (MFG) 2) Standard care (SC) *Completers*	MSANS 1) 7.9 (3.1) N=21 2) 8.7 (3.3) N=21 p=NR (ns)	MSANS[1] **1) 7.2 (2.0) N=21** **2) 8.4 (3.1) N=21** **p<0.05**		
Mueser[2], in press[100] 1) Family Intervention for Dual Disorders (FIDD) 2) Family Psychoeducation (FPE) *Completers*	Brief Psychiatric Rating Scale BPRS (Total) 1) 2.0 (0.6) N=52 2) 2.0 (0.5) N=56 p=NR	BPRS Total at month 12 1) 1.9 (0.5) N=39 2) 2.0 (0.6) N=45 p=NR	BPRS Total at month 18 1) 1.7 (0.4) N=28 2) 1.9 (0.5) N=34 p=NR	BPRS Total at month 36 (FINAL) 1) 1.9 (0.5) N=23 2) 1.9 (0.5) N=25 p=NR **Linear regression, ANCOVA models (differences between groups 1) and 2) over time:** **F 3.8, df 1,86 p=0.05** Effects over time, groups 1) and 2) combined: **F 8.0, df 1,390 p=0.005**
	Brief Psychiatric Rating Scale BPRS (Psychosis) 1) 2.1 (1.0) N=52 2) 2.1 (1.4) N=56 p=NR	BPRS Psychosis at month 12 1) 1.9 (1.0) N=39 2) 2.1 (0.1) N=45 p=NR	BPRS Psychosis at month 18 1) 1.8 (0.8) N=28 2) 1.6 (0.7) N=34 p=NR	BPRS Psychosis at month 36 FINAL) 1) 1.9 (0.8) N=23 2) 1.9 (0.9) N=25 p=NR **Linear regression, ANCOVA models (differences between groups 1) and 2) over time:** **F 7.1, df 1,86 p=0.009** Effects over time, groups 1) and 2) combined: F 3.4, df 1,390 p=0.07
	Days drinking, past 6 months 1) 45.5 (50.2) N=52 2) 37.1 (37.8) N=56 p=NR	Days drinking, past 6 months at month 12 1) 16.7 (28.2) N=39 2) 32.8 (47.0) N=45 p=NR	Days drinking, past 6 months at month 18 1) 25.1 (40.2) N=28 2) 22.3 (32.3) N=34 p=NR	Days drinking, past 6 months at month 36 (FINAL) 1) 36.0 (45.4) N=23 2) 32.3 (55.7) N=25 p=NR Effects over time, groups 1) and 2) combined: F 0.24, df 1,283 p=0.63

174

Family Involved Psychosocial Treatments for Adult Mental Health Conditions: A Review of the Evidence

Study, Year Interventions *Sample*	Pre-treatment (baseline)	During-treatment	Post-Treatment	Long-term follow up
	Days drug use, past 6 months N=52 1) 49.9 (55.8) N=52 2) 50.0 (47.9) N=56 p=NR	Days drug use, past 6 months at month 12 1)25.0 (45.9) N=39 2)44.2 (59.4) N=45 p=NR	Days drug use, past 6 months at month 18 1) 28.4 (46.8) N=28 2) 32.3 (49.3) N=34 p=NR	Days drug use, past 6 months at month 36 (FINAL) 1) 43.4 (67.6) N=23 2) 30.6 (57.1) N=25 Effects over time, groups 1) and 2) combined: F 3.05, df 1,290 p=0.08
GLOBAL FUNCTIONING				
McFarlane 1996[29] 1) Assertive Community Treatment (ACT) + MFG 2) ACT + Crisis intervention with families *ITT*			Employment rate during 2 year study period 1) 32% N=37 2) 19% N=31 p<0.07	
Mueser[2], in press[100] 1) Family Intervention for Dual Disorders (FIDD) 2) Family Psychoeducation (FPE) *Completers*	Global Assessment Scale 1) 43.4 (10.1) N=52 2) 42.7 (8.2) N=56 p=NR	Global Assessment Scale at month 12 1) 49.0 (12.6) N=39 2) 47.2 (10.9) N=45 p=NR	Global Assessment Scale at month 18 1) 49.8 (12.9) N=28 2) 48.4 (11.2) N=34 p=NR	Global Assessment Scale at month 36 (FINAL) 1) 48.3 (12.0) N=23 2) 47.5 (9.0) N=25 p=NR **Effects over time, groups 1) and 2) combined: F 11.9, df 1,388 p<0.001** Linear regression, ANCOVA models (differences between groups 1) and 2) over time: F 2.9, df 1,86 p=0.08
	% stable days in community, past 6 months 1) 84% N=52 2) 87% N=56 p=NR	% stable days in community, past 6 months at month 12 1) 86% N=39 2) 85% N=45 p=NR	% stable days in community, past 6 months at month 18 1) 97% N=28 2) 89% N=34 p=NR	% stable days in community, past 6 months at month 36 (FINAL) 1) 92% N=23 2) 93% N=25 p=NR **Effects over time, groups 1) and 2) combined: F 5.68, df 1,387 p=0.02**

Family Involved Psychosocial Treatments for Adult Mental Health Conditions: A Review of the Evidence

Study, Year Interventions Sample	Pre-treatment (baseline)	During-treatment	Post-Treatment	Long-term follow up
HEALTH CARE UTILIZATION				
Dyck, 2002[102] 1) Multiple Family Groups 2) Standard care *ITT*	% hospitalized in year prior[3] 1) 29% N=16/55 2) 38% N=19/51 p=0.15	% hospitalized in year prior[1] **1) 9% N=5/55** **2) 22% N=11/51** **p=0.03[5]**		
		% received crisis/urgent care in year prior[1] 1) 13% N=7/55 2) 22% N=11/51 p=0.09		
	Outpatient Service Utilization (hours) in year prior[3] 1) 16.0 (24.7) N=55 2) 23.3 (34.4) N=51 p=0.21	Outpatient Service Utilization (hours) in year prior[1] 1) 15.8 (27.4) N=55 2) 14.1 (21.8) N=51 p=0.40		
McDonnell, 2006[103] 1) Multiple Family Groups 2) Standard Care *Modified ITT*	% hospitalized (all psychiatric) in year prior[3] 1) 31% N=16/53 2) 37% N=16/44 p=NR (ns)	% hospitalized (all psychiatric) in year prior[1] 1) 8% N=4/53 2) 21% N=9/44 p=NR (ns)	% hospitalized (all psychiatric) in year prior[4] 1) 23% N=12/53 2) 16% N=7/44 p=NR (ns)	% hospitalized (all psychiatric) in year prior[6] 1) 8% N=4/53 2) 19% N=8/44 p=NR (ns)
	% hospitalized (community hospitals) in year prior[3] 1) 25% N=13/53 2) 33% N=14/44 p=NR (ns)	% hospitalized (community hospitals) in year prior[1] **1) 4% N=2/53** **2) 19% N=8/44** **p<0.05**	% hospitalized (community hospitals) in year prior[4] 1) 21% N=11/53 2) 12% N=5/44 p=NR (ns)	% hospitalized (community hospitals) in year prior[6] 1) 8% N=4/53 2) 14% N=6/44 p=NR (ns)
	% hospitalized (state hospitals) in year prior[3] 1) 8% N=4/53 2) 9% N=4/44 p=NR (ns)	% hospitalized (state hospitals) in year prior[1] 1) 4% N=2/53 2) 7% N=3/44 p=NR (ns)	% hospitalized (state hospitals) in year prior[4] 1) 6% N=3/53 2) 9% N=4/44 p=NR (ns)	% hospitalized (state hospitals) in year prior[6] **1) 2% N=1/53** **2)14% N=6/44** **p<0.05**
	Outpatient Service Utilization (hours) in year prior[3,7] 1) 55.8 (88.1) N=53 2) 57.6 (85.3) N=44 p=NR (ns)	Outpatient Service Utilization (hours) in year prior[1] **1) 79.3 (94.6) N=55** **2) 53.6 (74.2) N=51** **p<0.05**	Outpatient Service Utilization (hours) in year prior[4] **1) 39.9 (71.0) N=53** **2) 27.2 (51.9) N=44** **p<.05**	Outpatient Service Utilization (hours) in year prior[6] 1) 14.0 (15.8) N=53 2) 25.2 (33.5) N=44 p=NR (ns)

Family Involved Psychosocial Treatments for Adult Mental Health Conditions: A Review of the Evidence

Study, Year Interventions *Sample*	Pre-treatment (baseline)	During-treatment	Post-Treatment	Long-term follow up
Schooler, 1997[24] 1) Applied Family Management 2) Supportive Family Management *Patients who stabilized, and were in maintenance only*			Days to re-hospitalization 1) 515 N=157 2) 504 N=156 p=NR (ns)	
			% re-hospitalized 1) 29% N=157 2) 35% N=156 p=0.28	
			Days to first rescue medication 1) 323 N=157 2) 351 N=156 p=NR (ns)	
			Days to psychotic relapse 1) 524 N=157 2) 544 N=156 p=NR (ns)	

Outcomes reported as mean (standard deviation) unless otherwise noted.

Short-term follow up = 6 months post-treatment, unless otherwise noted; Long term=12 months post-treatment, unless otherwise noted. Measures listed in the study descriptive tables but not reported here if either 1) the authors did not report beyond 12 months, it is reported in long term follow up column and noted. Measures listed in the study descriptive tables but not reported here if either 1) the authors did not report findings from these measures or 2) they did not test for differences between conditions on these measures.

ns = not significant (at 5% level); NR = not reported; N/A = not applicable; Completers = findings for analyses conducted only with treatment completers; ITT = findings for analyses using an intent-to-treat approach; MSANS = Modified Scale for Assessment of Negative Symptoms;

[1]Timepoint = Year 1 of two year intervention.
[2]FIDD arm treatment duration = 9-18 months; FPE = 3 months.
[3]Timepoint = one year prior to baseline.
[4]Timepoint = Year 2 of two year intervention.
[5]MFG versus SC significantly correlated with hospitalization year after baseline. Cochran-Mantel-Haenszel procedure that controlled for hospitalization year before randomization, yielded a significant association between group membership and hospitalization (p<0.04).
[6]Timepoint = One year after two year intervention.
[7]McDonell appears to contradict Dyck (2002); however, crisis utilization services were not included in estimate of outpatient utilization in Dyck, but were included in McDonell figures. MFG treatment group utilization increase during utilization period due to addition of 24 90 minute MFG sessions in year 1, and 12 in year 1 (post baseline). When these sessions are removed, no group differences observed.

Family Involved Psychosocial Treatments for Adult Mental Health Conditions: A Review of the Evidence

Table 11. Family Outcomes - Schizophrenia Spectrum Disorder Studies

Study, Year Interventions *Sample*	Baseline	Mid-treatment (one year)[1]	Post-treatment (two years)[1]
FAMILY FUNCTIONING			
Mueser, 2001[104] 1) Applied Family Management 2) Supportive Family Management *Patients who stabilized, and were in maintenance only*	SAS: Social/leisure factor 1) 2.8 (0.6) N=157 2) 2.7 (0.6) N=156 p=NR	SAS: Social/leisure factor 1) 2.7 (0.7) N=157 2) 2.6 (0.6) N=156 p=NR	SAS: Social/leisure factor 1) 2.8 (0.7) N=157 2) 2.6 (0.6) N=156 Mixed effects model:[2] Test of differences between groups over time: F(2,299)=0.29 p=NR (ns)
	SAS: Family relationships factor 1) 1.8 (0.7) N=157 2) 1.9 (0.6) N=156 p=NR	SAS: Family relationships factor 1) 1.9 (0.6) N=157 2) 1.8 (0.6) N=156 p=NR	SAS: Family relationships factor 1) 1.9 (0.6) N=157 2) 1.9 (0.6) N=156 Mixed effects model:[2] Test of differences between groups over time: F(2,299)=0.92 p=NR (ns)
	Patient Rejection Scale[3] 1) 61.0 (22.1) N=157 2) 57.3 (19.6) N=156 p=NR	Patient Rejection Scale[3] 1) 59.2 (21.5) N=157 2) 58.9 (21.7) N=156 p=NR	Patient Rejection Scale[3] 1) 61.2 (23.0) N=157 2) 60.2 (23.0) N=156 Mixed effects model:[2] Test of differences between groups over time: **F(2,288)=3.07** **p<0.01** Effect size (r): 0.30
			SAS Family friction[4] **B=-0.187 SE 0.063** **p<0.01** Effect size (r): 0.24
COUPLE FUNCTIONING			
Mueser, 2001[104] 1) Applied Family Management 2) Supportive Family Management *Patients who stabilized, and were in maintenance only*	SAS: romance / sexual factor 1) 2.8 (1.1) N=157 2) 2.9 (0.9) N=156 p=NR	SAS: romance / sexual factor 1) 2.7 (1.0) N=157 2) 2.6 (1.0) N=156 p=NR	SAS: romance / sexual factor 1) 2.7 (1.1) N=157 2) 2.6 (1.0) N=156 Mixed effects model:[2] Test of differences between groups over time: F(2,236)=0.71 p=NR (ns)

Outcomes reported as mean (standard deviation) unless otherwise noted. Short-term follow up = 6 months post-treatment, unless otherwise noted. Long term=12 months post-treatment, unless otherwise noted. If an outcome had a final measure reported beyond 12 months, it is reported in long term follow up column and noted. Measures listed in the study descriptive tables but not reported here if either 1) the authors did not report findings from these measures or 2) they did not test for differences between conditions on these measures.
ns = not significant (at 5% level); NR = not reported; N/A = not applicable; SAS = Social Adjustment Scale
[1]Family outcomes for this study calculated at baseline, year 1, and year 2 of two year treatment.
[2]Mixed effects model included covariates diagnosis, gender, site, Brief Psychiatric Rating scale.
[3]Patient rejection scale, high scores indicate more negative family attitudes toward the patient.
[4]Based on random effects models; effects sizes computed by averaging outcomes for months 18-24.

178

Table 12. Intermediate Outcomes – Schizophrenia Spectrum Disorder Studies

Study, Year Interventions Sample	Baseline / Short Term	During treatment	During treatment/post-treatment	Final
ATTENDANCE				
Mueser, 2009[99] and in press[100] 1) Family Intervention for Dual Disorders (FIDD) 2) Family Psychoeducation (FPE) ITT			Engagement in treatment (≥ 2 sessions, either arm) 1) 88% N=46/52 2) 84% N=47/56 p=NR (ns) Exposed to treatment (≥ 3sessions FIDD; ≥6 sessions FPE) 1) 62% N=32/52 2) 55% N=31/56 p=NR (ns)	Relatives attending family support group (between end of treatment and month 36) 1) 15% N=6/40 2) 11% N=5/46 p=NR (ns)
Schooler, 1997[24] 1) Applied Family Management 2) Supportive Family Management Completers	Attendance, initial workshop[1] 1) 75.2% N=272 2) 79.2% N=256 p=NR (ns) Attendance, monthly treatment [1] 1) 53.5% N=272 2) 60.3% N=256 p=NR (ns)	Attendance, monthly treatment[2] 1) 60.4% N=157 2) 66.2% N=156 p=NR (ns)	% Attendance, monthly treatment[3] 1) 50.2% N=157 2) 50.9% N=156 p=NR (ns)	- Attendance, monthly treatment[4] 1) 39.3%N=157 2) 33.3% N=156 p=NR (ns)
ADHERENCE				
Mueser[2], in press[100] 1) Family Intervention for Dual Disorders (FIDD) 2) Family Psychoeducation (FPE) Completers	Days medication non-adherence (in past 30) at baseline 1) 4.5 (8.1) N=52 2) 2.6 (6.4) N=56 p=NR (ns)	Days medication non-adherence (in past 30) at month 12 1) 2.6 (8.1) N=39 2) 5.2 (9.0) N=45 p=NR (ns)	Days medication non-adherence (in past 30) at month 18 1) 4.0 (6.9) N=28 2) 3.1 (7.8) N=34 p=NR (ns)	Days medication non-adherence (in past 30) at month 36 (FINAL) 1) 2.5 (3.0) N=23 2) 1.2 (1.9) N=25 p=NR (ns) Time effects, combined groups: F 3.34, df 1,350 p=0.07

Outcomes reported as mean (standard deviation) unless otherwise noted. Short-term follow up = 6 months post-treatment, unless otherwise noted. Long term=12 months post-treatment, unless otherwise noted. If an outcome had a final measure reported beyond 12 months, it is reported in long term follow up column and noted. ns = not significant (at 5% level); NR = not reported; N/A = not applicable; Completers = findings for analyses conducted only with treatment completers; ITT = findings for analyses using an intent-to-treat approach.

[1]During 16-24 week stabilization phase.

[2]For subjects that stabilized, attendance during months 1-6 of maintenance phase.

[3]For subjects that stabilized, attendance during months 7-12 of maintenance phase.

[4]For subjects that stabilized, attendance during months 18-24 of maintenance phase (final).

[5]FIDD arm treatment duration = 9-18 months; FPE = 3 months.

Table 13. Study Descriptive Information – Post Traumatic Stress Disorder (PTSD) Studies

Study, Year Funding Source	Sample Characteristics	Inclusion and Exclusion Criteria	Treatment Groups	Intervention	Outcomes Assessed	Quality
Glynn, 1999[8] Government	N = 36 Gender: 100% male Age: 46.6 (3.1) yrs Race/ethnicity: White 45% African American: 29% Hispanic 26% Marital Status: NR - Education (years): 13.5 (2.5) yrs Veterans: 100% Family Characteristics: Wife/conjugal partner 90% Sibling 5% Parent 5% Recruitment Method: All current patients at Veterans Affairs Hospital (inpatient and outpatient), recruited from Los Angeles, CA area.	MH Condition: PTSD Assessed by: Clinician-Administered PTSD Scale SO: Any family member Inclusions: 1) military service during the Vietnam conflict, 2) clinical diagnosis of combat PTSD, 3) stable psychiatric medication regimen at randomization, 4) willingness to provide informed consent Exclusions: 1) medical condition contraindicating use of exposure therapy (e.g., severe cardiovascular disease), 2) history or present evidence of an organic brain, psychotic, or severe dissociative disorder, 3) current substance dependence, 4) evidence of overt physical aggression to self or others within preceding year	1) Exposure Therapy + Behavioral Family Therapy (BFT) N = 17 (11 completed) 2) Exposure Therapy N = 12 (12 completed) 3) 2 month wait list + BFT if desired N = 13 (13 completed) Randomized: N=42 Analysis: Baseline N=36 Post-treatment N=36 Short term (final) 6 months N=20	1) Format: Exposure Therapy + BFT Manualized: Yes Sessions: 18 exposure sessions followed by 16 sessions of BFT Txt Length: 9 weeks for exposure therapy then 11-12 weeks of BFT weekly, then 2 biweekly BFT meetings, then 2 monthly BFT meetings Approach: Repeated exposure to trauma memory followed by cognitive restructuring + skills training in BFT for education on the disorder, communication training, anger management, and problem-solving skills. 2) Format: Exposure Therapy Manualized: Yes Sessions: 18 Txt Length: 9 weeks Approach: Exposure therapy with cognitive restructuring 3) Format: wait list + BFT if desired Manualized: Yes Sessions: 16 Txt Length: 11-12 weeks of BFT weekly, then 2 biweekly BFT meetings, then 2 monthly BFT meetings Approach: Psychoeducation, communication training, anger management, problem-solving skills training	Patient Outcomes Symptom Improvement a. M-PTSD b. Impact of Events Scale c. CAPS Global functioning a. SAS-SR Family Outcomes Family functioning: a. SPSI Intermediate Outcome Attendance a. # dropouts Outcome time-frame: Baseline Post-treatment Short term (Final) – 6 months	Allocation concealment: NR Blinding: NR Intention to treat analysis: No Withdrawals adequately described: Yes Treatment Integrity: Therapists met weekly with supervisors; supervisors reviewed progress notes; sessions audiotaped and PI listened to random 20% for protocol adherence (then provided feedback to therapists) Study Quality: Fair

Family Involved Psychosocial Treatments for Adult Mental Health Conditions: A Review of the Evidence

Evidence-based Synthesis Program

Study, Year Funding Source	Sample Characteristics	Inclusion and Exclusion Criteria	Treatment Groups	Intervention	Outcomes Assessed	Quality
Weine, 2008[105] Government	N = 197 Gender: 48% male Age: 37.7 years Race/ethnicity: Bosnia refugees 100% Marital Status: Married 82% Divorced or separated 11% Single, never married 4% Widowed 3% Education: HS graduate 62% Veterans: NR Family Characteristics: N=166 Gender: 40% male Age: 35.5 yrs Marital Status: Married 87% Divorced or separated 3% Single, never married 10% Education: HS graduate 56% Recruitment Method: community based organizations	MH Condition: PTSD Assessed by: PTSD Symptoms Scale SO: Any family member(s) >17 age living in same household Inclusions: Bosnian refugees who screened positive for PTSD; not currently receiving mental health services. Exclusions: Those who screened positive for an acute confusional state, active psychosis, or substance intoxication or withdrawal	1) Coffee and Family Education and Support (CAFES) N = 110 2) No treatment control group N = 87 Analysis: Baseline N=197 Short term (6 months) N=197 Long term (12 months) N=197 Final (18 months) N=197	1) Format: Groups for the patient and family members (all family members > 17 yrs old invited; 7 families/group) Manualized: Yes Sessions: 9 Txt Length: 16 weeks Approach: Community-based, family focused program aimed at improving access to mental health services by impacting family processes intervention included support, psychoeducation, and communication training among other topics 2) No treatment	Patient Outcome Health Care Utilization a. # of mental health visits Intermediate Outcome Attendance a. attrition rate Outcome timeframe: Baseline Short term: 6 months Long term: 12 months Final: 18 months	Allocation concealment: NR Blinding: NR Intention to treat analysis: NR Withdrawals adequately described: Yes Treatment Integrity: 20 hrs implementation training, weekly group and individual supervision, monthly videotaping of CAFES sessions Study Quality: Fair

NR = not reported; PI = Principal Investigator; HS = high school; SO = significant other or family member included; M-PTSD = Mississippi Scale for Combat-Related PTSD; CAPS = Clinician Administered PTSD Scale; SAS-SR = Social Adjustment Scale-Self-report; SPSI = Social Problem-Solving Inventory

Family Involved Psychosocial Treatments for Adult Mental Health Conditions: A Review of the Evidence

Table 14. Patient Outcomes - Post Traumatic Stress Disorder Studies

Study, Year Interventions Sample	Outcome Baseline	Post-Treatment	Short-term Follow-up	Long-term Follow-up
SYMPTOM IMPROVEMENT				
Glynn, 1999[8] 1) Exposure therapy + Behavioral Family Therapy (BFT) 2) Exposure therapy 3) 2 month wait list + then BFT if desired *Completers only*	Positive symptoms[a] 1) 0.03 (0.10) N=11 2) -0.03 (0.15) N=12 3) 0.01 (0.14) N=13 p=ns Negative symptoms[a] 1) -0.04 (0.12) N=11 2) -0.05 (0.12) N=12 3) 0.01 (0.11) N=13 p=ns	Positive symptoms[a] 1) **-0.06 (0.15) N=11** 2) **-0.07 (0.12) N=12** 3) **0.02 (0.09) N=13** **p < 0.05** ***Groups 1) & 2) significantly < 3)** Negative symptoms[a] 1) -0.11 (0.23) N=11 2) -0.15 (0.17) N=12 3) -0.02 (0.17) N=13 p=ns	Positive symptoms[a] 1) -0.07 (0.12) N=10 2) -0.09 (0.16) N=10 3) NR p=ns Negative symptoms[a] 1) -0.10 (0.21) N=10 2) -0.15 (0.21) N=10 3) NR p=ns	
GLOBAL FUNCTIONING				
Glynn, 1999[8] 1) Exposure therapy + BFT 2) Exposure therapy 3) 2 month wait list + then BFT if desired *Completers only*	Social Adjust Scale (SAS-SR)[b] 1) 2.64 (0.47) N=11 2) 2.73 (0.25) N=12 3) 2.84 (0.71) N=13 p=ns	Social Adjust Scale (SAS-SR)[b] 1) 2.40 (0.61) N=11 2) 2.48 (0.43) N=12 3) 2.72 (0.69) N=13 p=ns	Social Adjust Scale (SAS-SR)[b] 1) 2.32 (0.55) N=10 2) 2.55(0.61) N=10 3) NR p=ns	
HEALTH CARE UTILIZATION				
Weine, 2008[105] 1) Coffee and Family Education and Support (CAFES) 2) No treatment (control) *ITT analyses*	# mental health visits in prior 6 months 1) 0.1 N=110 2) 0.1 N= 87 p=NR		# mental health visits in prior 6 months 1) 5.2 N=110 2) 2.2 N=87 p=NR *(6months)*	# mental health visits in prior 6 months 1) 6.3 N=110 2) 2.3 N=87 p=NR *(12 months)* # mental health visits in prior 6 months 1) 6.0 N=110 2) 1.7 N=87 p=NR *(18 months- final)* *Random effects regression model:* **Significant between group differences: β = 3.17, p<0.005**

Outcomes reported as mean (standard deviation) unless otherwise noted. Short-term follow up = 6 months post-treatment, unless otherwise noted. Long term=12 months post-treatment, unless otherwise noted. If an outcome had a final measure reported beyond 12 months, it is reported in long term follow up column and noted.

ns = not significant (at 5% level); NR = not reported; N/A = not applicable; Completers = findings for analyses conducted only with treatment completers; ITT = findings for analyses using an intent-to-treat approach.

[a] Composite of Clinician Administered PTSD Scale (CAPS) scores; Mississippi Scale for Combat-Related PTSD scale scores; and Impact of Events Scale; Higher score indicates more severe symptoms or worse social adjustment.

[b] Higher score indicates more severe symptoms or worse social adjustment.

Table 15. Family Outcomes – Post Traumatic Stress Disorder Studies

Study, Year Interventions *Sample*	Outcome Baseline	Post-Treatment	Short-term Follow-up	Long-term Follow-up
FAMILY FUNCTIONING				
Glynn, 1999[8] 1) Exposure therapy + Behavioral Family Therapy (BFT) 2) Exposure therapy 3) 2 month wait list + then BFT if desired	Social Problem-Solving Inventory (SPSI) NR	Social Problem-Solving Inventory (SPSI) No group comparisons on family functioning outcomes *Subgroup comparison* *(change scores from baseline to post)* **(a) BFT completers:** **6.00 (22.61) N=NR** **(b) No BFT participation** **-9.10 (21.70) N=NR** **p<0.05**		

Outcomes reported as mean (standard deviation) unless otherwise noted. Short-term follow up = 6 months post-treatment, unless otherwise noted; Long term=12 months post-treatment, unless otherwise noted. If an outcome had a final measure reported beyond 12 months, it is reported in long term follow up column and noted.
NR = not reported

Table 16. Intermediate Outcomes – Post Traumatic Stress Disorder Studies

Study, Year Interventions *Sample*	Outcome Baseline	Post-Treatment	Short-term Follow-up	Long-term Follow-up
ATTENDANCE				
Glynn, 1999[8] 1) Exposure therapy + Behavioral Family Therapy (BFT) 2) Exposure therapy 3) 2 month wait list + then BFT if desired *Completers only*	# of dropouts N/A	# of dropouts 1) 6 N=17 2) 0 N=12 3) 0 N=13 **p < 0.01**		
Weine, 2008[105] 1) Coffee and Family Education and Support (CAFES) 2) No treatment (control) *ITT analyses*	Attrition Rate N/A	Attrition Rate NR	Attrition Rate 1) 17% 2) 14% p=NR	Attrition Rate 1) 6% 2) 10% p=NR *(12 months)* Attrition Rate 1) 4% 2) 1% p=NR *(18 months - final)*

Outcomes reported as mean (standard deviation) unless otherwise noted. Short-term follow up = 6 months post-treatment, unless otherwise noted. If an outcome had a final measure reported beyond 12 months, it is reported in long term follow up column and noted; Long term=12 months post-treatment, unless otherwise noted.
NR = not reported; N/A = not applicable; Completers = findings for analyses conducted only with treatment completers; ITT = findings for analyses using an intent-to-treat approach

Table 17. Study Descriptive Information – Sexual Functioning Disorders Studies

Study, Year Funding Source	Sample Characteristics	Inclusion and Exclusion Criteria	Treatment Groups	Intervention	Outcomes Assessed	Quality
Aubin, 2009[106] Funding source not reported	N = 44 Gender: 100% male Age: 52.4 yrs Race/ethnicity: White 86% Non-white 14% Marital Status: Married 68% Cohabitating or dating 32% Relationship length: 18.4 yrs Education: 25% High school 75% College or greater Veterans: NR Family Characteristics: Female partners 100% Wives 68% Girlfriend/SO 32% Age: 50.0 years Recruitment Method: Newspaper advertisements, referrals from practitioners, flyers	MH Condition: Erectile dysfunction (ED) Assessed by: NR SO: Female intimate partner Inclusions: 20-80 yrs old; ED for ≥6 months (due to a medical condition or not); absence of medical condition that prohibits Sildenafil intake or compromises study completion; stable heterosexual relationship ≥1 year; men consent to pre-tx medical evaluation to establish level of organic involvement of ED and safety of Sildenafil dosage; both partners read, write, and speak English fluently; provide informed consent Exclusions: Fair-to-severe mood disorders (BDI-II > 19), substance-related disorders (≥3 drinks a day), lifetime female sexual dysfunction except pain related to lubrication; inability to interrupt psychotherapy during study; spousal abuse; extra-marital affair in last year; recent discussion of or separation plans; gender identity disorder in last 5 years	1) Medication (Sildenafil) + sex therapy N = 27 (24 completed) 2) Medication (Sildenafil) only N = 24 (20 completed) Randomized: N =51 Analysis: Baseline N= 44 Post-treatment: N = 44 Short term (Final-2 months): N = 44	1) Format: medication + couple sex therapy Manualized: Yes Sessions: 8 sex therapy sessions (weekly for weeks 1-4; biweekly thereafter) Txt Length: 12 weeks Approach: "Sessions included an amalgam of existing couple and sex therapy strategies such as communication and emotional skills training, sensate focus, sexual fantasy training, and cognitive restructuring" with homework 2) Format: medication only with brief, typically individual, pick-up visits to assess side effects and medical concerns Manualized: NR Sessions: 8 (15 minute) sessions; weekly for weeks 1-4 and then biweekly Txt Length: 12 weeks Approach: NR	Patient Outcomes: Symptom Improvement a. International Index for Erectile Function (IIEF) Family Outcomes: Couple functioning: a. Dyadic Adjustment scale (DAS) b. Personal Assessment of Intimacy in Relationships (PAIR) Intermediate Outcomes Satisfaction with care a. Erectile Dysfunction Inventory of Treatment Satisfaction (EDITS) Attendance: a. Retention Outcome timeframe: Baseline Post-treatment Short term (final): 2 months	Allocation concealment: NR Blinding: NR Intention to treat analysis: No Withdrawals adequately described: Yes Treatment Integrity: all couples need by same therapist (Principal Investigator) **Study Quality: Poor**

Family Involved Psychosocial Treatments for Adult Mental Health Conditions: A Review of the Evidence

Study, Year Funding Source	Sample Characteristics	Inclusion and Exclusion Criteria	Treatment Groups	Intervention	Outcomes Assessed	Quality
Banner, 2007[107] Funding source not reported	N = 53 <u>Gender:</u> 100% male <u>Age:</u> 56.8 yrs <u>Race/ethnicity:</u> White 87% Asian 6% Other 7% <u>Marital Status:</u> NR <u>Relationship length:</u> 23.6 yrs <u>Education:</u> NR Veterans: NR *Family Characteristics:* 100% female partners *Recruitment Method:* Newspaper and radio advertisements, referrals from local practitioners	<u>MH Condition:</u> Erectile dysfunction without previously diagnosed medical etiology <u>Assessed by:</u> Psychologist telephone interview <u>SO:</u> Intimate partner of at least 6 months <u>Inclusions:</u> Heterosexual couples in the same relationship ≥6 months; Patient diagnosis of predominantly psychogenic ED confirmed by a urologist. <u>Exclusions:</u> Patient: diabetes mellitus, multiple sclerosis, spinal cord injury, prostate surgery or radiation, Peyronie's disease, or significant mental health problems requiring psychotropic drugs or hospitalization, or receiving medication for hypertension, heart disease/angina (especially nitrates) or vascular disease. Female partner: diagnosis of dyspareunia, primary anorgasmia or vaginimus.	1) Medication (Sildenafil) + cognitive behavioral sex therapy N = 30 (29 completed) 2) Medication (Sildenafil) only + sex therapy for non-responders after week 4 N = 27 (24 completed) <u>Randomized:</u> N = 57 <u>Analysis:</u> Baseline: N = 53 Post-treatment (4 weeks): N = 53 Final (8 weeks): N = 53	1) <u>Format:</u> Medication (Sildenafil) + cognitive behavioral sex therapy <u>Manualized:</u> NR <u>Sessions:</u> Weekly <u>Txt Length:</u> 4-8 weeks <u>Approach:</u> medication + cognitive-behavioral sex therapy 2) <u>Format:</u> Sildenafil + couple sex therapy for treatment non-responders <u>Manualized:</u> NR <u>Sessions:</u> 3-6 <u>Txt Length:</u> 4-8 weeks <u>Approach:</u> 1 pretreatment information session; follow-up visits with a psychologist at 4 and 8 weeks; 4 weeks of cognitive-behavioral sex therapy if non-responsive to medication at week 4; only 1 couple met the 'success' criteria after 4 weeks of medication only and all other couples (N = 23) we assigned to 4 weeks of sex therapy	<u>Patient Outcomes:</u> Symptom Improvement a. IIEF Patient Global functioning a. BDI <u>Family Outcomes:</u> Couple functioning: a. Revised DAS (Patient) Sexual satisfaction a. IIEF – sexual satisfaction (Patient) <u>Intermediate Outcomes</u> Attendance: a. Retention	<u>Allocation concealment:</u> NR <u>Blinding:</u> NR <u>Intention to treat analysis:</u> No <u>Withdrawals adequately described:</u> Yes <u>Treatment Integrity:</u> NR <u>**Study Quality: Poor**</u>

SO = significant other or family member included; NR = not reported; HS = high school; BDI = Beck Depression Inventory

Table 18. Patient Outcomes - Sexual Functioning Disorders Studies

Study, Year Interventions *Sample*	Outcome Baseline	Post-Treatment	Short-term Follow-up	Long-term Follow-up
SYMPTOM IMPROVEMENT				
Aubin, 2009[106] 1) Sildenafil + couple sex therapy 2) Sildenafil only *Completers only*	IIEF - Total Score 1) 33 (17) N=24 2) 40 (16) N=20 p=ns	IIEF - Total Score 1) 50.3 (16.4) N=24 2) 55 (13.7) N=20	IIEF - Total Score 1) 47.7 (19.6) N=24 2) 46.2 (14.2) N=20 *(at 2 months - final)* p=ns	
Banner, 2007[107] 1) Sildenafil + couple sex therapy 2) Sildenafil only (provided couple sex therapy for treatment non-responders after 4 week post-treatment assessment) *Completers only*	IIEF erectile function 1) 11.7 (7.2) N=29 2) 9.0 (7.2) N=24	IIEF erectile function 1) 17.4 (7.6) N = 29 2) 13.7 (8.4) N = 24 p = 0.10 *(week 4)* Clinical 'success' 1) 48% 2) 29% p=NR		
	IIEF erectile function *(% patients with score ≥ 19 - clinical success)* 1) 14% (4/29) p=ns 2) 17% (4/24) p=ns	IIEF erectile function 1) 48% (14/29) p=ns 2) 29% (7/24) p=ns p=NR *(week 4)*		

Outcomes reported as mean (standard deviation) unless otherwise noted. Short-term follow up = 6 months post-treatment, unless otherwise noted. If an outcome had a final measure reported beyond 12 months, it is reported in long term follow up column and noted. Measures listed in the study descriptive tables but not reported here if either 1) the authors did not report findings from these measures or 2) they did not test for differences between conditions on these measures.

ns = not significant (at 5% level); NR = not reported; N/A = not applicable; Completers = findings for analyses conducted only with treatment completers; ITT = findings for analyses using an intent-to-treat approach; IIEF = International Index for Erectile Function

[a]Between week 4 and week 8, Couple Sex Therapy was added to treatment group 2 non-responders.

Table 19. Family Outcomes - Sexual Functioning Disorders Studies

Study, Year Interventions Sample	Outcome Baseline	Post-Treatment	Short-term Follow-up	Long-term Follow-up
COUPLE FUNCTIONING				
Aubin, 2009[106] 1) Sildenafil + couple sex therapy 2) Sildenafil only *Completers only*	PAIR–Sexual Intimacy (Patient) 1) 68.3 (22.3) N=24 2) 67.6 (21.4) N=20 p=NR	PAI –Sexual Intimacy (Patient 1) 74.2 (23.7) N=24 2) 73.3 (20.0) N=20 p=NR	PAIR–Sexual Intimacy (Patient) 1) 73.0 (23.1) N=24 2) 71.6 (20.1) N=20 p=NR *(at 2 months – final)*	
	PAIR Emotional Intimacy (Patient) 1) 73.0 (18.0) N=24 2) 74.0 (18.0) N=20 p=NR	PAIR–Emotional Intimacy (Patient) 1) 73.0 (18.0) N=24 2) 70.0 (19.0) N=20 p=NR	PAIR–Emotional Intimacy (Patient) 1) 71.2 (20.6) N=24 2) 70.0 (23.2) N=20 p=NR *(at 2 months - final)*	
	DAS (Patient) 1) 113.8 (14.2) N=24 2) 113.4 (16.3) N=20 p=NR	DAS (Patient) 1) 115.2 (16.5) N=24 2) 115.2 (16.5) N=20 p=NR	DAS (Patient) 1) 112.4 (17.5) N=24 2) 112.4 (17.5) N=20 p=NR *(at 2 months – final)*	
SEXUAL FUNCTIONING				
Banner, 2007[107] 1) Sildenafil + couple sex therapy 2) Sildenafil + couple sex therapy for treatment non-responders *Completers only*	IIEF Sexual Satisfaction (Patient) 1) 4.8 (2.7) N=29 2) 4.2 (1.9) N=24 p=NR	IIEF Sexual Satisfaction (Patient) 1) 6.0 (1.9) N=29 2) 4.9 (2.0) N=24 p=NR *(week 4)*		
	IIEF Sexual Satisfaction *(% patients with score ≥6 - clinical success)* 1) 45% (13/29) 2) 29% (7/24) p=NR	IIEF Sexual Satisfaction *(% patients with score ≥6 - clinical success)* 1) 65.5% (19/29) 2) 37.5% (9/24) p=NR *(week 4)*		

Outcomes reported as mean (standard deviation) unless otherwise noted. Short-term follow up = 6 months post-treatment, unless otherwise noted. If an outcome had a final measure reported beyond 12 months, it is reported in long term follow up column and noted. Measures listed in the study descriptive tables but not reported here if either 1) the authors did not report findings from these measures or 2) they did not test for differences between conditions on these measures. ns = not significant (at 5% level); NR = not reported; N/A = not applicable; Completers = findings for analyses conducted only with treatment completers; ITT = findings for analyses using an intent-to-treat approach; IIEF = International Index for Erectile Function; DAS = Dyadic Adjustment Scale; PAIR = Personal Assessment of Intimacy in Relationships

[a]Between week 4 and week 8, Couple Sex Therapy was added to treatment group 2 non-responders.

Table 20. Intermediate Outcomes - Sexual Functioning Disorders Studies

Study, Year Interventions Sample	Outcome Baseline	Post-Treatment	Short-term Follow-up	Long-term Follow-up
ATTENDANCE				
Aubin, 2009[106] 1) Sildenafil + couple sex therapy 2) Sildenafil only Completers only	Retention (Pre-treatment - randomization) 1) N=24 2) N=27 p=NR	Retention NR	Retention 1) N=20 2) N=24 (at 2 months - final) p=NR	
Banner, 2007[107] 1) Sildenafil + couple sex therapy 2) Sildenafil + couple sex therapy for treatment non-responders Completers only	Retention (Pre-treatment -randomization) 1) N=30 2) N=27 p=NR	Retention 1) N=29 2) N=24 p=NR		
SATISFACTION WITH CARE				
Aubin,2009[106] 1) Sildenafil + couple sex therapy 2) Sildenafil only Completers only	EDITS (Patient) NR	EDITS (Patient) 1) 77.6 (12.8) N=24 2) 73.2 (17.5) N=20 p=ns	EDITS (Patient) **1) 71.9 (16.4) N=24** **2) 56.5 (22.8) N=18** * **1) vs. 2) p ≤0.01** (at 2 months - final)	

Outcomes reported as mean (standard deviation) unless otherwise noted. Short-term follow up = 6 months post-treatment, unless otherwise noted. If an outcome had a final measure reported beyond 12 months, it is reported in long term follow up column and noted. ns = not significant (at 5% level); NR = not reported; N/A = not applicable; Completers = findings for analyses conducted only with treatment completers; ITT = findings for analyses using an intent-to-treat approach; EDITS = Erectile Dysfunction Inventory of Treatment Satisfaction

Table 21. Study Descriptive Information – Depression, Eating Disorders, and Smoking Cessation Studies

Study, Year Funding Source	Sample Characteristics	Inclusion and Exclusion Criteria	Treatment Groups	Intervention	Outcomes Assessed	Quality
DEPRESSION						
Cohen, 2010[114] Government	N = 35 Gender: 100% female Age: 43.2 years Race/ethnicity: Caucasian 88% Black 3% Hispanic/Latino 6% Asian 3% Marital Status: Married 94% Education: High school or less 32% College 44% Post-bachelors 24% Veterans: NR *Family Characteristics:* Male partners Age: 45.1 yrs *Recruitment Method:* Newspaper, radio, TV, flyers, and pamphlets at local clinics	MH Condition: Depression in heterosexual women Assessed by: SCI for DSM-IV Axis I Disorders SO: Male partner Inclusions: Married or living together for 1+ yrs; both partners 21+ yrs; fluent in English; women score ≥21 on BDI-II; women met diagnostic criteria and, if taking concurrent medication for depression, were in individual psychotherapy for ≥12 wks or taking stable dose of medication for ≥8 wks; male partners could not meet diagnostic criteria for depression Exclusions: Severely discordant couples (DAS of ≤75); act of infidelity in preceding 6 months or more than 2 acts of physical aggression in preceding year by 1 or both partners; already receiving couples therapy; male partners in individual psychotherapy or on antidepressant medication	1) Treatment (Brief Couple Therapy, BCT) (N = 18 couples) 2) Wait list control (N = 17 couples) Randomized: N = 35 couples Analysis: Post-treatment: N = 30 Final: N = 27	Format: Brief Couple therapy Manualized: Yes Sessions: 5 (weekly for 2 hours) Txt Length: 5 weeks with 3 month follow-up evaluation Approach: combination of psychoeducational and cognitive-behavioral marital therapy	Patient Outcomes: Symptom improvement: a. BDI-II b. HAM-D Intermediate Outcomes: None Family Outcomes: Relationship satisfaction a. DAS Outcome timeframe: Baseline Post-treatment Short term (Final): 3 months	Allocation concealment: unclear Blinding: Yes (treating clinicians and outcome assessors) Intention to treat analysis: No Withdrawals adequately described: Yes Treatment Integrity: session audiotapes coded for therapy adherence and therapist competence Study quality: Fair

Study, Year Funding Source	Sample Characteristics	Inclusion and Exclusion Criteria	Treatment Groups	Intervention	Outcomes Assessed	Quality
EATING DISORDERS						
Gorin, 2003[115] Foundation	N = 94 Gender: 0% male Age: 45.2 yrs Race/ethnicity: 86% Caucasian Marital Status: NR Veterans: 0% *Family Characteristics:* spouse or cohabiting partner *Recruitment* *Method:* newspaper advertisements	MH Condition: Binge eating disorder Assessed by: DSM-IV research criteria for binge eating disorder SO: spouse or cohabiting partner Inclusions: women; 18-65 yrs, BMI≥25; spouse or cohabitating partner willing to participate Exclusions: engaged in purging behaviors more than 1x/month; met DSM-IV criteria for anorexia nervosa, bulimia nervosa or EDNOS; receiving concurrent treatment for weight loss; currently taking appetite suppressants; pregnancy	1) Standard group cognitive behavioral therapy (CBT-SD) (N = 32) 2) Group CBT with spouse involvement (CBT-SI) (N = 31) 3) Wait-list control group (N = 31) Randomized: N =94 Analysis: N = 62 (completed all assessments; no additional information about when withdrawals occurred)	1) Format: Group therapy (patients only) Manualized: Yes Sessions: 12, 90 min each Txt Length: 12 weeks Approach: cognitive behavioral therapy 2) Format: Group therapy (patient and spouse) Manualized: Yes (modified to actively include spouses) Sessions: 12, 90 min each Txt Length: 12 weeks Approach: cognitive behavioral therapy with spouse involvement (attend all group meetings)	Patient Outcomes: Symptom improvement: a. 7-day calendar recall of binges b. EDEQ Patient global functioning a. BDI Intermediate Outcomes a. Attendance at weekly meetings Family Outcomes: Couple functioning: a. DAS b. Author-developed 7-point Likert scale - understanding of binge eating, level of agreement about re-ducing binge eating Outcome timeframe: Baseline Post-treatment Short term (Final): 6 months	Allocation concealment: Unclear Blinding: Unclear Intention to treat analysis: completed ITT and found results did not differ from treatment completer analysis; only completer analysis reported Withdrawals adequately described: 34% of entire sample failed to complete assessments (groups comparable); unclear if other withdrawals Treatment Integrity: Adherence checklist completed by therapist at the end of each group meeting Study quality: Fair

Family Involved Psychosocial Treatments for Adult Mental Health Conditions: A Review of the Evidence

Study, Year Funding Source	Sample Characteristics	Inclusion and Exclusion Criteria	Treatment Groups	Intervention	Outcomes Assessed	Quality
SMOKING CESSATION						
McBride, 2004[118] Government NOTE: study conducted at an Army Medical Center	N = 625 Gender: 0% male (enrolled pregnant women) Age: 24 yrs Race/ethnicity: White 77% Marital Status: Married 96% Veterans: 0% Family Characteristics: intimate partners Recruitment Methods: introductory letter sent to all women scheduled for first prenatal visit	MH Condition: smoking Assessed by: self-report via screening survey (telephone) of all women with scheduled first prenatal visit SO: intimate partner Inclusions: ≤20 weeks pregnant, age ≥18 yrs, current smoker or recent quitter (smoker in 30 days prior to pregnancy), living with intimate partner, willing to have partner contacted for participation Exclusions: no additional criteria reported	1) Woman-only (WO) – usual care + late-pregnancy relapse prevention kit, 6 health advisor counseling calls 2) Partner-assisted (PA) – WO + booklet and videos about support behaviors, 6 calls to partner from health advisor, written agreement regarding support behaviors, stop smoking assistance to partner (if appropriate) 3) Usual care – provider advice at first prenatal visit; self-help guide mailed to patient Randomized: N = 625 Analysis: N = 583 (all randomized except women who miscarried) at all assessment times	1) Format: individual therapy via telephone Manualized: standard protocol Sessions: 6 calls (3 in pregnancy, 3 in post-partum) Txt Length: from first prenatal visit through 4 months post-partum Approach: motivational interviewing 2) Format: individual therapy via telephone (separate calls to woman and partner) Manualized: standard protocol Sessions: 6 calls (3 in pregnancy, 3 in post-partum) Txt Length: not stated Approach: motivational interviewing 3) Format: individual Manualized: not stated (standard self-help guide provided) Sessions: 1 Txt Length: first prenatal visit Approach: provider advice	Patient Outcomes: a. Smoking status: self report of smoking in past 7 days Intermediate Outcomes: a. Smoking-specific support: Partner interaction Questionnaire (10 item version) b. General interpersonal support: 1. emotional support 2. instrumental support Family/Couple Outcomes: NR Outcome timeframe: Baseline (first prenatal visit) Post-treatment: 2-months post-partum Short term: 6-months post-partum Long terms – 12 months post-partum *Treatment continued to 4 months post-partum	Allocation concealment: Unclear Blinding: NR Intention to treat analysis: Yes after excluding patients who miscarried – missing values imputed to be "smoker" Withdrawals adequately described: Yes Treatment Integrity: NR **Study quality: Poor**

NR = not reported; SCI = structured clinical interviews; SO = significant other or family member included; DSM = Diagnostic and Statistical Manual of Mental Disorders; BDI-II = Beck Depression Inventory 2nd Edition; DAS = Dyadic Adjustment Scale; HAM-D = Hamilton Rating Scale for Depression; EDEQ = Eating Disorder Examination Questionnaire; ED-NOS = Eating Disorders Not Otherwise Specified

Table 22. Patient Outcomes - Depression, Eating Disorders, and Smoking Cessation Studies

Study, Year Interventions Sample	Baseline	Post-Treatment	Short-term Follow-up	Long-term Follow-up
SYMPTOM IMPROVEMENT – DEPRESSION				
Cohen, 2010[114] 1) Brief Couple Therapy 2) Wait list *Completers*	BDI-II 1) 31.4 (9.3) N=18 2) 30.2 (11.1) N=17 p=ns HAM-D 1) 26.9 (6.8) N=18 2) 28.5 (6.9) N=17 p=ns	BDI-II 1) 20.3 (13.5) N=16 2) 25.3 (13.9) N=14 p=ns HAM-D 1) 18.4 (10.8) N=16 2) 26.3 (10.6) N=14 p=ns	BDI-II 1) 14.4 (10.6) N=15 2) 26.9 (17.2) N=12 All univariate comparisons: p=ns Hierarchical linear modeling: **Effect size d=0.54** **β=-0.41, p<0.01** **Improvement (>50% reduction from baseline)** 1) 67% 2) 20% p<0.01 Recovery (BDI-II<11) 1) 40% 2) 8% p<0.01 HAM-D 1) 13.6, (11.4) N=15 2) 26.4 (12.3) N=12 Univariate: p<0.01 Hierarchical linear modeling: **Effect size d=0.72** **β=-0.47, p<0.001** **Improvement (>50% reduction from baseline)** 1) 67% 2) 17% p<0.01 Recovery (HAM-D<6) 1) 47% 2) 8% p<0.01	

Family Involved Psychosocial Treatments for Adult Mental Health Conditions: A Review of the Evidence

Study, Year Interventions Sample	Baseline	Post-Treatment	Short-term Follow-up	Long-term Follow-up
SYMPTOM IMPROVEMENT – EATING DISORDERS				
Gorin, 2003[115] 1) Group Cognitive Behavioral Therapy (CBT) with spouse 2) Group CBT 3) Wait List Control* *Completers*	Days Binged (7-day recall) 1) 3.4 (2.1) 2) 3.8 (1.7) 3) 3.8 (1.8) All comparisons: p=ns Days Binged (EDEQ) 1) 9.6 (6.1) 2) 7.6 (5.7) 3) 8.5 (5.2) All comparisons: p=ns	Days Binged (7-day recall) 1)1.2 (1.8) 2) 1.8 (2.0) 3) 3.0 (1.8) All comparisons: p=ns Days Binged (EDEQ) 1) 3.3 (4.4) 2) 2.4 (2.8) 3) 5.9 (4.6) All comparisons: p=ns	Days Binged (7-day recall) 1) 0.7 (0.9) 2) 1.1 (1.4) All comparisons: p=ns Days Binged (EDEQ) 1) 3.5 (4.6) 2) 1.6 (2.1) All comparisons: p= ns	
SYMPTOM IMPROVEMENT – SMOKING CESSATION				
McBride, 2004[118] 1) Partner assisted + women-only care 2) Women-only care 3) Usual care *All, excluding miscarriages*	Current Smoker 1) 46% 2) 45% 3) 46% All comparisons: p=ns	Abstinence 1) 42% 2) 37% 3) 38% All comparisons: p=ns	Abstinence 1) 37% 2) 36% 3) 33% All comparisons: p=ns	Abstinence 1) 35% 2) 32% 3) 29% All comparisons: p=ns
GLOBAL FUNCTIONING – EATING DISORDERS				
Gorin, 2003[115] 1) Group CBT with spouse 2) Group CBT 3) Wait list control *Completers*	BDI 1) 20.4 (10.0) 2) 18.7 (8.9) 3) 17.4 (9.9) All comparisons: p=ns	BDI 1) 11.8 (9.4) 2) 14.8 (9.3) 3) 16.8 (9.5) All comparisons: p=ns	BDI 1) 12.2 (9.2) 2) 12.9 (8.1) All comparisons: p=ns	

Outcomes reported as mean (standard deviation) unless otherwise noted. Short-term follow up = 6 months post-treatment, unless otherwise noted. Long term=12 months post-treatment, unless otherwise noted. If an outcome had a final measure reported beyond 12 months, it is reported in long term follow up column and noted.

ns = not significant (at 5% level); NR = not reported; N/A = not applicable; Completers = findings for analyses conducted only with treatment completers; ITT = findings for analyses using an intent-to-treat approach; BDI-II = Beck Depression Inventory – Second Edition; CBT = Cognitive Behavioral Therapy; EDEQ = Eating Disorder Examination Questionnaire; HAM-D = Hamilton Rating Scale for Depression

Table 23. Family Outcomes – Depression, Eating Disorders, and Smoking Cessation Studies

Study, Year Interventions Sample	Baseline	Post-treatment	Short-term Follow-up	Long-term Follow-up
COUPLE FUNCTIONING – DEPRESSION				
Cohen, 2010[114] 1) Brief Couple Therapy 2) Wait list *Completers*	DAS 1) 96.6 (17.4) N=18 2) 90.3 (18.4) N=17 p=ns	DAS 1) 100.6 (20.5) N=16 2) 91.9 (23.5) N=14 p=ns	DAS 1) 102.1, (22.7) N=15 2) 92.9 (19.8) N=12 All univariate comparisons: p= ns Hierarchical linear modeling: **Effect size d= 0.43, β=0.55, p<0.01**	
COUPLE FUNCTIONING – EATING DISORDERS				
Gorin, 2003[115] 1) Group Cognitive Behavioral Therapy (CBT) with spouse 2) Group CBT 3) Wait list controls *Completers*	DAS 1) 95.1 (28.0) 2) 98.4 (21.0) 3) 99.0 (19.8) All comparisons: p=ns	DAS 1) 99.1 (24.7) 2) 101.4 (26.0) 3) 100.0 (20.1) All comparisons: p=ns	DAS 1) 99.1 (22.8) 2) 99.2 (23.5) All comparisons: p=ns	

Outcomes reported as mean (standard deviation) unless otherwise noted. Short-term follow up = 6 months post-treatment, unless otherwise noted. If an outcome had a final measure reported beyond 12 months, it is reported in long term follow up column and noted. ns = not significant (at 5% level); NR = not reported; N/A = not applicable; Completers = findings for analyses conducted only with treatment completers; ITT = findings for analyses using an intent-to-treat approach; CBT = Cognitive Behavioral Therapy; DAS = Dyadic Adjustment Scale

Table 24. Intermediate Outcomes – Depression, Eating Disorders, and Smoking Cessation Studies

Study, Year Interventions Sample	Baseline	Short-term Follow-up	Long-term Follow-up
ATTENDANCE – EATING DISORDERS			
Gorin, 2003[115] 1) Group CBT with spouse 2) Group CBT 3) Wait list controls *Completers*		At Weekly Meetings Completers (N=62) 1) 9/12 2) 9/12 3) Not applicable p=0.45	
SOCIAL SUPPORT – SMOKING CESSATION			
McBride, 2004[118] 1) Partners assisted + woman-only care 2) Woman-only care 3) Usual care *All, excluding miscarriages*		No differences between groups - results not reported by treatment group **For all participants** **Significant linear decline over time for:** 1) Smoking-specific support (Positive) 2) Instrumental support 3) Emotional support **Significant U-shaped function for:** **Smoking-specific support (Negative)**	

Outcomes reported as mean (standard deviation) unless otherwise noted. Short-term follow up = 6 months post-treatment, unless otherwise noted. If an outcome had a final measure reported beyond 12 months, it is reported in long term follow up column and noted. Completers = findings for analyses conducted only with treatment completers; CBT = Cognitive Behavioral Therapy

APPENDIX E. FOREST PLOTS FROM POOLED ANALYSES FOR ALCOHOL AND DRUG USE STUDIES

Figure 1a. Percent Days Abstinent, Differences between BCT and ICBT: Studies Not Conducted with Data from Fals-Stewart.

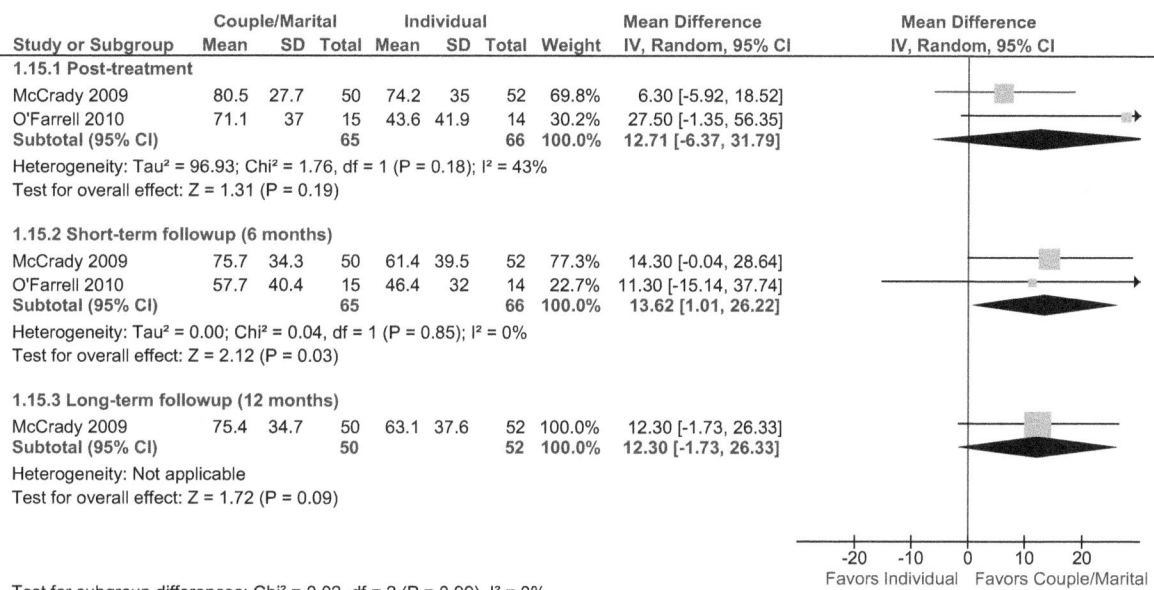

*Horizontal bars for each study represent the study's confidence interval. Confidence intervals extending below 0 indicate non-significant differences. Size of box or diamond reflects sample size.

BCT = Behavioral Couple or Marital Therapy; ICBT = Individual Cognitive-Behavioral Therapy

Figure 1b. Percent Days Abstinent, Differences between BCT and ICBT: Studies Conducted with Data from Fals-Stewart.

Study or Subgroup	Couple/Marital			Individual			Weight	Mean Difference IV, Random, 95% CI	Mean Difference IV, Random, 95% CI
	Mean	SD	Total	Mean	SD	Total			
1.13.1 Post-treatment									
Fals-Stewart 1996	95.4	15.4	40	91.1	14.1	40	12.9%	4.30 [-2.17, 10.77]	
Fals-Stewart 2006	96.3	16.3	46	93.6	17.7	46	11.1%	2.70 [-4.25, 9.65]	
Fals-Stewart 2008	94.1	13.4	46	88.3	13	46	18.5%	5.80 [0.40, 11.20]	
Kelley 2002 (Drug)	85.9	22.7	22	81.8	26.2	21	2.5%	4.10 [-10.58, 18.78]	
Kelley 2002 (EtOH)	90.2	21.9	25	86.6	17.4	22	4.3%	3.60 [-7.65, 14.85]	
Lam 2009	92.3	15.2	10	88.3	16.7	10	2.7%	4.00 [-10.00, 18.00]	
Winters 2002	94.2	6.4	36	90.2	8	36	48.0%	4.00 [0.65, 7.35]	
Subtotal (95% CI)			225			221	100.0%	4.21 [1.89, 6.53]	

Heterogeneity: Tau² = 0.00; Chi² = 0.54, df = 6 (P = 1.00); I² = 0%
Test for overall effect: Z = 3.56 (P = 0.0004)

Study or Subgroup	Mean	SD	Total	Mean	SD	Total	Weight	Mean Difference	
1.13.2 Short-term followup (6 months)									
Fals-Stewart 1996	81.5	28.6	40	70.4	24.5	40	13.3%	11.10 [-0.57, 22.77]	
Fals-Stewart 2006	85.9	18.1	46	75	20.3	46	29.3%	10.90 [3.04, 18.76]	
Fals-Stewart 2008	84.1	26.5	46	70.3	27.1	46	15.1%	13.80 [2.85, 24.75]	
Kelley 2002 (Drug)	77.6	25.8	22	63.6	42.3	21	4.1%	14.00 [-7.06, 35.06]	
Kelley 2002 (EtOH)	80.6	27.2	25	71.4	26.2	22	7.8%	9.20 [-6.08, 24.48]	
Lam 2009	85.1	20.7	10	78.2	22.6	10	5.0%	6.90 [-12.09, 25.89]	
Winters 2002	81.9	16.3	31	71.9	17.9	32	25.4%	10.00 [1.55, 18.45]	
Subtotal (95% CI)			220			217	100.0%	10.93 [6.67, 15.19]	

Heterogeneity: Tau² = 0.00; Chi² = 0.61, df = 6 (P = 1.00); I² = 0%
Test for overall effect: Z = 5.03 (P < 0.00001)

Study or Subgroup	Mean	SD	Total	Mean	SD	Total	Weight	Mean Difference	
1.13.3 Long-term followup (12 months)									
Fals-Stewart 1996	73.2	29.8	40	65.1	26.9	40	11.9%	8.10 [-4.34, 20.54]	
Fals-Stewart 2003	59.6	26.4	62	49.3	28.4	62	19.8%	10.30 [0.65, 19.95]	
Fals-Stewart 2006	79.3	29.7	46	60.2	20.9	46	16.8%	19.10 [8.61, 29.59]	
Fals-Stewart 2008	74.1	25.8	46	60.2	27.3	46	15.7%	13.90 [3.05, 24.75]	
Kelley 2002 (Drug)	66.9	35.6	22	53.4	24.8	21	5.5%	13.50 [-4.77, 31.77]	
Kelley 2002 (EtOH)	70.9	25.6	25	60.4	22.4	22	9.8%	10.50 [-3.22, 24.22]	
Lam 2009	77.8	20.2	10	70.2	18.6	10	6.4%	7.60 [-9.42, 24.62]	
Winters 2002	74.2	22.2	33	65.4	26.1	35	14.0%	8.80 [-2.70, 20.30]	
Subtotal (95% CI)			284			282	100.0%	11.89 [7.59, 16.19]	

Heterogeneity: Tau² = 0.00; Chi² = 3.00, df = 7 (P = 0.89); I² = 0%
Test for overall effect: Z = 5.42 (P < 0.00001)

Test for subgroup differences: Chi² = 13.78, df = 2 (P = 0.001), I² = 85.5%

(forest plot x-axis: -20, -10, 0, 10, 20; Favors Individual — Favors Couple/Marital)

*Horizontal bars for each study represent the study's confidence interval. Confidence intervals extending below 0 indicate non-significant differences. Size of box or diamond reflects sample size.
BCT = Behavioral Couple or Marital Therapy; ICBT = Individual Cognitive-Behavioral Therapy; EtOH = alcohol

Figure 2. Percent Days Abstinent, Differences between BCT and ICBT: Alcohol Use Disorder Studies Only

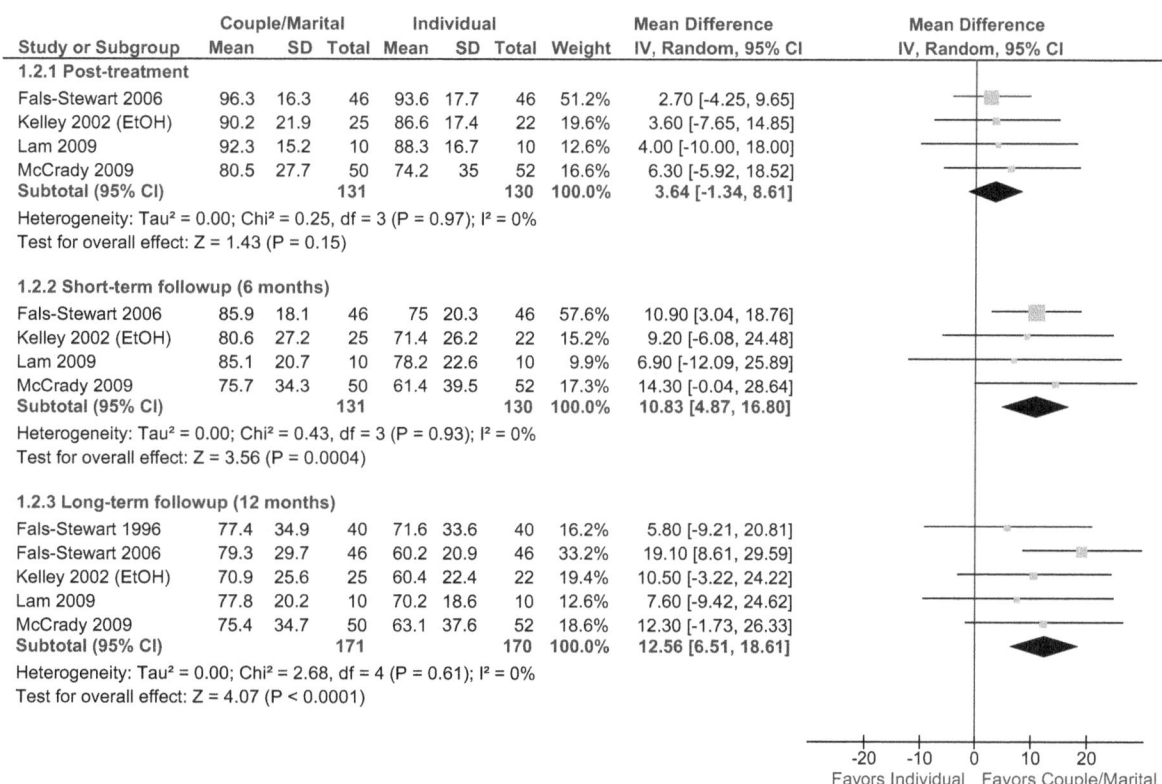

Study or Subgroup	Couple/Marital			Individual			Weight	Mean Difference IV, Random, 95% CI
	Mean	SD	Total	Mean	SD	Total		
1.2.1 Post-treatment								
Fals-Stewart 2006	96.3	16.3	46	93.6	17.7	46	51.2%	2.70 [-4.25, 9.65]
Kelley 2002 (EtOH)	90.2	21.9	25	86.6	17.4	22	19.6%	3.60 [-7.65, 14.85]
Lam 2009	92.3	15.2	10	88.3	16.7	10	12.6%	4.00 [-10.00, 18.00]
McCrady 2009	80.5	27.7	50	74.2	35	52	16.6%	6.30 [-5.92, 18.52]
Subtotal (95% CI)			131			130	100.0%	3.64 [-1.34, 8.61]

Heterogeneity: Tau² = 0.00; Chi² = 0.25, df = 3 (P = 0.97); I² = 0%
Test for overall effect: Z = 1.43 (P = 0.15)

1.2.2 Short-term followup (6 months)								
Fals-Stewart 2006	85.9	18.1	46	75	20.3	46	57.6%	10.90 [3.04, 18.76]
Kelley 2002 (EtOH)	80.6	27.2	25	71.4	26.2	22	15.2%	9.20 [-6.08, 24.48]
Lam 2009	85.1	20.7	10	78.2	22.6	10	9.9%	6.90 [-12.09, 25.89]
McCrady 2009	75.7	34.3	50	61.4	39.5	52	17.3%	14.30 [-0.04, 28.64]
Subtotal (95% CI)			131			130	100.0%	10.83 [4.87, 16.80]

Heterogeneity: Tau² = 0.00; Chi² = 0.43, df = 3 (P = 0.93); I² = 0%
Test for overall effect: Z = 3.56 (P = 0.0004)

1.2.3 Long-term followup (12 months)								
Fals-Stewart 1996	77.4	34.9	40	71.6	33.6	40	16.2%	5.80 [-9.21, 20.81]
Fals-Stewart 2006	79.3	29.7	46	60.2	20.9	46	33.2%	19.10 [8.61, 29.59]
Kelley 2002 (EtOH)	70.9	25.6	25	60.4	22.4	22	19.4%	10.50 [-3.22, 24.22]
Lam 2009	77.8	20.2	10	70.2	18.6	10	12.6%	7.60 [-9.42, 24.62]
McCrady 2009	75.4	34.7	50	63.1	37.6	52	18.6%	12.30 [-1.73, 26.33]
Subtotal (95% CI)			171			170	100.0%	12.56 [6.51, 18.61]

Heterogeneity: Tau² = 0.00; Chi² = 2.68, df = 4 (P = 0.61); I² = 0%
Test for overall effect: Z = 4.07 (P < 0.0001)

Test for subgroup differences: Chi² = 5.97, df = 2 (P = 0.05), I² = 66.5%

*Horizontal bars for each study represent the study's confidence interval. Confidence intervals extending below 0 indicate non-significant differences. Size of box or diamond reflects sample size.
BCT = Behavioral Couple or Marital Therapy; ICBT = Individual Cognitive-Behavioral Therapy; EtOH = alcohol

Figure 3. Percent Days Heavy Drinking, Differences between BCT and ICBT: Alcohol Use Disorder Studies Only

Study or Subgroup	Couple/Marital			Individual			Weight	Mean Difference IV, Fixed, 95% CI	Mean Difference IV, Fixed, 95% CI
	Mean	SD	Total	Mean	SD	Total			
1.9.1 Post-treatment									
Fals-Stewart 2005	5.2	14.3	25	4.9	15.1	25	65.5%	0.30 [-7.85, 8.45]	
McCrady 2009	10.5	22.2	50	18.7	34.6	52	34.5%	-8.20 [-19.44, 3.04]	
Subtotal (95% CI)			75			77	100.0%	-2.63 [-9.23, 3.97]	
Heterogeneity: Chi² = 1.44, df = 1 (P = 0.23); I² = 31%									
Test for overall effect: Z = 0.78 (P = 0.43)									
1.9.2 Short-term followup (6 months)									
Fals-Stewart 2005	14.1	19.3	25	23.6	15	25	63.8%	-9.50 [-19.08, 0.08]	
McCrady 2009	12.3	27.4	50	23.8	37.6	52	36.2%	-11.50 [-24.23, 1.23]	
Subtotal (95% CI)			75			77	100.0%	-10.22 [-17.88, -2.57]	
Heterogeneity: Chi² = 0.06, df = 1 (P = 0.81); I² = 0%									
Test for overall effect: Z = 2.62 (P = 0.009)									
1.9.3 Long-term followup (12 months)									
Fals-Stewart 2005	19.2	21.3	25	38.2	25.6	25	44.9%	-19.00 [-32.05, -5.95]	
McCrady 2009	12.8	26.2	50	22.7	34.2	52	55.1%	-9.90 [-21.70, 1.90]	
Subtotal (95% CI)			75			77	100.0%	-13.99 [-22.74, -5.24]	
Heterogeneity: Chi² = 1.03, df = 1 (P = 0.31); I² = 3%									
Test for overall effect: Z = 3.13 (P = 0.002)									

```
                                                    -20  -10   0   10   20
                                                   Favors couple  Favors individual
```

Test for subgroup differences: Chi² = 4.66, df = 2 (P = 0.10), I² = 57.1%

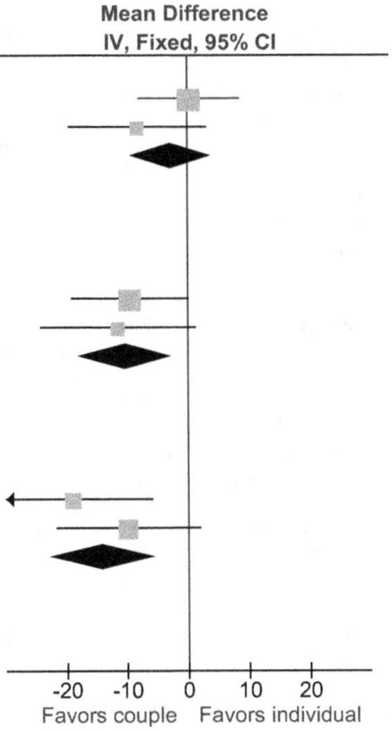

*Horizontal bars for each study represent the study's confidence interval. Confidence intervals extending below 0 indicate non-significant differences.
Size of box or diamond reflects sample size.
BCT = Behavioral Couple or Marital Therapy; ICBT = Individual Cognitive-Behavioral Therapy

Figure 4. Percent Days Abstinent, Differences between BCT and ICBT: Drug Use Disorder Studies Only

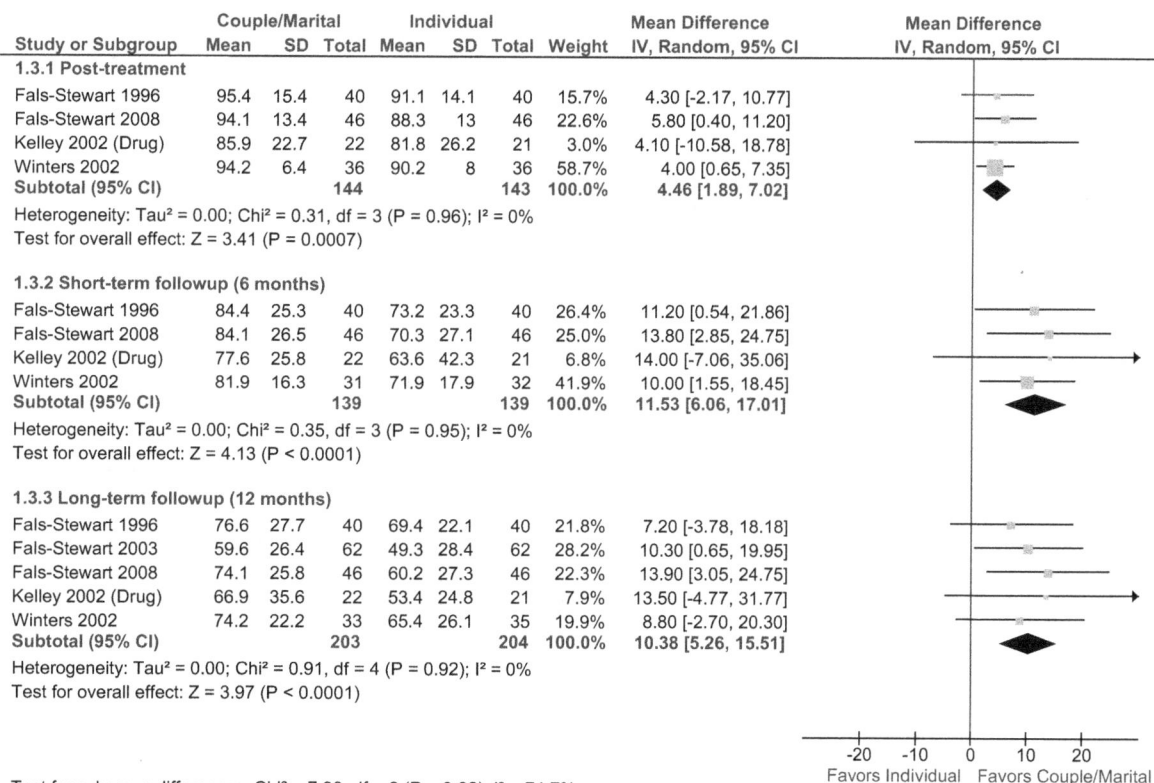

Study or Subgroup	Couple/Marital			Individual			Weight	Mean Difference IV, Random, 95% CI
	Mean	SD	Total	Mean	SD	Total		
1.3.1 Post-treatment								
Fals-Stewart 1996	95.4	15.4	40	91.1	14.1	40	15.7%	4.30 [-2.17, 10.77]
Fals-Stewart 2008	94.1	13.4	46	88.3	13	46	22.6%	5.80 [0.40, 11.20]
Kelley 2002 (Drug)	85.9	22.7	22	81.8	26.2	21	3.0%	4.10 [-10.58, 18.78]
Winters 2002	94.2	6.4	36	90.2	8	36	58.7%	4.00 [0.65, 7.35]
Subtotal (95% CI)			144			143	100.0%	4.46 [1.89, 7.02]

Heterogeneity: Tau² = 0.00; Chi² = 0.31, df = 3 (P = 0.96); I² = 0%
Test for overall effect: Z = 3.41 (P = 0.0007)

1.3.2 Short-term followup (6 months)								
Fals-Stewart 1996	84.4	25.3	40	73.2	23.3	40	26.4%	11.20 [0.54, 21.86]
Fals-Stewart 2008	84.1	26.5	46	70.3	27.1	46	25.0%	13.80 [2.85, 24.75]
Kelley 2002 (Drug)	77.6	25.8	22	63.6	42.3	21	6.8%	14.00 [-7.06, 35.06]
Winters 2002	81.9	16.3	31	71.9	17.9	32	41.9%	10.00 [1.55, 18.45]
Subtotal (95% CI)			139			139	100.0%	11.53 [6.06, 17.01]

Heterogeneity: Tau² = 0.00; Chi² = 0.35, df = 3 (P = 0.95); I² = 0%
Test for overall effect: Z = 4.13 (P < 0.0001)

1.3.3 Long-term followup (12 months)								
Fals-Stewart 1996	76.6	27.7	40	69.4	22.1	40	21.8%	7.20 [-3.78, 18.18]
Fals-Stewart 2003	59.6	26.4	62	49.3	28.4	62	28.2%	10.30 [0.65, 19.95]
Fals-Stewart 2008	74.1	25.8	46	60.2	27.3	46	22.3%	13.90 [3.05, 24.75]
Kelley 2002 (Drug)	66.9	35.6	22	53.4	24.8	21	7.9%	13.50 [-4.77, 31.77]
Winters 2002	74.2	22.2	33	65.4	26.1	35	19.9%	8.80 [-2.70, 20.30]
Subtotal (95% CI)			203			204	100.0%	10.38 [5.26, 15.51]

Heterogeneity: Tau² = 0.00; Chi² = 0.91, df = 4 (P = 0.92); I² = 0%
Test for overall effect: Z = 3.97 (P < 0.0001)

Test for subgroup differences: Chi² = 7.90, df = 2 (P = 0.02), I² = 74.7%

*Horizontal bars for each study represent the study's confidence interval. Confidence intervals extending below 0 indicate non-significant differences. Size of box or diamond reflects sample size.
BCT = Behavioral Couple or Marital Therapy; ICBT = Individual Cognitive-Behavioral Therapy

Figure 5. Relationship Adjustment using Dyadic Adjustment Scale, Difference in Mean Scores between BCT and ICBT: Alcohol Use Disorder Studies Only

Study or Subgroup	Couple/Marital Mean	SD	Total	Individual Mean	SD	Total	Weight	Mean Difference IV, Fixed, 95% CI	Mean Difference IV, Fixed, 95% CI
1.18.1 Post-treatment									
Fals-Stewart 2005	119.3	11.9	25	104.6	11.6	25	35.2%	14.70 [8.19, 21.21]	
Fals-Stewart 2006	123	12.1	46	111.2	18.6	46	36.4%	11.80 [5.39, 18.21]	
Kelley 2002 (EtOH)	115.4	18.2	25	102.2	19.1	22	13.0%	13.20 [2.49, 23.91]	
Lam 2009	114.6	16.8	10	98.1	17.9	10	6.5%	16.50 [1.28, 31.72]	
Walitzer 04 CAF+BCT	108.4	14.4	19	105.4	26.2	21	8.9%	3.00 [-9.94, 15.94]	
Subtotal (95% CI)			125			124	100.0%	12.52 [8.66, 16.39]	
Heterogeneity: Chi² = 2.84, df = 4 (P = 0.59); I² = 0%									
Test for overall effect: Z = 6.35 (P < 0.00001)									
1.18.2 Short-term followup (6 months)									
Fals-Stewart 2005	112.6	16.2	25	98.4	11.6	25	25.5%	14.20 [6.39, 22.01]	
Fals-Stewart 2006	117.2	13.7	46	102.2	14.4	46	47.1%	15.00 [9.26, 20.74]	
Kelley 2002 (EtOH)	103.9	16.2	25	86.7	19.2	22	14.8%	17.20 [6.97, 27.43]	
Lam 2009	105.9	19.6	10	93.9	20.2	10	5.1%	12.00 [-5.44, 29.44]	
Walitzer 04 CAF+BCT	107.8	12.7	16	108.3	25.6	15	7.5%	-0.50 [-14.87, 13.87]	
Subtotal (95% CI)			122			118	100.0%	13.80 [9.86, 17.75]	
Heterogeneity: Chi² = 4.45, df = 4 (P = 0.35); I² = 10%									
Test for overall effect: Z = 6.87 (P < 0.00001)									
1.18.3 Long-term followup (12 months)									
Fals-Stewart 2005	109.3	17.2	25	96	19.3	25	20.8%	13.30 [3.17, 23.43]	
Fals-Stewart 2006	112.4	14	46	98	18.8	46	46.6%	14.40 [7.63, 21.17]	
Kelley 2002 (EtOH)	91.4	19.9	25	82.1	20.7	22	15.8%	9.30 [-2.35, 20.95]	
Lam 2009	99.8	20.3	10	88.9	22	10	6.2%	10.90 [-7.65, 29.45]	
Walitzer 04 CAF+BCT	101.2	15.9	17	113.6	23	14	10.6%	-12.40 [-26.62, 1.82]	
Subtotal (95% CI)			123			117	100.0%	10.32 [5.69, 14.94]	
Heterogeneity: Chi² = 11.56, df = 4 (P = 0.02); I² = 65%									
Test for overall effect: Z = 4.37 (P < 0.0001)									

-20 -10 0 10 20

Favors Individual   Favors Couple/Marital

Test for subgroup differences: Chi² = 1.27, df = 2 (P = 0.53), I² = 0%

*Horizontal bars for each study represent the study's confidence interval. Confidence intervals extending below 0 indicate non-significant differences. Size of box or diamond reflects sample size.
BCT = Behavioral Couple or Marital Therapy; ICBT = Individual Cognitive-Behavioral Therapy; EtOH = alcohol

Figure 6. Relationship Adjustment using Dyadic Adjustment Scale, Difference in Mean Scores between BCT and ICBT: Drug Use Disorder Studies Only

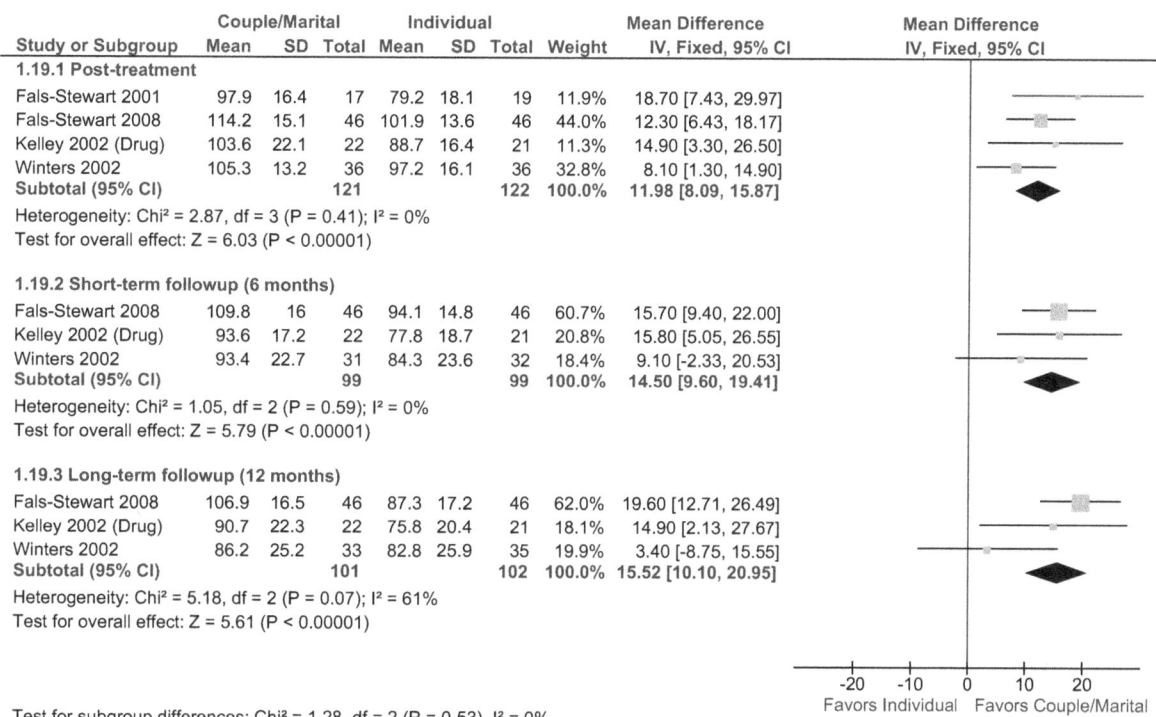

*Horizontal bars for each study represent the study's confidence interval. Confidence intervals extending below 0 indicate non-significant differences. Size of box or diamond reflects sample size.
BCT = Behavioral Couple or Marital Therapy; ICBT = Individual Cognitive-Behavioral Therapy

Figure 7. Percent Days Abstinent, Differences between BCT and ICBT: Studies with Female Subjects Only

Study or Subgroup	Couple/Marital Mean	SD	Total	Individual Mean	SD	Total	Weight	Mean Difference IV, Random, 95% CI
1.7.1 Post-treatment								
Fals-Stewart 2006	96.3	16.3	46	93.6	17.7	46	17.7%	2.70 [-4.25, 9.65]
McCrady 2009	80.5	27.7	50	74.2	35	52	5.7%	6.30 [-5.92, 18.52]
Winters 2002	94.2	6.4	36	90.2	8	36	76.5%	4.00 [0.65, 7.35]
Subtotal (95% CI)			132			134	100.0%	3.90 [0.97, 6.83]

Heterogeneity: Tau² = 0.00; Chi² = 0.27, df = 2 (P = 0.88); I² = 0%
Test for overall effect: Z = 2.61 (P = 0.009)

Study or Subgroup	Mean	SD	Total	Mean	SD	Total	Weight	MD
1.7.2 Short-term followup (6 months)								
Fals-Stewart 2006	85.9	18.1	46	75	20.3	46	46.2%	10.90 [3.04, 18.76]
McCrady 2009	75.7	34.3	50	61.4	39.5	52	13.9%	14.30 [-0.04, 28.64]
Winters 2002	81.9	16.3	31	71.9	17.9	32	40.0%	10.00 [1.55, 18.45]
Subtotal (95% CI)			127			130	100.0%	11.01 [5.67, 16.35]

Heterogeneity: Tau² = 0.00; Chi² = 0.26, df = 2 (P = 0.88); I² = 0%
Test for overall effect: Z = 4.04 (P < 0.0001)

Study or Subgroup	Mean	SD	Total	Mean	SD	Total	Weight	MD
1.7.3 Long-term followup (12 months)								
Fals-Stewart 2006	79.3	29.7	46	60.2	20.9	46	41.8%	19.10 [8.61, 29.59]
McCrady 2009	75.4	34.7	50	63.1	37.6	52	23.4%	12.30 [-1.73, 26.33]
Winters 2002	74.2	22.2	33	65.4	26.1	35	34.8%	8.80 [-2.70, 20.30]
Subtotal (95% CI)			129			133	100.0%	13.92 [7.14, 20.71]

Heterogeneity: Tau² = 0.00; Chi² = 1.75, df = 2 (P = 0.42); I² = 0%
Test for overall effect: Z = 4.02 (P < 0.0001)

Test for subgroup differences: Chi² = 10.36, df = 2 (P = 0.006), I² = 80.7%

*Horizontal bars for each study represent the study's confidence interval. Confidence intervals extending below 0 indicate non-significant differences. Size of box or diamond reflects sample size.
BCT = Behavioral Couple or Marital Therapy; ICBT = Individual Cognitive-Behavioral Therapy

Figure 8. Relationship Adjustment using Dyadic Adjustment Scale, Difference in Mean Scores between BCT and ICBT: Studies with Female Subjects Only

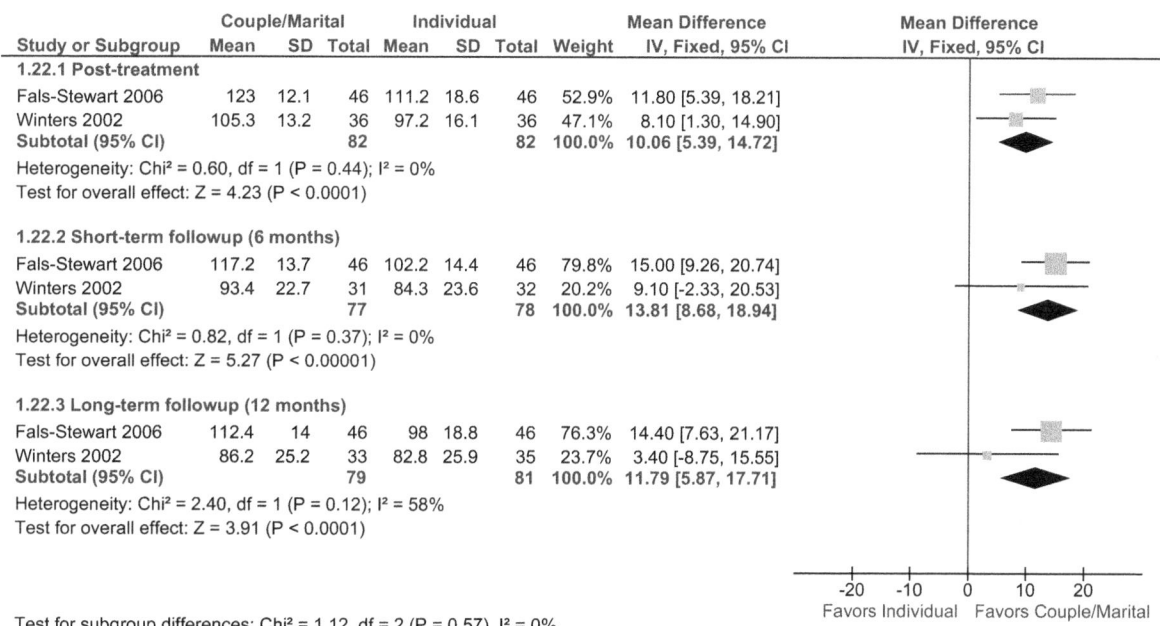

*Horizontal bars for each study represent the study's confidence interval. Confidence intervals extending below 0 indicate non-significant differences. Size of box or diamond reflects sample size.
BCT = Behavioral Couple or Marital Therapy; ICBT = Individual Cognitive-Behavioral Therapy

Figure 9. Percent Days Abstinent, Differences between BCT and ICBT: Studies with Male Subjects Only

Study or Subgroup	Couple/Marital			Individual			Weight	Mean Difference IV, Random, 95% CI	Mean Difference IV, Random, 95% CI
	Mean	SD	Total	Mean	SD	Total			
1.6.1 Post-treatment									
Fals-Stewart 1996	95.4	15.4	40	91.1	14.1	40	57.5%	4.30 [-2.17, 10.77]	
Kelley 2002 (Drug)	85.9	22.7	22	81.8	26.2	21	11.2%	4.10 [-10.58, 18.78]	
Kelley 2002 (EtOH)	90.2	21.9	25	86.6	17.4	22	19.0%	3.60 [-7.65, 14.85]	
Lam 2009	92.3	15.2	10	88.3	16.7	10	12.3%	4.00 [-10.00, 18.00]	
Subtotal (95% CI)			97			93	100.0%	4.11 [-0.80, 9.01]	

Heterogeneity: Tau² = 0.00; Chi² = 0.01, df = 3 (P = 1.00); I² = 0%
Test for overall effect: Z = 1.64 (P = 0.10)

Study or Subgroup	Couple/Marital			Individual			Weight	Mean Difference IV, Random, 95% CI	
	Mean	SD	Total	Mean	SD	Total			
1.6.2 Short-term followup (6 months)									
Fals-Stewart 1996	81.5	28.6	40	70.4	24.5	40	44.1%	11.10 [-0.57, 22.77]	
Kelley 2002 (Drug)	77.6	25.8	22	63.6	42.3	21	13.5%	14.00 [-7.06, 35.06]	
Kelley 2002 (EtOH)	80.6	27.2	25	71.4	26.2	22	25.7%	9.20 [-6.08, 24.48]	
Lam 2009	85.1	20.7	10	78.2	22.6	10	16.6%	6.90 [-12.09, 25.89]	
Subtotal (95% CI)			97			93	100.0%	10.30 [2.56, 18.05]	

Heterogeneity: Tau² = 0.00; Chi² = 0.28, df = 3 (P = 0.96); I² = 0%
Test for overall effect: Z = 2.61 (P = 0.009)

Study or Subgroup	Couple/Marital			Individual			Weight	Mean Difference IV, Random, 95% CI	
	Mean	SD	Total	Mean	SD	Total			
1.6.3 Long-term followup (12 months)									
Fals-Stewart 1996	73.2	29.8	40	65.1	26.9	40	22.3%	8.10 [-4.34, 20.54]	
Fals-Stewart 2003	59.6	26.4	62	49.3	28.4	62	37.1%	10.30 [0.65, 19.95]	
Kelley 2002 (Drug)	66.9	35.6	22	53.4	24.8	21	10.3%	13.50 [-4.77, 31.77]	
Kelley 2002 (EtOH)	70.9	25.6	25	60.4	22.4	22	18.3%	10.50 [-3.22, 24.22]	
Lam 2009	77.8	20.2	10	70.2	18.6	10	11.9%	7.60 [-9.42, 24.62]	
Subtotal (95% CI)			159			155	100.0%	9.85 [3.98, 15.73]	

Heterogeneity: Tau² = 0.00; Chi² = 0.31, df = 4 (P = 0.99); I² = 0%
Test for overall effect: Z = 3.29 (P = 0.001)

Test for subgroup differences: Chi² = 2.93, df = 2 (P = 0.23), I² = 31.7%

*Horizontal bars for each study represent the study's confidence interval. Confidence intervals extending below 0 indicate non-significant differences. Size of box or diamond reflects sample size.
BCT = Behavioral Couple or Marital Therapy; ICBT = Individual Cognitive-Behavioral Therapy; EtOH = alcohol

Figure 10. Relationship Adjustment using Dyadic Adjustment Scale, Difference in Mean Scores between BCT and ICBT: Studies with Male Subjects Only

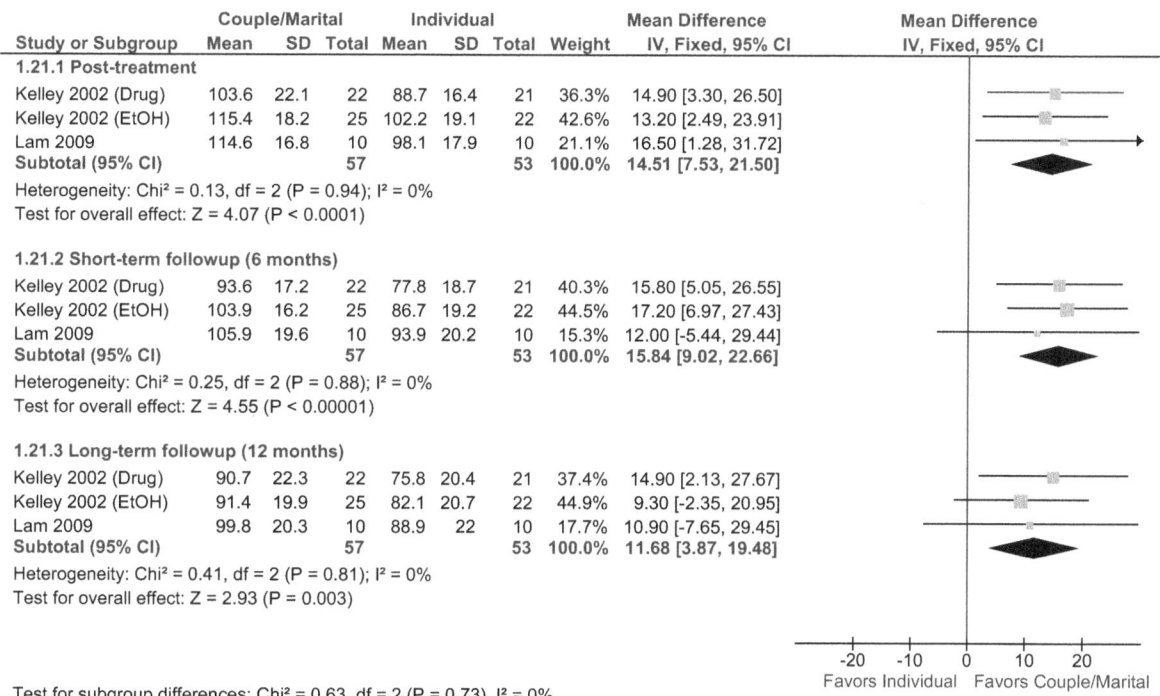

Study or Subgroup	Couple/Marital Mean	SD	Total	Individual Mean	SD	Total	Weight	Mean Difference IV, Fixed, 95% CI
1.21.1 Post-treatment								
Kelley 2002 (Drug)	103.6	22.1	22	88.7	16.4	21	36.3%	14.90 [3.30, 26.50]
Kelley 2002 (EtOH)	115.4	18.2	25	102.2	19.1	22	42.6%	13.20 [2.49, 23.91]
Lam 2009	114.6	16.8	10	98.1	17.9	10	21.1%	16.50 [1.28, 31.72]
Subtotal (95% CI)			57			53	100.0%	14.51 [7.53, 21.50]

Heterogeneity: Chi² = 0.13, df = 2 (P = 0.94); I² = 0%
Test for overall effect: Z = 4.07 (P < 0.0001)

Study or Subgroup	Couple/Marital Mean	SD	Total	Individual Mean	SD	Total	Weight	Mean Difference IV, Fixed, 95% CI
1.21.2 Short-term followup (6 months)								
Kelley 2002 (Drug)	93.6	17.2	22	77.8	18.7	21	40.3%	15.80 [5.05, 26.55]
Kelley 2002 (EtOH)	103.9	16.2	25	86.7	19.2	22	44.5%	17.20 [6.97, 27.43]
Lam 2009	105.9	19.6	10	93.9	20.2	10	15.3%	12.00 [-5.44, 29.44]
Subtotal (95% CI)			57			53	100.0%	15.84 [9.02, 22.66]

Heterogeneity: Chi² = 0.25, df = 2 (P = 0.88); I² = 0%
Test for overall effect: Z = 4.55 (P < 0.00001)

Study or Subgroup	Couple/Marital Mean	SD	Total	Individual Mean	SD	Total	Weight	Mean Difference IV, Fixed, 95% CI
1.21.3 Long-term followup (12 months)								
Kelley 2002 (Drug)	90.7	22.3	22	75.8	20.4	21	37.4%	14.90 [2.13, 27.67]
Kelley 2002 (EtOH)	91.4	19.9	25	82.1	20.7	22	44.9%	9.30 [-2.35, 20.95]
Lam 2009	99.8	20.3	10	88.9	22	10	17.7%	10.90 [-7.65, 29.45]
Subtotal (95% CI)			57			53	100.0%	11.68 [3.87, 19.48]

Heterogeneity: Chi² = 0.41, df = 2 (P = 0.81); I² = 0%
Test for overall effect: Z = 2.93 (P = 0.003)

Test for subgroup differences: Chi² = 0.63, df = 2 (P = 0.73), I² = 0%

*Horizontal bars for each study represent the study's confidence interval. Confidence intervals extending below 0 indicate non-significant differences. Size of box or diamond reflects sample size.
BCT = Behavioral Couple or Marital Therapy; ICBT = Individual Cognitive-Behavioral Therapy; EtOH = alcohol